The History of a
Genetic Disease

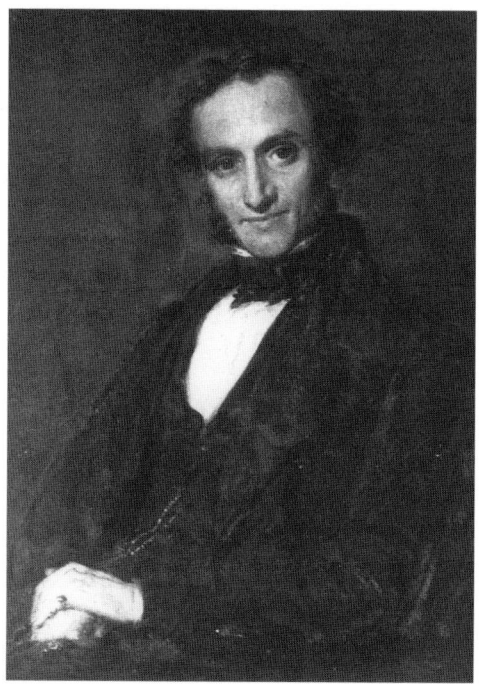

Dr. Meryon (1850) by John Linnell. Oil on Canvas, 184 cm × 243 cm. *Private Collection.*

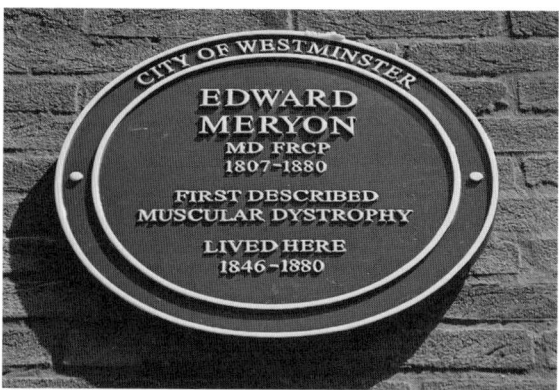

Plaque on the site of Edward Meryon's former home at 14 Clarges Street, Piccadilly, London by Westminster City Council. Metal, 45 cm diameter. *London, Clarges Street.*

The History of a Genetic Disease
Duchenne muscular dystrophy or Meryon's disease

SECOND EDITION

Alan E. H. Emery & Marcia L. H. Emery

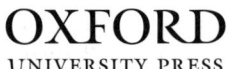

OXFORD
UNIVERSITY PRESS

Great Clarendon Street, Oxford OX2 6DP

Oxford University Press is a department of the University of Oxford.
It furthers the University's objective of excellence in research, scholarship,
and education by publishing worldwide in

Oxford New York

Auckland Cape Town Dar es Salaam Hong Kong Karachi
Kuala Lumpur Madrid Melbourne Mexico City Nairobi
New Delhi Shanghai Taipei Toronto

With offices in

Argentina Austria Brazil Chile Czech Republic France Greece
Guatemala Hungary Italy Japan Poland Portugal Singapore
South Korea Switzerland Thailand Turkey Ukraine Vietnam

Oxford is a registered trade mark of Oxford University Press
in the UK and in certain other countries

Published in the United States
by Oxford University Press Inc., New York

© Oxford University Press, 2011

The moral rights of the author have been asserted

Database right Oxford University Press (maker)

First published by the Royal Society of Medicine Press Limited 1995

All rights reserved. No part of this publication may be reproduced,
stored in a retrieval system, or transmitted, in any form or by any means,
without the prior permission in writing of Oxford University Press,
or as expressly permitted by law, or under terms agreed with the appropriate
reprographics rights organization. Enquiries concerning reproduction
outside the scope of the above should be sent to the Rights Department,
Oxford University Press, at the address above

You must not circulate this book in any other binding or cover
and you must impose the same condition on any acquirer

British Library Cataloging in Publication Data

Data available

Library of Congress Cataloging in Publication Data

Data available

Typeset in Minion by Glyph International, Bangalore, India
Printed in Great Britain
on acid-free paper by
CPI Antony Rowe, Chippenham, Wiltshire

ISBN 978–0–19–959147–3

10 9 8 7 6 5 4 3 2 1

Oxford University Press makes no representation, express or implied, that the drug dosages in
this book are correct. Readers must therefore always check the product information and clinical
procedures with the most up-to-date published product information and data sheets provided
by the manufacturers and the most recent codes of conduct and safety regulations. The authors
and the publishers do not accept responsibility or legal liability for any errors in the text or for
the misuse or misapplication of material in this work. Except where otherwise stated, drug
dosages and recommendations are for the non-pregnant adult who is not breastfeeding.

λαμπάδια ἔχοντες διαδώσουσιν ἀλλήλοις

Those having torches will pass them on to others
Plato's *Republic* (4th century BC)

Contents

Acknowledgements *xi*
Foreword to the first edition *xiii*
Preface *xv*
About the authors *xvii*
List of illustrations *xix*

1 The history of muscular dystrophy: a unique story *1*
   A mirror of developments in medical science *1*
   The history involves several 'firsts' *5*
   Individuals involved in the history *6*
   The importance of nineteenth-century medical science *7*

2 Early history of muscular dystrophy *11*
   Charles Bell (1774–1842) *13*
   Gaetano Conte (1798–1858) *18*
   Richard Partridge (1805–1873) *20*
   William J. Little (1810–1894) *22*

3 Edward Meryon's contribution to muscular dystrophy *27*
   Society and medicine in Victorian times *27*
   The constitution of man *30*
   Edward Meryon and Charles Darwin *32*
   How did Meryon first become interested in muscle disease? *33*
   Granular degeneration of muscle *35*
   Knowledge of heredity at the time *41*
   Why has Meryon's contribution to muscular dystrophy been largely neglected? *44*
   Meryon's other contributions *48*

4 The life of Edward Meryon (1807–1880) *53*
   Charles Lewis Meryon (1783–1877) *55*
   John Meryon (1776–1857) *57*
   Edward Meryon (1807–1880) *58*

5 Duchenne de Boulogne (1806–1875) *73*
   Duchenne's life *73*
   La Salpêtrière *77*
   Paralysie hypertrophique de l'enfance *81*
   Muscle pathology *84*
   Duchenne's views on aetiology and pathogenesis *86*
   Duchenne's attitude to Meryon's work *88*
   An assessment of Duchenne's contribution *90*

6 Refining the clinical picture *93*
   Increasing interest in muscle disease *93*
   William Richard Gowers (1845–1915) *94*
   Gowers' contribution to medicine and neurology *96*
   Pseudohypertrophic muscular paralysis *97*
   Treatment *103*
   Clinical heterogeneity *103*

7 Resolution of heterogeneity *105*
   Early studies of the problem—Leyden and Möbius *105*
   Wilhelm Heinrich Erb (1840–1921) *106*
   Erb's contributions to neurology *107*
   Dystrophia muscularis progressiva *108*
   Facioscapulohumeral muscular dystrophy of Landouzy and Dejerine *109*

8 Nosology of the dystrophies *115*
   Genetic heterogeneity *116*
   Nosology based on clinical and genetic differences *118*
   The classification of Walton and Nattrass *120*
   Discriminant and segregation analysis *125*

9 Recognition of other types of muscular dystrophy *131*
   Becker muscular dystrophy *131*
   Emery–Dreifuss muscular dystrophy *133*
   Other rare forms of X-linked muscular dystrophy *136*
   Limb girdle muscular dystrophies *138*
   Distal muscular dystrophies *142*
   Ocular and oculopharyngeal muscular dystrophies *144*
   Congenital muscular dystrophies *145*
   Conclusions *148*

10 Biochemical diagnosis and carrier detection *153*
   Serum enzymes *154*
   Carrier detection *156*
   Bayesian statistics *158*

11 Pathogenesis of Duchenne dystrophy *163*
   Neurogenic basis of dystrophy *163*
   Vascular hypothesis *164*
   Muscle biochemistry *165*
   Contribution of muscle pathology *167*
   A defect in membranes *171*

12 The search for the gene *177*
   Recombinant DNA technology *177*
   Localizing the Duchenne gene *180*
   Duchenne and Becker muscular dystrophies shown to be allelic *185*
   DNA markers for carrier detection and prenatal diagnosis *187*
   Isolation of the Duchenne gene *188*
   Dystrophin—the gene product *194*
   Dystrophin-associated glycoproteins *196*
   Genotype–phenotype correlations *198*
   Some unanswered questions *200*

13 Current trends and the future *207*
   Genetic and clinical heterogeneity *207*
   Pathogenesis *207*
   Clinical variation *210*
   Infection and muscular dystrophy *212*
   Treatment *213*
   The future *216*

Author index *221*

Subject index *225*

Acknowledgements

In researching material for this book we have had a great deal of encouragement and help from many individuals. Those who have played an important role in the history of the disease have generously contributed much scientific and biographical data. The many individuals and organizations that have helped us with bibliographic and genealogical research include: Joan Fergusson and Iain Milne and colleagues of the Royal College of Physicians of Edinburgh Library; Geoffrey Davenport and Julie Allum and colleagues of the Royal College of Physicians Library, London; The Librarian and Mr Greenwood, and Mira Gogova and Elizabeth A. Rogers, Archivists, Royal Society of Medicine; Gill Furlong and Susan Stead, Manuscripts and Rare Books Library, University College London; Rosemary Clarkson, Cambridge University Library; Devon and Exeter Institute; Alina Ozimek, Librarian, Historical Library, Harvey Cushing/John Hay Whitney Medical Library, Yale University, New Haven, Connecticut; Helen Young, Librarian, Paleography Room, University of London Library; Katrina Sinclair and staff of the Medical Library, St Thomas' Hospital; staff of the Manuscripts Section and the Printed Books Section, Guildhall Library, London; staff of the Greater London Record Office; Stephen Wilson, Librarian, National Hospital for Neurology and Neurosurgery, Queen Square, London; Bill Hopkins and Gillian Kidd, Department of Medical Illustration, Edinburgh University; John Gibson, Worcester; Dr Denis Harriman; Dr Angelo Cerracchio of Naples; Giancarlo Izzo (Italian Consul, Edinburgh); Sarah Dodgson, Librarian, The Athenaeum; Roger Davey and staff, East Sussex Record Office; Jean Tsushima, Honorary Editor, Huguenot & Walloon Research Association; Mary Bayliss, Honorary Secretary, The Huguenot Society; Joyce Crow, Honorary Librarian, Sussex Archaeological Society; the late Alma Fabes, Rye; Rosemary Allan, Oxford; and Professors Tiemo Grimm, Giovanni Nigro, and Reinhardt Rüdel.

With regard to illustrations of the prominent individuals involved in this history, we have retained those relevant at the time of their contributions, and not replaced them by possibly more recent images from later life which some might perhaps have preferred!

One person we especially wish to acknowledge is David Easton, a direct descendant of Edward Meryon. He has generously provided much interesting information about Meryon's personal life which he has collected and preserved over the years.

Finally we should like to thank Lord Walton for permission to reproduce his Foreword to the original publication, and to Nicola Wilson and staff at Oxford University Press for their valued support and encouragement.

Foreword to the first edition

I was delighted to be asked by Alan and Marcia Emery to write a Foreword to this fascinating volume. It is a remarkably comprehensive and scholarly account of the progressive development of knowledge of a tragic crippling disease and, as such, I believe will prove to be of great interest not just to medical historians but to all of those working in neuromuscular disease. As the tale of discovery unfolds, innumerable messages emerge, bringing with them lessons for all clinical investigators, irrespective of the field of research in which they are involved. If I may paraphrase the wise saying of John Clare, written many centuries ago: 'Out of old books comes all this new knowledge that men can learn.' All doctors and scientists must on occasions have experienced that blinding flash of inspiration, perhaps even of presumed achievement, in believing that they have discovered something new and raising the hope that it might constitute a significant contribution to the developing jigsaw of knowledge, only to find that someone else had made the identical discovery many years earlier.

I was touched by reading in this splendid account that the authors regard my contributions, first with Nattrass and subsequently with others, as having added significantly to our store of knowledge on the form of muscular dystrophy which we entitled in 1954 the Duchenne type because of our dissatisfaction with the previous label of 'pseudohypertrophic muscular dystrophy'. At that time we referred to the contributions of Edward Meryon in passing, but did not, I believe, recognize their seminal importance. If we had done so at the time, perhaps in the light of the persuasive case now made by the Emerys, we would have preferred the eponymous title of Meryon muscular dystrophy. It is good to see that this book pays due tribute to the important clinical delineations and pathological observations made by Meryon in the 1850s, which antedated those made by the great French neurologist, Duchenne. As the authors rightly point out, Duchenne's personal and extensive observations took the matter a considerable stage further, so that perhaps after all posterity may agree that Duchenne muscular dystrophy is an apposite term. I was also touched to read that Alan Emery felt that at a chance meeting I may have inspired him to work on this topic.

I shall not be the first, nor the last, invitee requested to produce a Foreword to an important publication (often at very short notice!) to confess that it was originally my intention to skim through the pages of this book and to write an account based largely upon my personal knowledge of the subject and of the authors. However, I must admit that once I began to read, I found that this historical account dealing successively with the early history of muscular dystrophy, refinements of its clinical picture, heterogeneity and nosology, and moving on to consider biochemistry, pathogenesis and the molecular genetics of the disorder, gripped me from the beginning, so that in the end I could not resist continuing to read on and on. Surely this must be one of the most comprehensive historical accounts of the birth and subsequent growth of knowledge of a single disease ever to have been written. Some of the material it contains is inevitably familiar to me, but there are innumerable nuggets of information of which I was quite unaware, not least relating to the very early contributions of Bell, Conte, Partridge, and Little; many other gems are scattered throughout the pages. The Emerys have done us all a significant service in writing this book, which will prove of very great interest not just to those working in neuromuscular disease worldwide but also, I believe, to medical historians now and in the future.

John Walton
(Lord Walton of Detchant TD, MA, MD, DSc, FRCP)

Oxford, December 1994

Preface

Since the first publication of this book in 1995, Edward Meryon's life and work has attracted much attention. In 1996 the Meryon Society was inaugurated at the Royal Society of Medicine in London. The aim was to encourage research into the history of neuromuscular disorders through meetings held each year in Oxford attended by international authorities in the field, and to include an invited lecture. To date 13 lectures have been presented, most subsequently published in the journal *Neuromuscular Disorders*[1].

Some might argue that the ultimate accolade was to have Edward Meryon's life and work selected for inclusion in the new edition of the *Oxford Dictionary of National Biography*[2].

A further development was the erection of a commemorative plaque in 2005 on the site of Meryon's former home at 14 Clarges Street, Piccadilly, London at an unveiling ceremony attended by several living descendants of Meryon.

The subject of muscular dystrophy in general has progressed considerably since the book was first published. These developments have centred on defining clinically and genetically many other forms of dystrophy, advances in understanding the details of pathogenesis and, perhaps most importantly, new approaches to treatment through various forms of gene therapy. Some of these developments will be briefly discussed. However, this is not meant to be a textbook on the subject but rather a detailed account of the life and work of Edward Meryon and the extension of his observations into the present day.

1. Emery, A. E. H., Emery, M. A brief history of the Meryon Society. *Neuromuscular Disorders*, 2007; **17**: 723–4.
2. Emery, A. E. H., Emery, M. L. H. Meryon, Edward (bap .1807, d. 1880). In: Oxford Dictionary of National Biography, H. C. G. Matthew & B. Harrison (eds). Oxford: Oxford University Press, 2004.

About the authors

Alan E. H. Emery is Emeritus Professor of Human Genetics, University of Edinburgh and Honorary Fellow, Green Templeton College, Oxford.

Over a long career he has published some 400 articles and written or edited 24 books, mainly, but not exclusively, concerned with genetics and neuromuscular disorders. In 1989 he helped found the European Neuromuscular Centre and was its first Research Director; later, in 2001, he established the Section of Medical Genetics of the Royal Society of Medicine, and became its Founding President. He has received many national and international awards and honorary degrees. In retirement he now has more time for his hobbies of oil painting and writing poetry.

Marcia L. H. Emery was born in Cleveland, Ohio and graduated in Clinical Psychology at Wooster College with an honours year at St Andrew's University; she later gained an MSc in Information Sciences from Case Western Reserve University.

In more recent years her interests have centred on medical history and art history and she has published several articles on these subjects. Like her husband she now has a little more time for her hobbies of needlework and identifying and studying butterflies.

The authors live in Devon but retain strong associations with Green Templeton College, Oxford.

List of illustrations

Figure 1.1 Number of articles on muscular dystrophy published each year. Note the increase in the mid 1970s following evidence of a membrane defect in Duchenne dystrophy, and again some 10 years later when the gene was identified. *3*

Figure 2.1 Drawings from a tomb at Beni Hasan (circa 2800–2500 BC). *12*

Figure 2.2 Egyptian relief painting from the Eighteenth Dynasty. (Reproduced by kind permission of Professor P. E. Becker.) *12*

Figure 2.3 Portion of Raphael's *Transfiguration* (1520). *13*

Figure 2.4 *Beggars*. Engraving by Hieronymus Cock. (Reproduced by kind permission of the Philadelphia Museum of Art.) *14*

Figure 2.5 Sir Charles Bell, 1774–1842. (Reproduced by kind permission of the National Galleries of Scotland, Edinburgh.) *15*

Figure 2.6 Illustrations from Charles Bell's *Essays on the Anatomy of Expression in Painting*. Above: laughter; below: hydrophobia. *16*

Figure 2.7 Memorial tablet to Sir Charles Bell in Hallow Church, Worcester. *17*

Figure 2.8 Richard Partridge, 1805–1873. (Reproduced by kind permission of The President and Council of the Royal College of Surgeons of England.) *22*

Figure 2.9 William J. Little, 1810–1894. (Reprinted from The Lancet, Vol. 63, Biographical sketch of William J. Little, M.D., Physician to the London Hospital, etc., pp.16–22, Copyright (1854), with permission from Elsevier.) *23*

Figure 3.1 Soho, London around 1850. (From a drawing in *Punch* entitled *A Court for King Cholera* by John Leech.) *28*

Figure 3.2 London University, 1831. (From *The Public Buildings of Westminster Described*, London: John Harris.) *33*

Figure 3.3 The illustrations of muscle tissue accompanying Meryon's 1852 publication. A, Diseased muscles, the transverse striæ appearing faintly in places. Drawn from the preparation.

B, Diseased muscle from the upper extremities, the transverse striæ beginning to disappear and granules taking their place. C, Diseased muscle from the lower extremities, the transverse striæ having disappeared. D, Diseased muscle from the lower extremities, shewing little more than granular matter. (Reproduced by kind permission of the Royal Society of Medicine.) *37*

Figure 3.4 Title page of Meryon's monograph, published in 1864. *39*

Figure 3.5 The Royal Medical & Chirurgical Society at 53 Berners Street. (Reproduced by kind permission of the Royal Society of Medicine.) *46*

Figure 4.1 An abbreviated Meryon family tree. Square, male; circle, female; diamond with number, number of males/females. *54*

Figure 4.2 Charles Lewis Meryon, MD, FRCP (1783–1877); Edward Meryon's paternal uncle. (Reproduced by permission of the Royal College of Physicians.) *56*

Figure 4.3 Mermaid Street, Rye, as it is today. (Author's photograph, 1994.) *59*

Figure 4.4 Edward Meryon's election to Fellowship, the Royal Medical and Chirurgical Society, 1846. (Reproduced by kind permission of the Royal Society of Medicine.) *64*

Figure 4.5 Edward Meryon's residence from 1847 to 1880 at 14 Clarges Street, Piccadilly (house on the right hand side). The building was destroyed in the Second World War and a new building on the site now bears a plaque to Meryon's former home. (Reproduced by kind permission of the Greater London Photograph Library.) *65*

Figure 4.6 Catherine Meryon (née Baily) (1811–1897), *c*. 1861. (Reproduced by kind permission of Mr David Easton.) *67*

Figure 4.7 Edward Meryon. (Engraving by J. R. Black of London, *c*. 1862.) (Reproduced by kind permission of Mr. David Easton.) *68*

Figure 4.8 Edward Meryon in later years, *c*. 1880. (From *Epigrams, Epitaphs, Personal Anecdotes, &tc.*, London: for private circulation [188?].) *69*

Figure 4.9 Rediscovery in 1993 of Edward Meryon's long neglected grave in Brompton Cemetery, London, being cleaned by one of the authors. The inscription simply reads 'In memory of Edward Meryon, MD who died November 8th 1880 aged 73 years'. *69*

Figure 5.1 Rue de L'Ecole de Médecine, 1861 (showing the Tourelle, the house in which Charlotte Corday assassinated Jean-Paul Marat). (Etching by Charles Meryon.) *75*

Figure 5.2 Duchenne around the time he began his research into muscle disease. (Reproduced with permission from *The Founders of Neurology*, edited by Webb Haymaker, 1953. Courtesy of Charles C. Thomas, Publishers, Springfield, Illinois.) *76*

Figure 5.3 The entrance to the Hôpital de la Salpêtrière as it is today. (Author's photograph, 1994.) *77*

Figure 5.4 'An electro-physiological experiment' from Duchenne's *Mécanisme de la Physionomie Humaine. 78*

Figure 5.5 Duchenne in middle age. (Kindly provided by Professor Fernando Tomé, Paris.) *79*

Figure 5.6 Duchenne's case number 68, published in 1861. Note the lordosis and enlarged calves. *82*

Figure 5.7 Duchenne's own photograph of his patient with *Paralysie hypertrophique* (Figure 13 in Ref. 16). *83*

Figure 5.8 The patient studied by Griesinger. Note the enlarged calves. *86*

Figure 5.9 An illustration from Duchenne's 1868 publication. *87*

Figure 6.1 Sir William Gowers, (1845–1915). (Reproduced by kind permission of Dr. Macdonald Critchley.) *95*

Figure 6.2 Gowers' manoeuvre or sign. (From W. R. Gowers' *Pseudo-hypertrophic Muscular Paralysis*, 1879.) *100*

Figure 7.1 Wilhelm Heinrich Erb (1840–1921). (Reproduced with permission from *The Founders of Neurology*, ed. by Webb Haymaker, 1953. Courtesy of Charles C. Thomas, publishers, Springfield, Illinois.) *107*

Figure 7.2 One of Duchenne's cases illustrated in Figure 16 of his *Album de Photographies Pathologiques*[14]. Note the facial weakness and winging of the scapula. *110*

Figure 7.3 Louis Théophile Joseph Landouzy (1845–1917). (Reproduced with permission from *The Founders of Neurology*, edited by Webb Haymaker, 1953. Courtesy of Charles C. Thomas, publishers, Springfield, Illinois.) *111*

Figure 7.4 Joseph Jules Dejerine (1849–1917). (Reproduced from *The Founders of Neurology*, ed. by Webb Haymaker, 1953. Courtesy of Charles C. Thomas, publishers, Springfield, Illinois.) *112*

Figure 8.1 Ade T. Milhorat. (Reproduced by kind permission of his son, Thomas H. Milhorat, MD.) *117*

Figure 8.2 Frederick John Nattrass. (Reproduced by kind permission of Lord Walton.) *121*

Figure 8.3 John Nicholas Walton. (The Right Honourable, Lord Walton of Detchant.) *123*

Figure 8.4 Newton Ennis Morton. *127*

Figure 9.1 Peter Emil Becker in his 76th year. (The eleven volumes of his *Handbook of Medical Genetics* can be seen at the left end of the top shelf.) *132*

Figure 9.2 A 6-year-old boy with preclinical Becker muscular dystrophy (note the enlarged calves) and his affected 26-year-old maternal uncle. *134*

Figure 9.3 Fritz E. Dreifuss. *135*

Figure 9.4 A 17-year-old male with Emery–Dreifuss muscular dystrophy. Note the flexion contractures of the elbows, and wasting of the lower legs. A cardiac pacemaker has been inserted. *137*

Figure 9.5 Victor Dubowitz. *140*

Figure 9.6 Limb girdle muscular dystrophy with onset in late adolescence. A sister was similarly affected. Note the winging of the scapulae and possible wasting of the thigh muscles. *142*

Figure 9.7 Distal muscular dystrophy. Note the wasting of the small muscles of the hands. *143*

Figure 9.8 Ocular muscular dystrophy. *144*

Figure 9.9 Congenital muscular dystrophy in a 3-year-old boy. He has generalized hypotonia and retarded motor development and still cannot sit without support. *146*

Figure 9.10 Professor Yukio Fukuyama and the author (AEHE) at a 1993 meeting of the European Neuromuscular Centre in Baarn, The Netherlands. *146*

Figure 10.1 Jean-Claude Dreyfus. *154*

Figure 10.2 Professor Setsuro Ebashi. *157*

Figure 10.3 Professor Hideo Sugita. *157*

Figure 10.4 E. A. (Tony) Murphy (left) and Victor A. McKusick, photographed in the Moore Clinic around 1964. *158*

Figure 10.5 Edmond A. (Tony) Murphy. *159*

Figure 11.1 Andrew G. Engel. *170*

Figure 11.2 Allen D. Roses. *173*

Figure 12.1 Kay E. Davies. *182*

Figure 12.2 Generation and identification of X chromosome probes and the detection of an X-linked restriction fragment length polymorphism. FACS, Fluorescent Activated Cell Sorter; RE, restriction enzyme; labelled probe. *183*

Figure 12.3 Peter S. Harper. *184*

Figure 12.4 Gene map of the X chromosome and its banding pattern. (Reproduced with kind permission of the late Dr. Victor McKusick.) *186*

Figure 12.5 Louis M. Kunkel. *190*

Figure 12.6 Ronald G. Worton. *192*

Figure 12.7 Eric P. Hoffman. *195*

Figure 12.8 Kevin P. Campbell. *197*

Figure 12.9 Skeletal muscle sections with immunolabelling for dystrophin. A, Normal: dystrophin located at the sarcolemma on all fibres. B, DMD with frame-shift deletion: no dystrophin is present (counterstained with haematoxylin and eosin). C, DMD with frame-shift deletion: single positive fibre ('revertant'). D, BMD with in-frame deletion: dystrophin labelling shows marked variation both between and within fibres. E, Manifesting carrier of DMD: dystrophin labelling shows variation between fibres. Magnification ×250; indirect immunoperoxidase labelling with a monoclonal antibody (Dy8/6C5) which recognizes an epitope at the extreme C-terminus of dystrophin. (Reproduced by kind permission of Dr. Margaret Johnson and the late Dr. Louise Anderson.) *199*

Figure 13.1 Distribution of predominant muscle weakness in different types of dystrophy. A, Duchenne-type and Becker-type; B, Emery–Dreifuss; C, limb girdle; D, facioscapulohumeral; E, distal; F, oculopharyngeal. Shaded areas are affected. (Reproduced from Emery, A.E.H., (1998), Fortnightly review: The muscular dystrophies, *BMJ*; **317**: 991–995 with permission from BMJ Publishing Group Ltd.) *208*

Figure 13.2 Diagrammatic representation of some of the proteins implicated in different forms of muscular dystrophy. bm, Basement membrane; pm, plasma membrane; NMJ, neuromuscular junction; AchR, acetylcholine receptor. *211*

Chapter 1

The history of muscular dystrophy: a unique story

Few would question the incredible advances in our understanding of inherited diseases that have occurred in recent years as a result of developments in molecular biology. The explosion of knowledge would have been quite unforeseen just a few years ago. The basic defect causing many of these diseases, which was previously completely unknown, has now been identified, and in some cases even treatment by genetic technology is becoming a real possibility.

This is perhaps an appropriate moment therefore to pause and consider the trail of historical events that has led us to this point in the case of a particular inherited disorder. This disorder is Duchenne muscular dystrophy, a serious condition and the second most common genetic disorder in many countries. Its cause was unknown until relatively recently and there has been no effective treatment. However, the responsible gene and its protein product have now been identified and gene therapy is under serious consideration. In many ways the history of the disease is unique because it encapsulates so many developments in medical science over the past 150 years, including microscopy, histopathology, nosology, biochemistry, medical genetics and, more recently of course, molecular biology.

A mirror of developments in medical science

In the middle of the nineteenth century, muscular dystrophy, or muscle paralysis as it was then often referred to, captured the interest of anatomists who wondered how the manifestations of the disease could be accounted for by the selective involvement of certain muscle groups. Later, pathologists and clinicians became interested in the disease and in this way the clinical features were defined. This was largely the result of the work of the English physician, Meryon, and the French physician, Duchenne. Gowers' monumental study of the disease refined the clinical picture even further. In retrospect it is now clear that Meryon made the first *systematic* detailed clinical and pathological study of the type of dystrophy with whose name Duchenne is usually associated. He showed that it was essentially a disease of muscle and *not* the nervous system and that it was familial with a predilection for males. His microscopic studies led him to suggest that the basic defect was a breakdown of the muscle fibre membrane. Some 135 years later this was shown to be true and to be caused by a defect in a membrane-associated protein, dystrophin. For all these reasons a case could therefore be made for now referring to the disorder as *Meryon's disease*. His observations, however, have been largely neglected and virtually nothing has been written about the man himself. We have therefore attempted to rectify the situation by providing some details of his life and work.

From the 1880s onwards the germ theory offered an explanation for many diseases whose cause had previously been unknown. This threw into greater prominence other disorders, including muscle diseases, which merited a different approach to their aetiology. Interest was also fuelled by improvements in the microscopic study of muscle tissue following the introduction of achromatic lenses and improved methods for fixing and mounting tissues which also occurred around this period. The result was the study of ever-increasing numbers of cases, and it soon became clear that muscular dystrophy was not a single disease. Many played a part in resolving this problem, which led to the identification of a number of specific disease entities. Apart from Duchenne muscular dystrophy, these included 'limb girdle' (Leyden, Möbius, Erb) and facioscapulohumeral types (Landouzy, Dejerine), and, later, the recognition of distal, oculopharyngeal, 'benign X-linked' (Becker), congenital, and other forms.

There followed an increasing interest in nosology and the classification of these disorders, based no longer on clinical grounds alone, but also on their different modes of inheritance. The most important contributions at this stage were those of Walton and Nattrass and Morton and Chung. The latter introduced the idea of using discriminant analysis in the delineation of specific diseases, which was an entirely new approach to the problem of resolving heterogeneity in a genetic disorder.

As the definition of specific types and their classification became clearer, developments in clinical chemistry led to the introduction of serum enzyme tests for detecting preclinical cases and female carriers of Duchenne dystrophy. Here the work of Ebashi and Sugita in Tokyo, and Dreyfus and Schapira in Paris, is particularly germane. Murphy can be credited with having introduced Bayesian statistics into medical genetics, and its first application in risk calculation was in Duchenne muscular dystrophy.

However, understanding the cause of the disease posed a very difficult problem. There was no shortage of ideas but little progress was made until the mid 1970s when biochemical and other evidence pointed to a membrane defect. Thereafter, scientific interest in muscular dystrophy revived with a

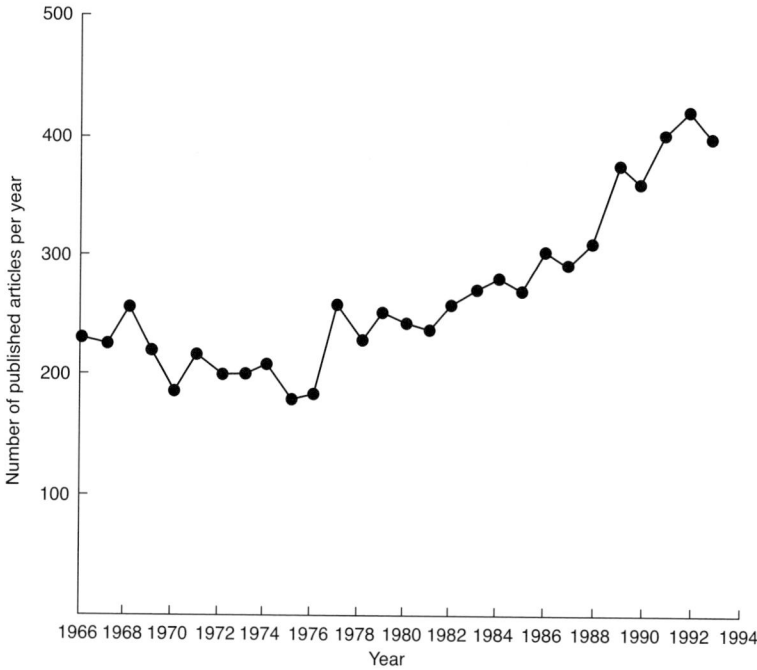

Fig. 1.1 Number of articles on muscular dystrophy published each year. Note the increase in the mid 1970s following evidence of a membrane defect in Duchenne dystrophy, and again some 10 years later when the gene was identified.

further increase in interest some 10 years later when the gene for Duchenne muscular dystrophy was identified (Figure 1.1). Since then there has been an explosion of research, with almost 1000 publications on muscular dystrophy alone in 2008.

However, not until the early 1980s did the technology become available to locate, isolate, and characterize the defective gene. This began with the localization of the gene through linkage to a DNA marker or restriction fragment length polymorphism (RFLP) by Kay Davies and Harper and their colleagues, and thereby provided a model for localizing the genes for other diseases whose cause was unknown. Subsequently, DNA studies showed that Duchenne and Becker dystrophies were allelic. Further developments involved international collaboration on a scale not previously seen in the biomedical sciences. For example, one paper at this time on the molecular pathology of Duchenne and Becker dystrophies listed no less than 77 authors from throughout the world.

In 1985 the work of Kunkel in the United States and Worton in Canada and their colleagues led to the isolation of the gene, and in 1987 the gene product was identified and named *dystrophin*. Here the defective protein had been identified by first locating and isolating the responsible gene and, from this, predicting the gene product. This was a complete reversal of previous approaches to understanding the basic defect in a metabolic disorder and was a triumph for 'reverse genetics'. From finding a linked DNA marker to isolating, cloning, and characterizing the responsible gene, and identifying the biochemical defect had taken less than 10 years and was a remarkable achievement. We are now entering the final phase in the history of the subject, with the possibility of curing the disorder through some form of gene therapy (Table 1.1).

Table 1.1 Landmarks in the history of Duchenne (DMD) and Becker muscular dystrophies (BMD)

1830–	Muscular dystrophy recognized as a disorder and DMD as a specific type of dystrophy
1860–1900	Microscopic myopathology defined
1930–1960	Resolution of heterogeneity by clinical and discriminant analysis. BMD defined (1955) X-linked inheritance confirmed by segregation analysis (1959)
1959–1960	Serum creatine kinase for diagnosis and carrier detection
1966–1968	Introduction of Bayesian statistics for risk estimation
1975–1980	Defect localized to muscle and other membranes by electron microscopy and biochemistry
1979–1982	Gene localized to Xp21 Linked restriction fragment length polymorphism (RFLP) identified (1982)
1983–1984	DMD and BMD shown to be allelic
1983–1985	Linked RFLPs first used for carrier detection (1983) and prenatal diagnosis (1985)
1985	Responsible gene isolated (gene-specific probes)
1987	Gene product (dystrophin) identified
1988	Dystrophin localized to sarcolemma, absent in DMD and abnormal in BMD
1989	First randomized controlled trials of glucocorticoids
1989–1990	Myoblast transfer in *mdx* mouse and humans Utrophin (dystrophin-like protein) identified Dystrophin-associated glycoprotein complex identified
1990–	Gene therapies in *mdx* mouse and later humans
1999–	Possibility of stem cell therapy
2003–	Antisense oligonucleotide therapeutic possibilities
2008–	Human trials of antisense oligonucleotide therapy

The history involves several 'firsts'

It is clear that this is more than a history of a disease. It involves many of the major developments in medical science and includes many 'firsts'. It was the first X-linked disease to be reported in a female with XO, Turner's syndrome (1957); discriminant analysis was applied to a large and complex body of medical data in this case to resolve clinical and genetic heterogeneity in muscular dystrophy (1959); Bayesian statistics were used in risk calculations in medical genetics (1966); a genetic disorder, in which the basic biochemical defect was completely unknown, was shown to be linked to a RFLP (1982) and then such linked RFLPs used in genetic counselling (1983) and prenatal diagnosis (1985); finally, the gene product (dystrophin) was the first to be identified (1987) by molecular genetic techniques alone when there was no prior knowledge as to the cause of the disease. The responsible gene remains one of the largest genes isolated and characterized in humans.

Although the story is presented as a continuous progression toward a solution, there were many occasions when lines of investigation ended abruptly for lack of new ideas or new technology. For example, in the nineteenth century it was recognized that only males were affected and transmission was through the maternal line. But it would be many years before the genetic mechanism for this was understood. Terms like 'heredo-familial' were often used and the curious transmission through females in haemophilia and muscular dystrophy was to many physicians a complete mystery even in the 1920s[1]. Only gradually did it become clear and accepted that the familial nature of these diseases was explicable in terms of Mendelian inheritance[2,3].

The identification of the defect in Duchenne muscular dystrophy is most unlikely ever to have been determined by conventional biochemical methods because it proved to represent only 0.002% of total muscle protein. In fact, the difficulties and frustrations of not being able to identify the defect resulted in many investigators of neuromuscular disorders up to the 1980s turning their attention to more accessible conditions such as the glycogen storage disorders and myoglobinuria[4]. The identification of the defect had to await the emergence of a new biotechnology in the early 1980s and with it an entirely different approach to the study of genetic diseases. This process continues. For example, preimplantation diagnosis is becoming a reality because DNA from a single cell can now be amplified with the polymerase chain reaction (PCR).

In describing the contribution made by the new molecular technologies, some detail has been included so that the elegance and ingenuity of this work can be better appreciated. However, an attempt has been made to keep such detail to a minimum, although hopefully without sacrificing accuracy.

Individuals involved in the history

Medical history reflects changes in attitudes to disease as well as changes in knowledge. It therefore inevitably involves considerations of social and cultural matters as well as the motivations of those involved. Apart from describing scientific developments in the history of Duchenne dystrophy, we have therefore included information about many of the individuals who have made significant contributions to the subject. But no uniform picture emerges; the participants in this history have come from varied backgrounds, each with their own particular interests, knowledge, abilities, and motivations.

Some became involved because a related disorder affected them (Little, and one of us [AEHE] wore callipers in childhood from osteomyelitis) or a close relative (Duchenne, Campbell). Some first became interested through the advice and guidance of a superior (Erb, Walton, Kay Davies, Hoffman), and others because of a general interest in the subject at the time (Meryon, Gowers, Harper). On occasions, some have been a major influence by spotting talent in others whom they have encouraged (Milhorat, Rowland, Walton, McKusick, Kakulas). Some became interested at an early stage in their careers and from then on it became a major commitment (Dreyfus, Sugita, Dubowitz, Fukuyama). Some have made many and important contributions to the subject of muscular dystrophy over many years (Duchenne, Erb, Becker, Walton, Dubowitz, Engel, Fardeau, Tomé). However, to others the subject was only of passing interest. They made a single and important observation but then turned to other interests and never returned to muscular dystrophy again (Bell, Morton, Murphy, Lindenbaum).

Most made their special contribution early in their careers. This has been particularly true in recent years. But in the past, the contrary was often the case (Duchenne, Erb, Becker). Many important advances have followed a great deal of planned and careful research, but sometimes it was the result of the immediate recognition of the importance of a chance observation (Dreyfus, Roses, Bakker).

In the past some continued their work despite severe financial problems (Duchenne). In recent times investigators have sometimes turned to muscular dystrophy because of the availability of research funding and only then became involved in the subject (Kunkel, Hoffman). In fact, the role of grant-giving bodies, such as MDA in America, MDC in Britain, and AFM in France, has been a major factor in encouraging and fostering research.

At this point, special mention should be made of Victor McKusick, a founder of medical genetics who, though not involved in muscular dystrophy himself, nevertheless encouraged and inspired many individuals in this history, including one of the authors [AEHE] in the early 1960s. For many years he was a medical professor and Director of Medical Genetics at Johns Hopkins Hospital. Throughout his retirement he maintained an interest in the subject and continued to produce scholarly work. He died in Baltimore in 2008 at the age of 86.

To return to muscular dystrophy, the technology has now become so complex and difficult that projects often require a whole team of investigators. It was, in a way, inevitable that emphasis would be given to the main contributors to this history. However, in almost all cases, certainly in recent years, many of these advances have only been made possible because of help provided by colleagues in the clinic and in the laboratory. Their consolation is knowing they have contributed their part to this exciting story. The single-authored paper, which so enlightened the early history of the disease, is nowadays very rare. Collaboration and cooperation on a national or even international scale has become the norm. Much of the success in recent years has been largely the result of such collaboration between many of those involved (Kay Davies, the late Louise Nicholson-Anderson, Kunkel, Worton, and Hoffman) who have generously made available their gene probes and dystrophin antibodies to others working in the field.

The importance of nineteenth-century medical science

We tend to assume that all significant advances in medicine have only occurred in recent times, but this is a mark of our intellectual arrogance. As Bynum has convincingly and eloquently argued, modern medicine is built on foundations that were firmly established in the nineteenth century[5]. France, Britain, and, later, America all played a part in this process, though many advances were largely pioneered in Germany. This is mirrored in the early history of muscular dystrophy. Duchenne himself emphasized that his observations had attracted more attention and were better acknowledged in Germany than in his own country. Almost all the previous studies of the disorder he reviewed in 1868 were from German publications. The history of muscular dystrophy from this period is replete with the names of German physician scientists (the term *scientist* first being used in 1833), and included Griesinger, Oppenheimer, Cohnheim, Friedrich, Erb, Leyden, Möbius, and Gräfe. They all had a significant influence on research at the time. Of course, others in France, most notably Duchenne himself and Charcot, and in Britain Meryon and Gowers, also played singularly important roles.

The emphasis then, as far as muscle disease was concerned, was largely clinical, physiological, and microscopical—that is, pathophysiological. This led to the delineation of Duchenne dystrophy as a specific disease of muscle and to the recognition that other types of muscular dystrophy also existed. These achievements were the result of inspired and careful observations almost always made by individuals with little more than a tendon hammer and microscope as aids to their research. From our vantage point their contributions now seem so obvious, but clearly they exhibited as much originality in their day as investigators do today.

Bynum[5] has pointed out that modern insights into the history of medicine make us sceptical, for example:

> about the easy assumption that the discovery of the tubercle bacillus by Robert Koch caused the decline in the prevalence of tuberculosis, or the invention of the stethoscope by R.T.H. Laënnec led to dramatic new ways of treating heart disease. (page xi)

As he argues throughout his book, the application of advances in medical research was never simple, instantaneous, or universal. These views were expressed mainly in the context of infectious diseases, but may nevertheless prove true in the case of recent advances in molecular genetics. Perhaps we should not be too surprised that the phenomenal success in recent years in isolating and cloning the Duchenne gene has translated into preventative measures, such as prenatal diagnosis, but which raise many ethical and social problems[6], and to a search for an effective treatment. As the late John Newsom-Davis[7] pointed out in an editorial in the *Journal of the Royal College of Physicians* concerning developments in neurology:

> The clinical [and genetic] approach to diagnosis remains a valid first step.... But it is no longer acceptable as an end in itself, for with these advances have come new opportunities for effective treatment

It would also be unwise to assume that all is now known about the disease. As discussed toward the end of the volume, many questions still remain unanswered. Nevertheless, there are now better reasons for being confident and optimistic than at any other time in the history of the disease.

The history of Duchenne muscular dystrophy has been a wonderful story to research and to relate. Some of the best scientific and medical minds have been involved. We hope this history will have served them well.

References

1. Rushton, A. R. *Genetics and Medicine in the United States 1800–1922*. Baltimore: Johns Hopkins University Press, 1994; 120–45.
2. Bateson, W. *Mendel's Principles of Heredity*. Cambridge: Cambridge University Press, 1909.

3. White, W. A. (ed.) *Modern Treatment of Nervous and Mental Diseases*. Philadelphia: Lea & Febiger, 1913. (On autosomal dominant 'ptosis') (See also Briggs, H. H. *Transactions of the American Ophthalmological Society* 1918; **16**: 255–76.)
4. Rowland, L. P. Preface. *Pathogenesis of Human Muscular Dystrophies*. Amsterdam: Excerpta Medica, 1977: xiii–xiv.
5. Bynum, W. F. *Science and the Practice of Medicine in the Nineteenth Century*. New York: Cambridge University Press, 1994.
6. Sulston, S., Ferry, G. *The Common Thread: A Story of Science, Politics, Ethics and the Human Genome*. London: Bantam Press, 2002.
7. Newsom-Davis, J. High hopes for neurology. *Journal of the Royal College of Physicians (London)*, 1994; **28**: 105.

Chapter 2

Early history of muscular dystrophy

Since the muscular dystrophies as a group are not uncommon and the most frequent form, namely Duchenne muscular dystrophy, is so distinctive it seems quite possible that it was observed and perhaps even recorded in earlier times. The ancient Egyptians often depicted physical abnormalities in their wall paintings with some care, and it is possible to identify cases of poliomyelitis as well as a variety of dwarfs[1]. However, evidence of muscular dystrophy in such paintings is less clear. Nevertheless, in searching through material in the Ashmolean Museum in Oxford, on the wall of a tomb (no. 17 in Newberry[2]) at Beni Hasan, dating from the Middle Kingdom (circa 2800–2500 BC), we found depicted a figure which could possibly demonstrate Duchenne muscular dystrophy (Figure 2.1).

The first figure on the left clearly has bilateral club foot. In the middle is a boy who could have muscular dystrophy: he has lost the normal arch of his feet (which is usually clear in Egyptian wall paintings); his calves are somewhat enlarged, and he may have some degree of pseudohypertrophy of certain upper limb muscles. On the other hand the hieroglyph above his head implies he may have been a dwarf. We have so far been unable to identify any other illustrations from early Egypt which might be interpreted as muscular dystrophy. However, Pöch and Becker[3] have suggested that a relief painting dating from the Eighteenth Dynasty of the New Kingdom (about 1500 BC) might portray a case of muscular dystrophy (Figure 2.2).

The subject depicted on the wall of the Temple of Hatshepsut is the Queen of Punt, who shows lumbar lordosis and may even have some calf enlargement. It may well be, however, that what we are seeing is no more than generalized obesity in a woman of Nubian origin.

In Raphael's *Transfiguration* (1520), which now hangs in the Musei Vaticani, a young boy in the foreground is being held up by his (?)father (Figure 2.3). This was interpreted by Vasari in his *Lives of the Artists* as a boy 'possessed':

> The possessed youth is shown in a distorted attitude stretching forth his limbs, crying, rolling his eyes and exhibiting in every movement the suffering he endures[4].

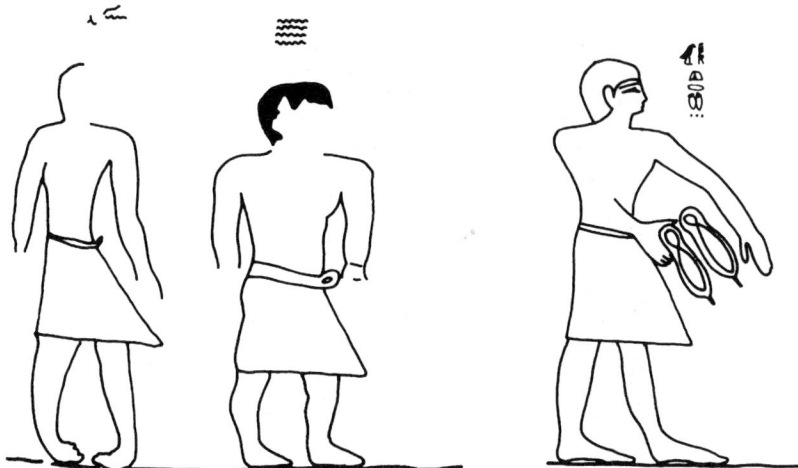

Fig. 2.1 Drawings from a tomb at Beni Hasan (circa 2800–2500 BC).

Many later writers have therefore suggested that it could illustrate a case of epilepsy. However, according to MacDonald Critchley[5], Gowers narrated that when Duchenne visited the National Hospital in London and saw an engraving of the painting in the board room, he was of the opinion that it represented a case of pseudohypertrophic muscular dystrophy.

Another illustration in which muscular dystrophy may have been portrayed is the engraving *Beggars* by Hieronymus Cock (*c.* 1520–1570), the Flemish artist.

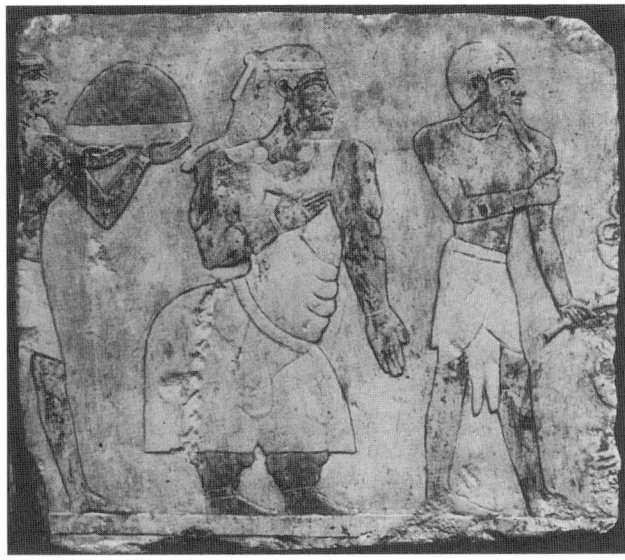

Fig. 2.2 Egyptian relief painting from the Eighteenth Dynasty. (Reproduced by kind permission of the late Professor P. E. Becker.)

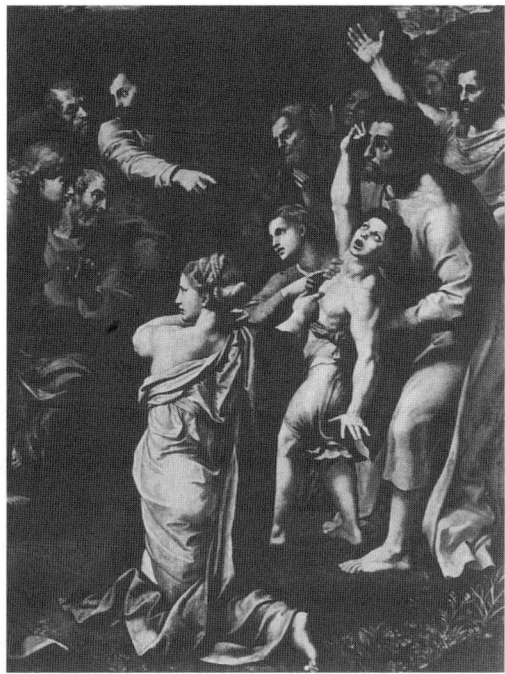

Fig. 2.3 Portion of Raphael's *Transfiguration* (1520).

It is based on an original drawing, now in Vienna, by Hieronymus Bosch. It shows 31 cripples with various deformities (Figure 2.4), which include wasted and stumped limbs, with an ingenious array of prostheses. With a little imagination it is possible to believe that at least one or two may have had some form of muscle disease.

A listing has been published of various abnormalities and genetic disorders in works of art with their locations[6]. However, unless an artist has specifically set out to depict a particular disorder (for example, muscular dystrophy in *The Sick Boy* (1915) by Karl Schmidt-Rottluff), the diagnosis in such cases can often only be speculative.

In tracing the early history of muscular dystrophy a study of its possible depiction by artists has therefore not been particularly helpful. More can be learned from clinical descriptions of the disease, the first of which, at least in the English language, can be attributed to Charles Bell.

Charles Bell (1774–1842)

Charles Bell (Figure 2.5) was born in Fountainbridge, then a suburb of Edinburgh, in 1774, but at the age of 5 his father died and the family moved to George Street in the centre of the city. He attended Edinburgh High School,

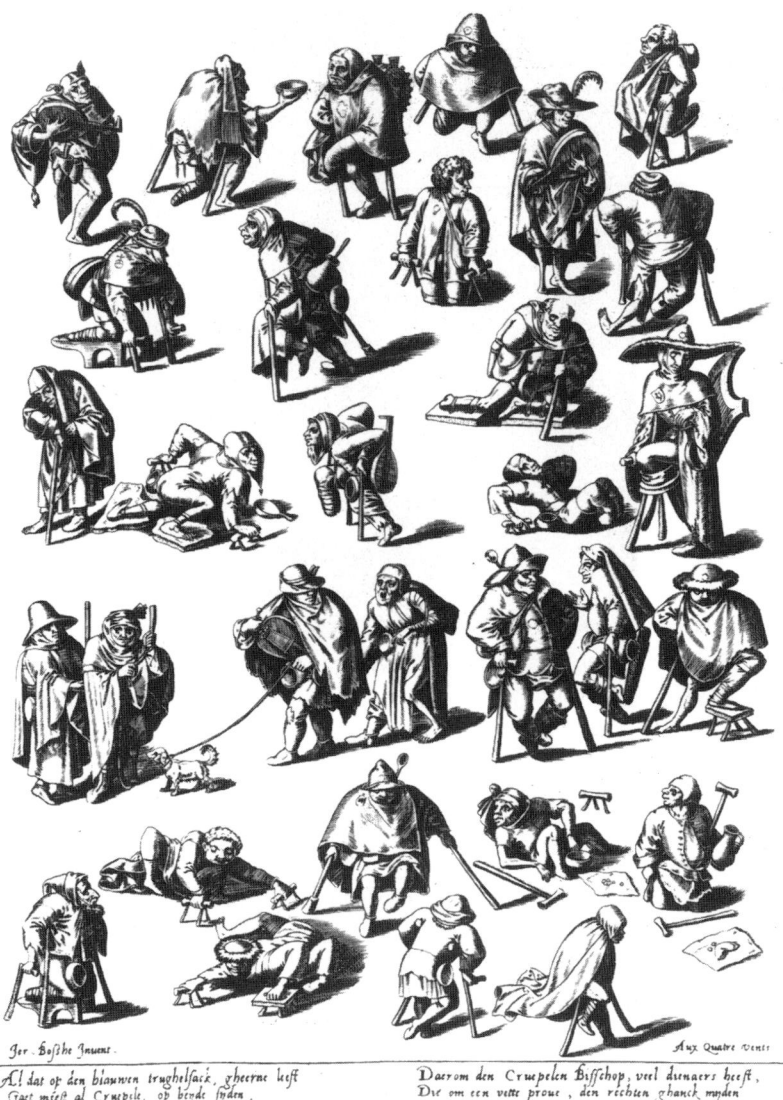

Fig. 2.4 *Beggars*. Engraving by Hieronymus Cock. (Reproduced by kind permission of the Philadelphia Museum of Art.)

which had a very good reputation although he was not happy there. His artistic talent was, however, soon recognized and developed under the tutelage of David Allan, the painter. Even while a youth he began to assist his brother John, a surgeon anatomist 11 years his senior, in his Anatomy School, while at the same time attending lectures at the university where Monro secundus was professor of anatomy. His first book, A *System* of *Dissections,* was published in

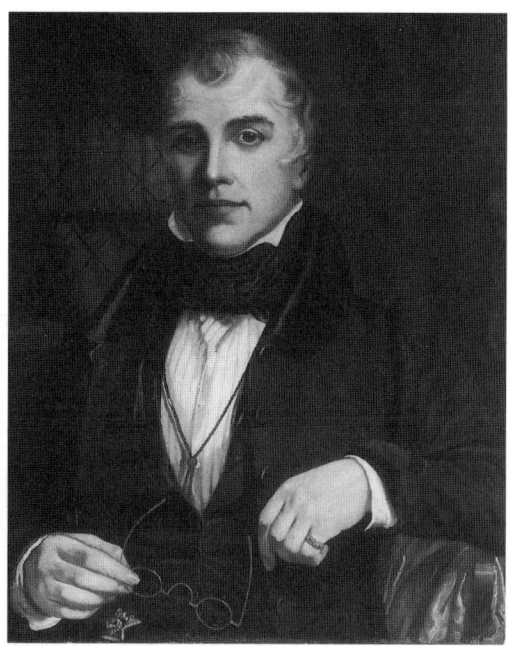

Fig. 2.5 Sir Charles Bell, 1774–1842. (Reproduced by kind permission of the National Galleries of Scotland, Edinburgh.)

1798 when he was only 24 years old, with plates engraved from his own careful drawings. The following year he was admitted as a member of the College of Surgeons in Edinburgh. However, he was urged by his brother George '… to go to London to see at least, what the world at large had to offer…' and so he left for the capital on 23 November, 1804 at the age of 30, where he then spent most of his working life as an anatomist-surgeon.

Within 2 years he published his famed *Essays on the Anatomy of Expression in Painting* (Figure 2.6), a work which Charles Darwin much admired and referred to in his own work *Expression of the Emotions*. In 1811, at this time living at 34 Soho Square, Bell married Marion Shaw of Ayr. The following year he became proprietor of the Windmill Street School of Anatomy, nowadays the Lyric Theatre, Shaftesbury Avenue, the present stage door formerly being the entrance for 'subjects for dissection'.

Bell joined the staff of the Middlesex Hospital in 1814, where he was to remain a surgeon for over 20 years; he was a founder of the Middlesex Medical School. In 1828 he was appointed professor of physiology and surgery at the newly established University of London, later known as University College. Two years later, however, he resigned over internecine disagreements among various members of the professoriate, a not uncommon situation at any time.

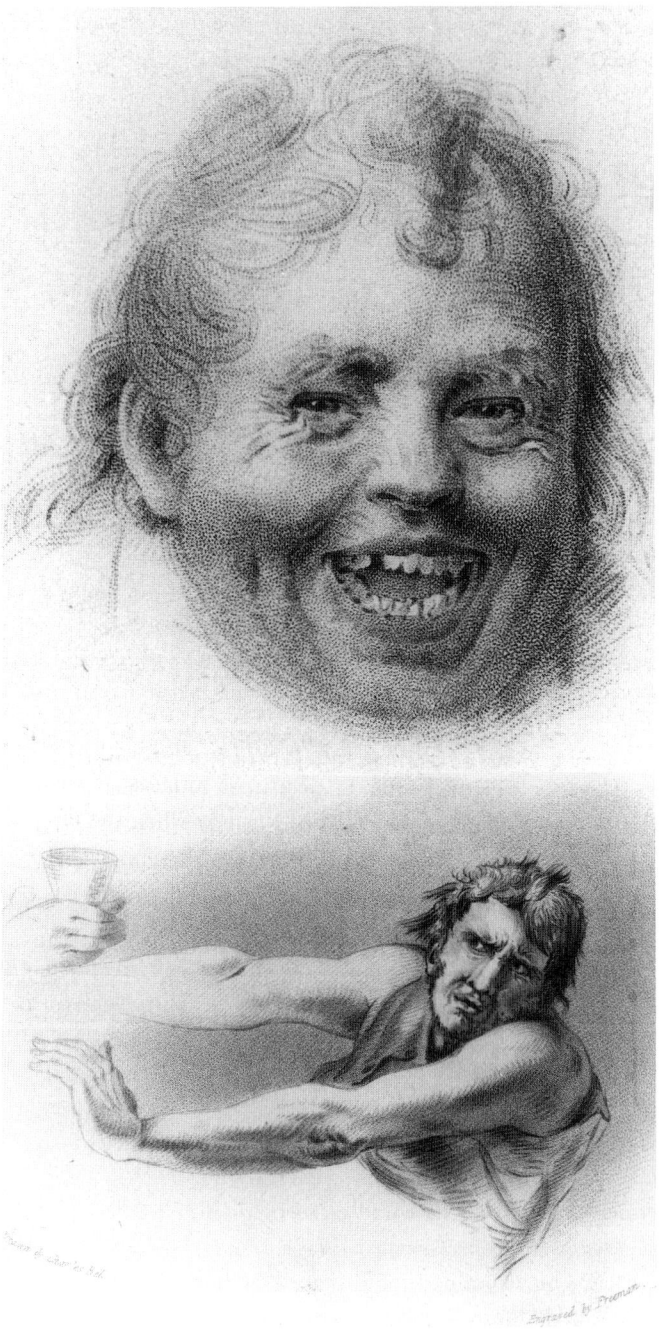

Fig. 2.6 Illustrations from Charles Bell's *Essays on the Anatomy of Expression in Painting*. Above: laughter; below: hydrophobia.

But this was the year in which he published his classical work, particularly germane to the history of muscular dystrophy, *The Nervous System of the Human Body*, which subsequently ran to several editions.

In 1836, at the age of 62, he returned to Edinburgh as professor of surgery and settled in Ainslie Place in the New Town. However, his return was not as happy as he had perhaps hoped. He had made his name and reputation in London and his colleagues in Edinburgh were possibly somewhat jealous. Whatever the reason, he turned increasingly to hobbies and working on new editions of his books. In fact, most of his correspondence at the time was concerned with the delights of fishing the streams of lowland Scotland[7].

His name is eponymously associated with facial palsy, but his main achievement was the elucidation, with the French experimental physiologist François Magendie, of the distinct functions of the posterior (sensory) and anterior (motor) nerve roots of the spinal cord. Unfortunately, his findings were somewhat soured by a controversy with Magendie over priorities, which has been detailed elsewhere[8]. Nevertheless, it is clear that he was well liked by most.

He was kind-hearted and sympathetic to his patients and genial and encouraging to his students. The latter eagerly attended his lectures, which were renowned for their clarity. He was one of those rare individuals who could have succeeded in several different careers: as an anatomist, surgeon, writer, or painter. He died on the 28th of April 1842 of angina while visiting friends at Hallow Park near Worcester, where he is buried (Figure 2.7).

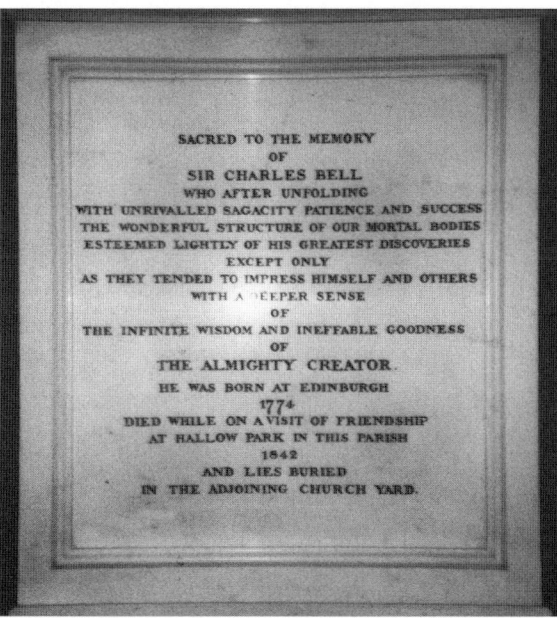

Fig. 2.7 Memorial tablet to Sir Charles Bell in Hallow Church, Worcester.

From the point of view of the history of muscular dystrophy, Bell described in *The Nervous System of the Human Body*[9] a number of individuals with various deformities resulting from muscle contractures, a subject which was to become the particular interest of Little nearly a quarter of a century later. Bell was especially concerned with the resultant effects of involvement of different muscle groups on function and deformity. Most of the cases he described seem likely to have had a neurogenic basis. But case number 89 (in the first edition published in 1830) is interesting because this seems likely to have been muscular dystrophy. This was a young man of 18 with muscle wasting which had first been noticed when he was around 10 years old:

> It began with a weakness in the thighs, which disabled him from rising; and it is now curious to observe how he will twist and jerk his body to throw himself upright from his seat. I use this expression, for it is a very different motion from that of rising from the chair.

This fits very well the description later eponymously associated with Gowers (Chapter 6) for the way in which individuals with weakness of the hip extensors rise from a sitting position.

In the details provided by Bell the emphasis, understandable in the light of his training and interest, is the involvement of different muscle groups. When the patient was aged 18, Bell records:

> All the muscles of the lower extremities, the hips, and the abdomen, are debilitated and wasted. The extensor quadriceps femoris of both limbs is wasted, and yet the vasti externi have not suffered in an equal degree. A firm ball, remarkably prominent just above the knee joint, marks the place of the vastus externus, while the rectus is quite wasted and gone…. There is a slight curvature or projection of the lumbar part of the spine. He is weak, and subject to palpitations on going up stairs….

There was no sensory loss.

This description would seem to agree with the diagnosis of muscular dystrophy and the fact that at 18 he could apparently still climb stairs suggests the possibility of Becker muscular dystrophy. Without muscle pathology, however, the diagnosis of muscular dystrophy cannot be certain. A review of Bell's other publications indicates that he did not seek nor write about any other cases like this.

Around this time, however, two Neapolitan physicians published a detailed account of two brothers who clearly would now be considered to have had muscular dystrophy.

Gaetano Conte (1798–1858)

Gowers, in his book *Pseudo-hypertrophic Muscular Paralysis*, published in 1879[10], refers to a report in 1838 by a Coste and Gioja of Naples of two brothers with possible muscular dystrophy. But this was a mistake perpetuated from Schmidt's *Jahrbücher*[11]. Research by Professor Giovanni Nigro of the University of Naples[12] has revealed that the cases in question were reported by Professor Gaetano Conte *(not* Coste) with the assistance of a Dr L. Gioja in 1836 (not 1838) in the *Annali Clinici dell' Ospedale degl' Incurabili di Napoli*[13]. The paper has now been reprinted in full in *Cardiomyology* in April 1986[12]. These same brothers had also been reported, though in much less detail, by Giovanni Semmola (1793–1865) in a lecture at the Accademia Pontaniana in late 1833 which was published the following year[14]. Semmola refers to this as a disease of voluntary muscle which in his opinion was unique and had not been described before. His report is particularly interesting because he mentions that there was also a younger brother who was just beginning to show signs of the disease. He therefore clearly recognized that this was a progressive condition. The family came from the town of Pescolamazza, south of Naples. Semmola makes a strong plea that the two older brothers should be brought to Naples and admitted to hospital so that this previously unknown disease could be thoroughly investigated and studied by experts, and appeals to the authorities to arrange this.

Gaetano Conte was born in Naples in 1798 at a time when the city was rapidly becoming a leading centre of medical learning. In the nineteenth century it was to boast no less than 50 medical and scientific journals and publications. From an early age Conte showed exceptional talent. In 1813 he was awarded highest honours in a public competition which later would allow him free access to the 'Collegio Medico-Chirurgico'. Five years later he took first place in a public competition for the chair of pathology in Salerno, a position he was unable to occupy until 1821, when he reached the legally prescribed age of 23. In his subsequent career he was instrumental in creating a Medical-Surgical-Pharmaceutical Institute and wrote widely on philosophy, pathology, public, and private hygiene as well as legal matters. He was apparently fluent in several languages, including English, French, Latin, and Greek. He became Professor at the Ospedale degl' Incurabili in Naples and in 1826 wrote a monograph on epilepsy which was translated into several languages. However, his most famous work of the period concerned the therapeutic value of thermal baths and sauna. In 1840 he suffered a stroke from which he partly recovered, although ill-health forced his retirement 3 years later. He moved then to Pozzuoli, where he had previously been medical director of the thermomineral baths. He died in 1858 in Capua, just north of Naples.

While head of the department at the Hospital for Incurables in Naples he was particularly interested in the care of patients with 'scrofola,' which at the time no doubt encompassed mainly tuberculosis *(Enciclopedia Italiana di Scienza,* ed. 1949, Roma), but probably also included other diseases with profound wasting such as muscular dystrophy. Certainly the two brothers he described could well have had the disease now referred to as Duchenne muscular dystrophy. They both manifested hypertrophy of the calf and deltoid muscles. Interestingly, it is recorded that '… the hypertrophied muscles had indeed lost that palpability typical of their fibres, yet they seemed to be invaded by a hard, earth-like substance, heterogeneous to their structure.' Nowadays, physicians often refer to the pseudohypertrophic calves in this condition as having a 'woody' consistency or feel. Weakness first became apparent at age 8 and was thereafter progressive, affecting particularly the lower limbs. The elder boy '…departed this life with signs of hypertrophy of the heart.' Cardiac failure is in fact not uncommon in various forms of muscular dystrophy. Two years later the other brother, then age 17, was admitted to the Hospital for Incurables. He was found to have widespread muscle weakness and his tongue was recorded as being enlarged (macroglossia occurs not infrequently in Duchenne muscular dystrophy). There were flexion contractures particularly of the hips and knees '…so much so that the heels could touch the buttocks…' and marked talipes. Such deformities commonly occur in the later stages of muscular dystrophy owing to weakness and resultant prolonged immobility. Sensation was normal as was mentation.

It seems very likely that these two brothers had muscular dystrophy and, in view of the early onset and relatively rapid progression, probably the Duchenne type of the disease. But since there was no report on muscle pathology, again the diagnosis cannot be entirely certain. As in the case of Charles Bell there is no evidence that Gaetano Conte made any attempt at a systematic study of such cases. Nevertheless, this appears to be the very first detailed clinical description of muscular dystrophy.

Richard Partridge (1805–1873)

Richard Partridge can be credited with having presented a case of what is very likely to have been muscular dystrophy to the Pathological Society of London in 1847 and with having also examined the muscle tissue at autopsy. It seems that he was the first to submit a case to pathological investigation.

Richard Partridge was born in January 1805 and studied medicine at St Bartholomew's Hospital, London, becoming a member of the Royal College of Surgeons in 1827. He then became a demonstrator at the Windmill Street School of Anatomy shortly after Charles Bell had relinquished his interest in the School. Later in his career he became professor of anatomy at King's College, London and subsequently surgeon at King's College Hospital. In 1831 he received publicity for having suspected the murder of an Italian boy whose body had been brought to the dissecting room of King's College by the notorious Bishop, Williams, and May. Partridge was aware of the methods employed by the infamous Edinburgh pair, Burke and Hare, and, suspecting foul play, delayed payment of the requested nine guineas by saying he had only a £50 note and no change, until the police arrived. Bishop and his accomplice Williams were found guilty and duly executed. Bishop's body, ironically, was in turn dissected at the Windmill Sheet School. May was reprieved and sentenced to transportation for life. This case was in large part responsible for the passing of the Anatomy Act the following year.

Partridge later achieved further publicity when he was sent to Spezzia to treat Garibaldi for a bullet wound (but failed to discover the bullet, the presence of which was subsequently demonstrated by the French surgeon, Auguste Nélaton). Partridge, like Charles Bell, was an accomplished artist and belonged to a family with artistic leanings; his brother, John, was a fashionable portrait painter, and his son (Bernard) later became a celebrated political cartoonist for *Punch*. Partridge was among those who in 1850 successfully proposed Edward Meryon for membership of the Athenaeum.

During his lifetime Partridge received many honours. He was elected a Fellow of the Royal Society in 1837 and held senior offices in no less than three organizations: vice-president of the Pathological Society, president of the Royal College of Surgeons (though '… it cannot be admitted that he was a great surgeon in the proper acceptation of that word.'[15]) and the Royal Medical & Chirurgical Society. His obituaries indicate that he was a much respected anatomist and teacher with a noted sense of humour: he referred to the half-starved-looking horses that drew his carriage as 'longissimus dorsi' and 'os innominatum'! He appears to have continued working right up to his death in March 1873 (Figure 2.8).

For the purposes of our historical study of muscular dystrophy, interest centres on a case he presented to the Pathological Society of London meeting on 15 November 1847[16,17]. The case was that of a 14-year-old boy who, from about the age of 9, had developed progressive muscle wasting and weakness, and enlarged calves and muscle contractures and who died from pneumonia following an attack of measles. At autopsy:

> The deltoid and sternomastoid muscles had undergone fatty degeneration. The calves (which were larger than natural, and had during the process of the paralysis, become permanently contracted) presented a greater degree of fatty degeneration in their muscular structure than the upper extremities, the soleus and gastrocnemius being more affected also than the flexor longus pollicis; neither the nerves or tendons had undergone change.

Partridge was puzzled by the case and was at a loss to explain it. Tissues were examined macroscopically but apparently not subjected to microscopic

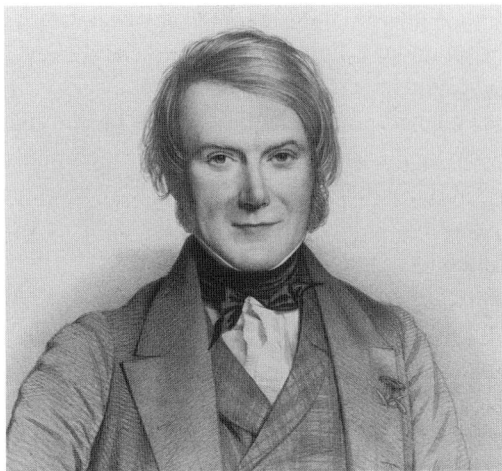

Fig. 2.8 Richard Partridge, 1805–1873. (Reproduced by kind permission of The President and Council of the Royal College of Surgeons of England.)

examination. Some 5 years later clinical details of this case, along with his affected brother, were reported by Edward Meryon in his 1852 paper[18].

However, the most detailed clinical description of the disease before Meryon and Duchenne was provided by Little.

William J. Little (1810–1894)

Willam J. Little is now perhaps best known for his eponymous association with spastic diplegia in children, so-called Little's disease, which he concluded was due to perinatal factors, most notably anoxia at birth[19,20]. But outside paediatrics, his name is associated among orthopaedic surgeons with his pioneering work on subcutaneous tenotomy for the relief of deformities, most notably club foot, from which he himself suffered and was successfully treated using this radical new procedure by Doctor Louis Stromeyer in Hanover. He also founded the Orthopaedic Institution of London, now the Royal Orthopaedic Hospital[21–24].

Little was born on 7 August 1810 in the East End of London not very far from the London Hospital where in later life he became senior physician. His childhood was dogged by ill-health, and an attack of infantile paralysis left him with a club foot. On the advice of Dr Algernon Frampton, who was later to become a colleague at the London Hospital, Little was sent to the country near Dover and later to the Jesuit College of St Omer in France. Here he developed a great love of the French language, in which he excelled and, as a schoolboy at St Omer, actually gained the prize in French composition. On returning to

England at the age of 16 he became apprenticed to an apothecary, but 2 years later surrendered his indentures to become a student at the London Hospital. In 1831, in the same year as Meryon, he became a Licentiate of the Apothecaries Company and the following year a member of the Royal College of Surgeons. As a result of being unsuccessful in an attempt to obtain a position as surgeon at the London Hospital, he turned to medicine, but this required further study. The Royal College of Physicians at that time required of all candidates for its licence a 2 year residence and graduation at a university. He decided to pursue further studies in Germany, partly to gain an additional qualification but also, one suspects, to learn more of Stromeyer's recently published technique of subcutaneous tenotomy, no doubt in the hope that it might in fact benefit himself. In the event he became a strong advocate of the technique, and his MD (Berlin) thesis was the first monograph on tenotomy for club foot to be published. This work led him to study the causes and treatment of various other deformities, his most important work on the subject being published in 1853[25].

His professional life mainly centred on the Royal Orthopaedic Hospital, the London Hospital, where he became senior physician, and private practice (Figure 2.9). He only retired from active medical work when he was well into his seventies. His remaining years were somewhat marred by increasing deafness, although he continued to take an active interest in medical matters until his death in 1894.

At the time most surgeons and physicians held only vague ideas as to the nature of deformities. Little's major contribution was the demonstration that

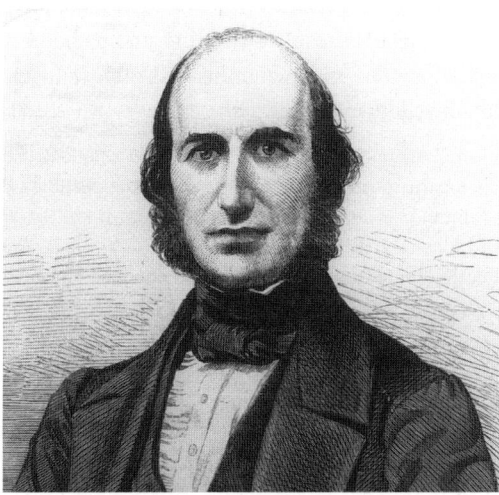

Fig. 2.9 William J. Little, 1810–1894. (Reprinted from The Lancet, Vol. 63, Biographical sketch of William J. Little, M.D., Physician to the London Hospital, etc., pp.16–22, Copyright (1854), with permission from Elsevier.)

such deformities could arise from abnormal muscular activity. In his book *Deformities of the Human Frame*[25], among other observations concerning the correction of such deformities, he provides a very careful and complete clinical description of two brothers with what would now be termed Duchenne muscular dystrophy. The details of these cases are more widely available now that they have been reprinted in full[26]. In essence, these two brothers (aged 14 and 12) presented very similar features. They had been normal at birth but were slow in learning to walk, with ambulation later becoming increasingly difficult.

Interestingly, in brother A (age 14) his gait '…was peculiar, his head and body having been inclined backwards…', what we would now refer to as lordosis. He walked on his toes and had enlarged calves. Both brothers ceased walking around age 11 and thereafter became confined to a lying position most of the day, only occasionally sitting in an armchair with support; they had both developed scoliosis. The shoulder girdle musculature was also affected: the shoulders appeared loose and upper arm very small, so that a stranger would fear to grasp him by the arms. This upper limb weakness in brother A is reflected in the observation:

> He can reach his mouth and feed himself by resting the elbows on table. He can touch his head by alternately helping each hand with the other.

This is a good description of trick movements, in which patients with muscle weakness can become quite adept. Both were very intelligent and there was no sensory loss.

However, Little was not content with providing a detailed clinical picture, but then proceeded to detail the autopsy findings in brother A, who died shortly after the consultation. The gastrocnemius and soleus muscles were uncommonly large, whitish yellow in colour with:

> …traces only of muscular tissue; the mass being composed of adipose matter, apparently occupying, for the most part, the areolar tissue; the posterior tibial, flex. long. poll. and flex. comm., presenting a slightly pink colour, were less degenerated than gastrocnemii and solei. The deltoids and sternomastoids as much changed as surales. Tendons unaffected. Spinal muscles small, but unchanged in structure. Interior of brain and medulla spinalis apparently healthy. (Ref. 25, page 16.)

And, more minutely:

> The degenerated muscles exhibited abundance of fat cells, with few traces of muscular fibre; in some fibrillae the transverse markings were scarcely distinguishable, in others they were quite distinct. (Ref. 25, page 16.)

There seems no doubt that these two brothers had muscular dystrophy, though the microscopic findings provide little detail and Little does not address the possibility that such weakness could perhaps have had a neurogenic basis.

Intriguingly, Little comments on an intracranial abnormality:

> Beneath squamous plate of right temporal bone and adjacent portion of parietal bone, a plate of bone, concave internally, convex externally, resembling squamous portion of a temporal bone, but thinner, was found. This abnormal plate was externally invested by layers of dura mater, to which it had remained attached on removal of calvarium; internally it was lined with arachnoid. Convolutions flattened and depressed, corresponding to the plate. Visceral arachnoid thickened, in many places opaque, with distinctly-organised deposit, as if from chronic inflammation. Numerous 'glandulae pacchioni.' (Ref. 25, page 16.)

This description is very similar indeed to that given by Partridge in his report[16], which also concerns a 14-year-old boy:

> On opening the cranium, a large plate of bone, corresponding to the squamous plate of the right temporal bone in situation and volume, was found between the dura mater and parietal arachnoid, the latter being thickened and opaque. The portion of brain beneath the plate of bone was slightly depressed. (Ref. 16, page 944.)

This same observation in both cases seems more than chance and raises the distinct possibility that they refer to one and the same case. This is supported by the fact that both were seen around the same time—November 1847 in Partridge's case and September 1847 in Little's case (although he actually reported it much later, in 1853).

If this is true then this would also be the same family later included by Meryon (Family H) among his cases. Finally, Little's case was first seen in consultation with a Mr Farish and Meryon admits that his case had previously been examined by Partridge and a Dr Farish!

By this time it is clear that among certain London physicians and surgeons there was already some interest in cases of muscle weakness in young boys for which there was no apparent and clear explanation. However, no systematic study of a series of such cases had been made. This was to be Meryon's unique contribution to the subject.

References

1. Dasen, V. *Dwarfs in Ancient Egypt and Greece*. Oxford: Clarendon Press, 1993.
2. Newberry, P. E. Beni Hasan, Part II. In: F. L. Griffith (ed.) *Archaeological Survey of Egypt*. London: Kegan Paul, Trench, Trübner & Co., 1893.
3. Pöch, W., Becker, P. E. Eine Muskeldystrophie auf einem altägyptischen Relief. *Nervenarzt*, 1955; **26**: 528–30.
4. Blashfield, E. H., Blashfield, E. W. & Hopkins, A. A. (eds.) Vasari, G.: *Lives of Seventy of the Most Eminent Painters, Sculptors and Architects*. London: George Bell, Vol. 3. 1897; 210–11.

5. Critchley, M. *Sir William Gowers (1845–1915): A Biographical Appreciation*. London: Heinemann, 1949.
6. Emery, A. E. H., Emery, M. Genetics in art. *Journal of Medical Genetics*, 1994; **31**: 420–2.
7. Bell, C. *Letters of Sir Charles Bell selected from his correspondence with his brother, George Joseph Bell*. London: Murray, 1870.
8. Gordon-Taylor, G., Walls, E. W. *Sir Charles Bell, His Life and Times*. Edinburgh and London: E. & S. Livingstone, 1958.
9. Bell, C. *The Nervous System of the Human Body*. London: Longman, 1830.
10. Gowers, W. R. *Pseudo-hypertrophic Muscular Paralysis—a Clinical Lecture*. London: J. & A. Churchill, 1879.
11. Schmidt, C. C. Krankhafte Hypertrophie des Muskelsystems. Mitteilung von den DDr. Coste und Gioja! In: *Schmidt's Jahrbücher der in- und ausländischen gesamten Medizin*, 1838; **24**: 176.
12. Nigro, G. Conte or Duchenne? *Cardiomyology*, 1986; **5**: 3–6.
13. Conte, G., Gioja, L. Scrofola del sistema muscolare. *Annali Clinici dell' Ospedale degl 'Incurabili di Napoli*, 1836; **2**: 66–79.
14. Semmola, G. 'Sopra due malattie...'. In: S. de Renzi (ed.) *Filiatre-Sebezio Giornale delle Scienze Mediche*, 1834; **8**: 58–68.
15. Obituary. Richard Partridge FRS FRCS. *Medical Times & Gazette*, 1873; **1**: 347–8.
16. Partridge, R. Fatty degeneration of muscle. (Report of Proceedings of the Pathology Society of London). *London Medical Gazette (New Series)*, 1847; **5**: 944.
17. Partridge, R. Fatty degeneration of voluntary muscle. *Transactions of the Pathological Society of London*, 1848; **1**: 334–5.
18. Meryon, E. On granular and fatty degeneration of the voluntary muscles. *Medico-Chirurgical Transactions*, 1852; **35**: 73–84.
19. Little, W. J. Course of lectures on the deformities of the human frame. Lecture IX, character of spastic rigidity of muscles and deformity in infants, young children and adults. *Lancet*, 1843/4; **1**: 350–4.
20. Little, W. J. On the influence of abnormal parturition, difficult labours, premature birth and asphyxia neonatorum, on the mental and physical condition of the child, especially in relation to deformities. *Transactions of the Obstetrical Society of London*, 1861; **3**: 293–345.
21. Siegel, I. M. Little big man: the life and genius of William John Little (1810–1894). *Orthopaedic Review*, 1988; **17**: 1160–6.
22. Schleichkorn, J. *The Sometime Physician*. New York: Farmingdale, 1987.
23. Biographical sketch. William J. Little, MD. *Lancet*, 1854; **1**: 16–22.
24. Obituary. William J. Little MD, FRCP. *Lancet*, 1894; **ii**: 168–9.
25. Little, W. J. *On the Nature and Treatment of the Deformities of the Human Frame: being a Course of Lectures delivered at the Royal Orthopaedic Hospital in 1843*. London: Longman, Brown, Green & Longmans, 1853.
26. Accardo, P. J. An early case report of muscular dystrophy—a footnote to the history of neuromuscular disorders. *Archives of Neurology*, 1981; **38**: 144–6.

Chapter 3

Edward Meryon's contribution to muscular dystrophy

The history of muscular dystrophy really begins with the first systematic study of the condition by Edward Meryon in the early 1850s. He lived during a very interesting period in English history, namely from 1807 to 1880. This was a time when much was changing in society and in the practice of medicine.

Society and medicine in Victorian times

Napoleon's ambitions had ended with the battle of Waterloo in 1815. Thereafter, apart from the Crimean War of 1854–6, which Trevelyan referred to as 'merely a foolish expedition to the Black Sea', the country was not to be engaged in any major war for a hundred years—that is, throughout Queen Victoria's reign (1837–1901). With peace there was rising prosperity, the driving force for which was the Industrial Revolution, with the British Empire providing much needed markets for its products. By the middle of the century, over 90% of British exports consisted of manufactured goods, whereas less than 10% of imports consisted of similar goods from elsewhere. Almost a quarter of world trade passed through British ports, most of it carried by British ships.

The need to convey manufactured and other goods within Britain required efficient means of transport and communication. George Stephenson's steam engine was introduced in 1814 and 227 miles of track had been built by 1836, which in 15 years alone had increased to 6802 miles. Steam replaced sail and the first steamer plied between Dover and Calais in 1821. Rowland Hill introduced the Penny Post in 1840 and the electric telegraph was installed in London 6 years later.

The manufacturing power and wealth of Britain increased enormously in the first half of Victoria's reign. But this was at a price. Factories and mills attracted people to the towns and cities where commercial business was also transacted. The population of London, for example, rose from 1.25 million in 1820 to 3.25 million in 1871. As a result there was much overcrowding and the development of squalid slum dwellings. In London, Lord Shaftesbury

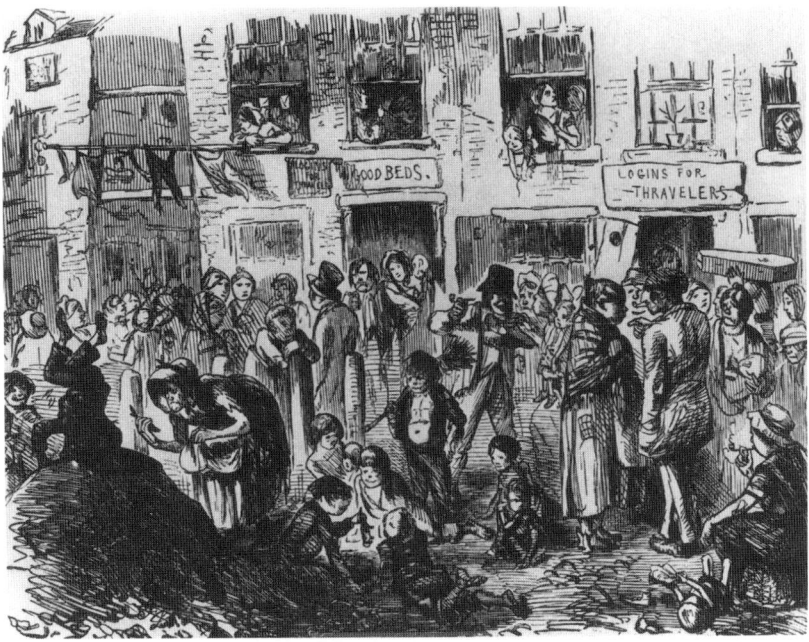

Fig. 3.1 Soho, London around 1850. (From a drawing in *Punch* entitled *A Court for King Cholera* by John Leech.)

discovered a room with a family in each of its four corners, and a room with a cesspool immediately below its boarded floor (Figure 3.1).

Among the underprivileged disease was rife, most notably tuberculosis, which remained a mystery, punctuated by periodic outbreaks of smallpox, typhoid, and cholera. Venereal disease and alcoholism were also all too common. Widespread famine occurred in Ireland in 1845–7 as a result of the failure of the potato crop. Many thousands died and others emigrated to Britain or North America.

Increasing awareness of these problems led to the Registration Act of 1836 whereby all births, marriages, and deaths were recorded and in this way the problems could begin to be quantified. There followed legislation in the 1830s and 1840s to protect workers, for example by prohibiting women and children from working underground or for more than 10 hours a day. The first Public Health Act dates from 1848. The many other Reform Bills of this period have been documented and discussed[1,2]. At the same time the 1858 Medical Act set up the General Medical Council which thereafter regulated entry into the profession at a time when there was also increasing specialization within the profession.

Great changes were taking place within medicine itself. The first half of the century saw the invention of a number of important diagnostic tools, such as the stethoscope (by René Laënnec in 1816), the ophthalmoscope (by Charles Babbage in 1847; later improved by Hermann von Helmholtz in 1851), the laryngoscope (by Manuel Garcia in 1854–5), the sphygmograph, the predecessor of the sphygmomanometer (by Etienne Jules Marey in 1860), and the clinical thermometer (by Thomas Allbutt around 1870). The medical journal *Lancet* was founded in 1823 and the British Medical Association in 1856. Photography as we now know it began in the 1840s and the first photomicrographs appeared around 1860.

At this time, along with developments in pathology and medical chemistry, there was also a growing interest in delineating specific disease entities, many of which still bear their discoverer's name, such as Parkinson's disease (James Parkinson, 1817), Bright's disease (Richard Bright, 1827), Hodgkin's disease (Thomas Hodgkin, 1832), Graves disease (Robert Graves, 1835), and Addison's disease (Thomas Addison, 1849).

However, the most dramatic new developments were to be seen in surgery, with the introduction of anaesthesia, most notably chloroform in obstetrics, by James Young Simpson in 1847, and the recognition that wound infections could be prevented by antiseptic surgery (Joseph Lister, 1867), later to be succeeded by aseptic surgery.

Previous to this period most believed that diseases like cholera were caused by noxious elements in the atmosphere (miasmic theories), outbreaks of which so outraged the Victorian novelist Charles Dickens. The frustration of physicians to find a cause for such diseases is exemplified by Dr Tertius Lydgate in George Eliot's *Middlemarch*. John Snow's demonstration that removal of the handle from the Broad Street pump curtailed an outbreak of cholera in Soho in 1854 is well known. This, and the work of others at the time, including William Farr and William Budd, demonstrated that the provision of clean water could eliminate the risk of cholera. As a result, the miasmic theory began to decline although it was not until toward the end of the century that Koch succeeded in culturing the causative *Vibrio cholerae*.

The idea of contagion causing puerperal fever proposed by the Hungarian physician Ignaz Semmelweiss and the American physician and author Oliver Wendell Holmes in the 1840s, and the later pioneering work of Louis Pasteur and Robert Koch, laid the foundation of the *germ theory* of disease. Later in the century, techniques were developed for culturing, staining, and identifying different disease-causing bacteria. These must therefore have been very exciting times for those working in medicine and searching for explanations for diseases.

The *Communist Manifesto* issued by Marx and Engels appeared in 1848 but it is much more likely that a little later Charles Darwin's theories would have attracted more attention. In 1858 papers were presented at the Linnean Society of London from Charles Darwin and Alfred Russel Wallace and the following year saw the publication of Darwin's *The Origin of Species*[3]. At the 1860 British Association for Advancement of Science meeting in Oxford there was the famous clash over Darwin's theory between Huxley and Bishop Wilberforce. The subject must have been a frequent topic of conversation, if not hotly debated, in many circles at the time.

No doubt Meryon, as an educated physician, would have been familiar with all these happenings.

The constitution of man

Meryon's first book[4], *The Constitution of Man*, was published in 1836 in the early years of his professional life. It is dedicated to Newman Smith, Esq., a governor of St Thomas' Hospital Medical School and later to become one of Meryon's mentors, and with whom he shared a common interest in natural history. In the dedication he states:

> During the leisure hours which usually attend the first few years of professional life, I have sought relaxation in accumulating materials for the following unpretending pages....

From this, and from various other sources of the period, it seems that the early years of a medical career were different from now. A private practice, for example, often took several years to develop, leaving more time at first for academic and other pursuits.

The main thesis of the book is a consideration of the factors which he believed influenced the physical and intellectual constitution of the various races of Man. As he states in the opening sentence, 'To know man unconnected with external nature, is to know him but half'.

There are six chapters. The first concerns the geology of the earth's surface. He considers the fossil evidence of the succession of life forms, from the simplest to the most complex. Meryon believed that Man appeared relatively recently and was a unique creation:

> ...that he is widely separated from all other beings.... (and) stands a distinct unconnected species in the animal chain. (Ref. 4, pages 39–40.)

In the second chapter he considers the animal world and in particular their various adaptations to the environment. But though some of his views on adaptations vaguely resemble those later expressed by Darwin, Meryon offers no explanation for how such adaptations may have come about, nor the succession of life forms, other than that they reflect '… the marks of a supreme and intelligent Power.'

He is clear, however, that the inheritance of acquired characteristics[5] is not supportable for a number of reasons. He cites, for example, the Chinese habit of binding the feet and of contracting the chest by tight lacing, neither of which, he emphasizes, has led to deformities in the offspring, and that the bowed shin bones of Africans is a reflection of the custom of squatting and is not hereditary. Yet a revered anatomist, Wood Jones, as late as 1943 persisted in the belief that the enlarged heel bones he observed in some races were caused by the inheritance of this character which had been acquired as a result of squatting[6].

It is clear in these discussions that Meryon was well read in natural history and comparative anatomy, in which he was later to become a lecturer at St Thomas' Hospital Medical School. For example, at one point he discusses the presence or absence in various animal species of the ligamentum teres of the hip joint and how this might be related to their differing ways of life.

In Chapter 3 he considers varieties of the human species and the classification of human races. He accepts the classification of Johann Friedrich Blumenbach (1752–1840), a distinguished professor of anatomy at the University of Göttingen at the time and the acknowledged founder of comparative anatomy[7]. His classification comprised[8,9] Caucasian, Mongolian, Ethiopian, American, and Malayan, to which Meryon adds as a sixth the so-called Hyperborean, for the inhabitants of the extreme northern latitudes.

Meryon admits, however, that such a classification '… can do but little in facilitating the study of man', and uses it merely to emphasize the features of different groups. He believed strongly that all the races of Man had a single origin. He then proceeds to describe the physical (and later, intellectual and temperamental) features of each group, and in the remaining three chapters attempts to explain how these are a reflection of diet and climate (humidity, temperature, sunlight). For example, when discussing Africans:

> Where the heat is most oppressive, there the colour of the skin is darkest; where the climate is most temperate and soil most fertile, there the tribes are the finest and tallest. The hair, moreover, is observed, generally speaking, to be woolly or not, according to the influence of climate; appearing black and straight in the Moors, Berbers and Arabs, as also in some tribes of Foulahs; universally woolly in the Negro…. (Ref. 4, page 156.)

There is no doubt in Meryon's mind, and in that of most Victorians of the period, that those from temperate countries (which included Britain) possessed the best qualities!

> In temperate countries where the action of the circulating system is rendered active by an invigorating atmosphere, the sanguine temperament generally prevails. A fair and ruddy complexion with bluish eyes, auburn hair, an enlivened countenance, firmness of muscle, and moderate plumpness, are the physical characteristics of this

temperament in its greatest purity; as goodness, generosity, intensity of feeling, and sincerity are its mental attributes. (Ref. 4, pages 185–6.)

In these discussions he makes special reference to goitre, owing to enlargement of the thyroid gland, being common in the mountainous regions of Austria and Switzerland for example, and also in Derbyshire where it was referred to as 'Derbyshire neck' (page 128), but for which he has no satisfactory explanation (it was not until 1918 that the cause was confirmed by David Marine of Cleveland, Ohio to be iodine deficiency). He also refers to albinism which he attributes to 'non-secretion of the *pigmentum nigrum*' in the skin (page 228) but does not mention that it can be familial.

Meryon must have put a great deal of thought and effort into writing *The Constitution of Man*. He makes reference to no less than 80 sources, ranging from the classical period (Theophrastus, Herodotus, Tacitus, Aristotle, Justin, and, of course, Hippocrates) to later times (Galen, Linnaeus, Buffon, Cuvier, Lamarck, and Lyell), as well as to philosophers such as Rousseau and Voltaire. Some of the quotations are given in Latin. He even refers to statistical data on mortality rates in various European countries. He mentions phrenology, then enjoying some popularity, but considers it has no foundation in fact!

On several occasions he refers to heredity in relation to 'whole families possessing some physical peculiarities' (page 100) and that 'we sometimes find the offspring assuming the characteristics of either one of its parents' (page 116), but he does not develop the topic further. And as we have seen, he can provide no satisfactory explanation for the succession of life forms found in fossil records. Furthermore, he refers to 'miasma as a known cause of fever', though he argues that this cannot be true in all cases (page 234), and he believed 'microscopic animals are generated spontaneously' (page 33). In expressing such opinions he was merely echoing those of the time. Nevertheless, the book is of historical interest because it encapsulates many of the views which were then held by educated people of mid-Victorian England. On several occasions he also strongly criticizes religious bigotry and intolerance, perhaps because of his own family's Huguenot origins.

Edward Meryon and Charles Darwin

Charles Darwin (1809–1882), whose celebrated work *On the Origin of Species by Means of Natural Selection* was published in 1859, was an avid reader of anything relating to natural variation. No doubt he therefore consulted Meryon's *The Constitution of Man*. Certainly the two men were well known to each other[10]. Both were members of the Geological Society, the Ethnological Society, and the Athenaeum. In fact it was Meryon in 1868, as a member of

Council, who proposed Darwin for Honorary Fellowship of the Royal Medical and Chirurgical Society (later the Royal Society of Medicine). The two men were also related: Darwin married a Wedgwood and Meryon's grandson also married a Wedgwood.

Both men, however, faced serious problems in their respective fields: Darwin was unable to explain how natural selection was possible, and Meryon was unable to explain how muscular dystrophy was inherited. Both ideas would have to await the emergence of Mendelian genetics in 1900.

How did Meryon first become interested in muscle disease?

In considering Meryon's work on muscular dystrophy the question arises as to how he might have become interested in the subject in the first place. Meryon was a medical student at London University (Figure 3.2), later to become University College London, from 1829 to 1831. The course outlines and introductory lectures were published at the time[11–13] and there is no mention of paralysis or muscle disease in the courses of anatomy (Prof. J. R. Bennett), comparative anatomy (Prof. R. E. Grant), surgery (Prof. Charles Bell), nature and treatment of diseases (Prof. J. Conolly), or materia medica (Prof. A. T. Thomson).

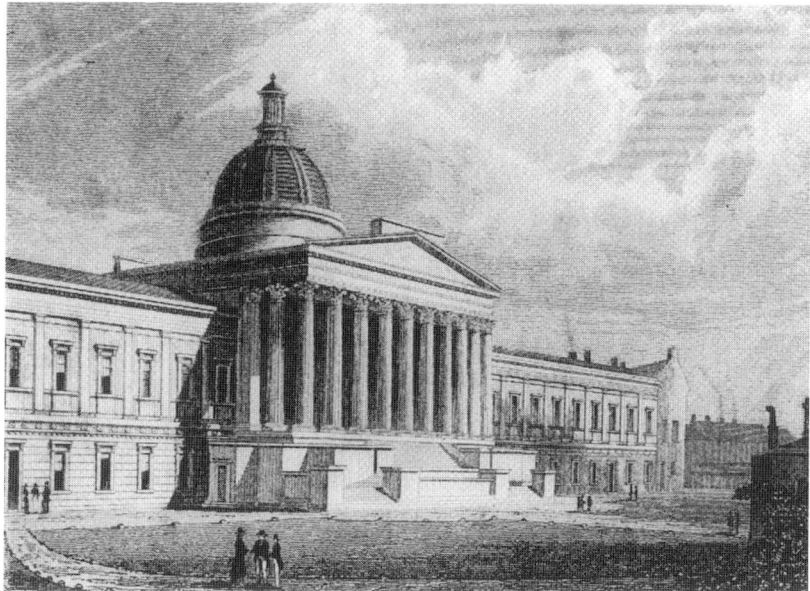

Fig. 3.2 London University, 1831. (From *The Public Buildings of Westminster Described*, London: John Harris.)

However, in Pattison's anatomy course he mentions 'changes produced in the structure of the muscular system from disease,' (Ref. 11, page 139), and this was actually the course in anatomy in which Meryon was awarded a gold medal. Charles Bell, in his course in physiology, specifically includes 'distinction in spasmodic and paralytic affections', and it was in this course that he was awarded a certificate of honour. It is therefore possible that Meryon's instruction as a student may have had a bearing on his later interest in muscle disease. But this is purely speculative.

The report of two affected brothers by Conte and Gioja of Naples in 1836 is most unlikely to have been familiar to Meryon when he presented his cases in 1851. We have seen that Charles Bell published details of a single case in 1830, but it seems somewhat unlikely that Meryon would have been aware of this or, if so, to have realized its significance. Duchenne's important contributions on muscle disease could not have been a guide either because they did not appear until the 1860s.

However, we have also seen that cases had been reported in 1847 quite independently by Partridge and by Little. Now Partridge and Little were both associated with the Royal Medical and Chirurgical Society. Richard Partridge FRS had been a Fellow since 1828 and in 1847 became vice president (and the following year vice president of the Pathological Society of London). William John Little had become a Fellow of the Society in 1845, 2 years before Meryon. Both Partridge and Little had presented material at Society meetings and Partridge's case was subsequently included among the cases reported by Meryon. It therefore seems quite likely that Partridge and Little may have been the source of Meryon's initial interest in the subject. Furthermore, Meryon's first case had been under the care of a Mr Tamplin (Richard Tamplin, Surgeon to the Royal Orthopaedic Hospital), who had earlier been Little's assistant.

Meryon mentions in his paper the names of several physicians and surgeons who had been involved in the care of some of his reported cases. We have identified all these individuals as being Fellows of the Society at the time. They include Sir Benjamin Brodie (1783–1862), who had been a Fellow of the Society since 1813 and had become president in 1839, Dr Bright (Richard Bright FRS, physician extraordinary to the Queen and consulting physician to Guy's Hospital), Mr Tatum (Thomas Tatum, surgeon to St George's Hospital), and Dr Barker (Thomas Barker, physician to St Thomas' Hospital, where Meryon lectured twice a week). At this time, William Withey Gull (1816–1890), noted for his particular interest and contributions on the causes of paralysis[14], was also a Fellow of the Society.

Thus, it seems that there was quite a lot of interest in such cases among members of the Society around 1850. However, it was Meryon's great contribution to realize the similarity among the various cases and, most significantly, that they represented a specific and unique disease entity. As Francis Bacon in 1620 so aptly wrote:

> the lofty and discursive mind recognizes and puts together the finest and most general resemblances.

Granular degeneration of muscle

Meryon's contributions to muscular dystrophy begin with a paper he presented at the Royal Medical and Chirurgical Society on 9 December 1851, in the presence of the president (Joseph Hodgson FRS) and the two secretaries (Seth Thompson and Campbell de Morgan). This was a well attended meeting, with no less than 90 Fellows being present, which included Sir James Syme and James Paget, as well as 19 visitors. There were three presentations at the meeting: a surgical paper, one on the alkalization of urine by Bence Jones, and, finally, Meryon's paper. The minutes of this meeting were reported in the *Lancet* at the time[15]. Full details appeared in the *Transactions* of the Society the following year[16]. Here he described in some detail nine boys (one of whom had died some years previously) in three different families, all affected with progressive muscle wasting and weakness. The clinical descriptions are detailed and would be consistent with the diagnosis of muscular dystrophy. In family (P) (with four affected brothers and at the time six unaffected sisters) and in family (H) (with two affected brothers and two unaffected sisters), onset was in early childhood with difficulty in running and jumping, a tendency to trip up and, later, difficulty in climbing stairs. Enlargement of the calf muscles was noted. Two brothers in the first family became chair-bound at ages 10 and 11, and death occurred at age 16 in one boy in the first family and at 14 in one boy in the second family (the case whose autopsy had been reported by Partridge in Chapter 2 and also by Little, also discussed in Chapter 2). Thus the disease in these two families strongly suggests Duchenne muscular dystrophy. However, in family (T) the disease appears to have been much milder, with onset around age 12 and ability to walk up to the age of 20. This description is therefore more compatible with Becker muscular dystrophy.

Family (P) appears to have been a noted county family and the eldest boy (The Hon. Geo P, born 1834) had been seen previously by Sir Benjamin Brodie, among others. On receiving a telegraphic message of his death, Meryon, with Mr Tatum, went to Bournemouth where they examined the body 22 hours after death and performed an autopsy. Meryon was aware that loss of muscle tissue could result from disease of the spinal cord but in the discussion of the paper reported in *Lancet*[15], in response to questioning, he repeatedly emphasized that in his opinion this was a disease of muscle and not the spinal cord. In the published paper he states that:

> the spinal cord itself and the membranes were perfectly sound and natural in appearance (Ref. 16, page 76).

and later:

> the spinal cord and nerves connected with it were carefully examined, and not the slightest trace of disease was detected. The relative proportion of the grey matter to the white in the cord, the ganglionic cells of the former, and the tubular structure of the latter, as well as of the nerves and the white substance within the neurolemma wherever examined by the microscope, all bore evidence of the healthy condition of the nervous system…. the only structural change observed was that which presented itself in the muscular fibres, which were broken down, and converted into granular and fatty matter (Ref. 16, page 78).

and thereafter refers to the condition as granular degeneration of the voluntary muscles.

This was a time when there was a great deal of interest in microscopy and no investigation of human tissues was now considered complete unless subjected to such study. It was no longer acceptable merely to describe macroscopic appearances. The Microscopical Society of London, of which Meryon was a founding member, had been formed in 1839[17]. Around the time Meryon was pursuing his studies of muscle the president (from 1850 to 1851) of the Microscopical Society was Arthur Farre MD FRS who was also a Fellow of the Royal Medical and Chirurgical Society, and who later became professor of midwifery at King's College. In fact, the Microscopical Society at this time boasted a high proportion of medical men among its members. This interest in microscopy among medical investigators had come about because of improvements in the technology which made the detailed study of tissues very much clearer.

The most important of these improvements was the introduction of achromatic lenses[18] by Joseph Jackson Lister (father of the famous surgeon) in the late 1820s. Other improvements around this time included the use of clearing agents which rendered tissues transparent, the use of very thin coverslips, and mounting in Canada balsam. By the mid-nineteenth century the microscope slide, coverslip, and mountant were much as we know them today[19]. Microscopy was rapidly moving away from being an amusing pastime to becoming an important scientific technique.

Illustrating the image, however, still depended usually on a camera lucida drawing. This might then be made into a lithographic print as was the case with the illustrations in Meryon's article (Figure 3.3). Photomicrography did

GRANULAR DEGENERATION OF MUSCLE | 37

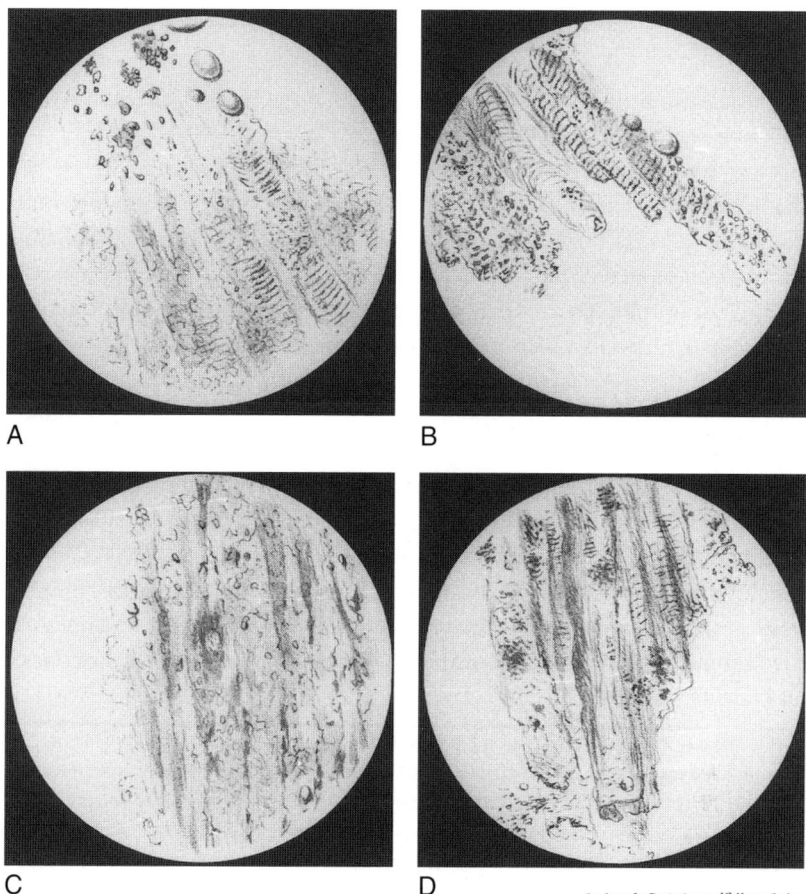

Fig. 3.3 The illustrations of muscle tissue accompanying Meryon's 1852 publication. A, Diseased muscles, the transverse striæ appearing faintly in places. Drawn from the preparation. B, Diseased muscle from the upper extremities, the transverse striæ beginning to disappear and granules taking their place. C, Diseased muscle from the lower extremities, the transverse striæ having disappeared. D, Diseased muscle from the lower extremities, shewing little more than granular matter. (Reproduced by kind permission of the Royal Society of Medicine.)

not appear until some years later and its first use in a publication of the Royal Medical and Chirurgical Society was not until 1867.

Meryon's description of his microscopical findings in affected muscle is quite precise:

> the striped elementary primitive fibres were found to be completely destroyed, the sarcous element being diffused, and in many places converted into oil globules and

granular matter, whilst the sarcolemma or tunic of the elementary fibre was broken down and destroyed (Ref. 16, page 76).

This last point is of singular interest now that the primary defect has been shown to reside in the muscle cytoskeleton.

A few years later, in 1864, he extended his observations on the disease in a chapter entitled 'Paralysis from granular degeneration of the voluntary muscles' in his book on various forms of paralysis[20]. Here, in addition to updating information on two of the previous families, he also includes a further family (no. 87) of four affected sons born to three sisters, an affected brother and sister (no. 89/90) and a seemingly sporadic case (no. 91). The family with an affected brother and sister is interesting because the onset was around age 7 and, when examined at ages 12 and 14 respectively, they both had a waddling gait with difficulty in walking and especially in climbing stairs. Later, he described another family with two affected sisters and an affected brother[21]. These families probably represent the condition now referred to as severe childhood autosomal recessive muscular dystrophy.

In his monograph (Figure 3.4), Meryon pursues further the question of the cause of the disease and again stresses that it is limited to muscle and does not have a neurogenic basis. For example, he compared the spinal cord of one of his patients with that of a control:

> On the day after the examination a youth of the same age (18) was kicked by a horse, and killed on the spot. My late friend, Mr Avery, who was then surgeon to the Charing Cross Hospital, procured for me the spinal cord, by which I was enabled to compare that of my patient with one that was known to be perfectly healthy, and I may state that in form, size, firmness, colour, and appearance under the microscope, the two corresponded in every respect (Ref. 20, page 201).

He also enlisted collaborative evidence from others:

> My friend the Hon and Rev Lord Sidney Godolphin Osborne, an accomplished microscopist, has for many years taken a lively interest in these cases of granular degeneration of the voluntary muscles, and has spent much time in examining the different tissues obtained at the post-mortem investigation made by Mr Savory. In a letter to me he observes, 'I am in my own mind quite satisfied that the peculiar paralysis about which you write to me, affords no direct evidence of lesion in any structure but the muscular' (Ref. 20, page 210).

and later:

> Notwithstanding an earnest desire to find a central nervous cause, I am induced to believe in an idiopathic disease of the muscles, dependent, perhaps, on defective nutrition, just as there is an idiopathic disease of the bones, dependent on the same cause. And I consider that the consequent degeneration of the muscles is characterized by a breaking up of the amorphous membrane which envelopes the primitive fibres, and

PRACTICAL

AND

PATHOLOGICAL RESEARCHES

ON THE

VARIOUS FORMS OF PARALYSIS.

BY

EDWARD MERYON, M.D.,

FELLOW OF THE ROYAL COLLEGE OF PHYSICIANS OF ENGLAND; LATE
LECTURER ON COMPARATIVE ANATOMY AT
ST. THOMAS'S HOSPITAL, ETC.

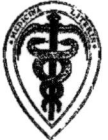

LONDON:
JOHN CHURCHILL AND SONS, NEW BURLINGTON STREET.

MDCCCLXIV.

Fig. 3.4 Title page of Meryon's monograph, published in 1864.

a dispersion of the contained granular matter; that the muscles affected lose their power, in direct proportion to the amount and progress of the degeneration; and that the disease is not apt to be accompanied with symptoms of nervous disturbance (Ref. 20, page 211).

Thus Meryon was convinced that this was a specific disorder, characterized by progressive muscle wasting and weakness, beginning in early childhood and leading to premature death in the late teens, and was not due to any involvement of the spinal neurones but was *essentially a disease of muscle*. But he also stressed the fact that the condition had a predilection for males and was frequently familial. In total he reported eight sibships, in seven of which only males were affected (Table 3.1). Furthermore, he was struck by the occurrence

Table 3.1 Sibships with muscular dystrophy (Meryon, 1852; 1864)

Family	Sibs		
	Affected (males)	Unaffected (females)	Affected sibships
I. (P)	4	7	1
II. (H)	2	2	1
III. (T)	3	1	1
IV. (87)	4	>3	3
V. (89/90)	1 (+ affected sister)	14 (?sex)	1
VI. (91)	1	?	1
Total	15 (+ affected sister)	>27	8
(delete V.)	14	>13	7

+, plus; ?, unknown

of the disease in the sons of three sisters (daughters being normal). Most intriguingly, he mentions:

> There is a marked peculiarity in all the members of the mother's family, which is a very uncommon development of the gastrocnemii muscles (Ref. 20, page 206).

Perhaps this indicates they were so-called *manifesting carriers*. Furthermore, in the reported discussion of the 1851 presentation[15], Sir Benjamin Brodie mentioned that the brother of the mother with affected sons had also suffered from the disease. It was further noted that a peculiar deficiency of vision (?colour blindness) could also be '… transmitted by daughters to their sons but not to their female children.' Finally, during Meryon's presentation of a case at a meeting of the Royal Medical and Chirurgical Society in February 1866[22], the comment was made regarding another case of granular degeneration of muscle that:

> the morbid changes were confined to the family of the father by his second marriage, thus exempting him from suspicion of personal taint. Supposing the disease to be hereditary, it seemed reasonable to infer that it was obtained through the maternal channel.

We now know that the disease is in fact inherited as a sex-linked or X-linked recessive trait and therefore only affects males. But it would be expected that in affected families there would also be some unaffected males. In Meryon's families, however, there were apparently *no* unaffected brothers of affected boys. This suggests that Meryon carefully selected the families to support his belief that the *familial peculiarity* was that *all* males in a family became affected with the disease. The question therefore arises as to what Meryon and his colleagues *at the time* would have concluded from these observations on the familial nature of the condition.

Knowledge of heredity at the time

How much understanding of human heredity might Meryon have had? The simple answer is probably not a great deal. He probably would have known of the theories of the early Greeks, such as Hippocrates, Anaxagoras, and Democritus, referred to as *pangenesis*[23]. According to this theory, male and female [sic] semen was believed to be formed from every part of the body, and in this way accounted for a child resembling its parents.

However, as Aristotle pointed out, this could not account for features from earlier ancestors, such as grandparents, being passed on. Nevertheless, the theory in one form or another persisted right up to the nineteenth century. In fact, Charles Darwin (1809–1882) proposed, in his provisional hypothesis of pangenesis in 1868[24], that every cell of the body was capable of producing countless tiny granules, which he referred to as *gemmules,* which were responsible for the formation of individual organs and features. He believed that these particles circulated in the body, passing into the reproductive cells, thus ensuring their transmission to subsequent generations. But this idea was later to be dealt a serious blow in 1876 by transfusion experiments carried out by his cousin, Francis Galton (1822–1911): transfusion of blood between different breeds of rabbits failed to affect their progeny. For this and various other reasons pangenesis was gradually rejected, later to be replaced by the germ plasm theory of August Weismann (1834–1914) which he developed in a series of publications in the 1880s. According to this theory, self-sustaining determinants in the germ plasm of the nuclei of the germ cells formed the basis of inheritance. This presaged the subsequent idea of discrete hereditary factors proposed by Gregor Mendel (1822–1884). However, the latter's seminal papers on inheritance and the segregation of hereditary factors, although first presented in 1865 and published the following year, remained virtually unknown in the scientific community until 1900. Thus, although it is possible that Meryon may have been familiar with earlier ideas of pangenesis at the time of his 1852 paper and later, this is perhaps as far as his knowledge of the mechanism of heredity may have gone.

By Meryon's time, however, there had already been published ideas about the *mode of inheritance* of certain human traits and diseases. Among the earliest of these were the works of the French polymath Pierre Louis Moreau de Maupertuis (1698–1759). Perhaps now more known for his refutation of preformationist theories and the vitriolic attacks on his mathematical work

(*The Principle of Least Action*) by Voltaire, he has also been considered by some[25,26] to have been a precursor of Mendel. For example, he studied a large family with polydactyly transmitted over several generations and concluded that the condition could be passed on by either males or females. He calculated that it was extremely unlikely that such a family could have occurred by chance. He also studied the transmission of polydactyly in the offspring of an affected bitch from which he bred.

To explain his observations he adapted the theory of pangenesis[27] and postulated that hereditary 'particles', present in the germ cells, had an affinity for a like particle, and each of a corresponding pair was transmitted by a parent to its offspring.

Furthermore, the particle from either the father or mother may dominate. Also, if there were too few particles (or they were too weakly attracted to each other) then a defect resulting from a deficiency of particles could occur (*monstre par defaut*). Alternatively, if there were too many particles (or attraction occurred more than usual) then a defect resulting from such an excess could occur (*monstre par excès*). Finally, he indicated that a sudden complete alteration of particles might occur and, if favoured, could account for the origin of a new species. Thus, in many ways Maupertuis anticipated many subsequent concepts of genetics which would now be referred to as single gene or unifactorial inheritance and multifactorial inheritance, and even new mutations and Darwinian evolution. But, as Sandler has pointed out[28], there are several fundamental differences between Maupertuis' ideas and those of Mendel. For example, Maupertuis associated dominance with the organization of particles, whereas Mendel associated it with the *expression* of one of the alternative forms of a trait.

Furthermore, Maupertuis' concept of the transmission of inherited traits is seen as resulting from the attraction of maternal and paternal particles for each other, whereas Mendel saw this as involving the separation or *segregation* of maternal and paternal factors during gamete formation. Nevertheless, there is no questioning the originality of Maupertuis' ideas. But perhaps because of their very originality his work was little appreciated until relatively recently. It therefore seems very unlikely that Meryon would have been aware of the work of this French scientist and there is no reference to him in any of Meryon's writings.

Since Meryon had had a good grounding in anatomy it might be imagined that he would have been familiar with the work of the embryologist Kaspar Friedrich Wolff (1733–1794), who is now best known for the structures which bear his name: the Wolffian body or mesonephros of the embryo and the Wolffian duct or kidney duct. Of particular interest for the present discussion,

Wolff distinguished between two different kinds of variability: those due to the environment and those (like polydactyly) which are inherited. However, much of this work was carried out while he was a professor in St Petersburg and most of our information concerning his ideas of variation comes from a study of his posthumous manuscripts[23]. It is therefore very unlikely that Meryon would have been acquainted with these ideas.

Joseph Adams (1756–1818), however, lived and worked most of his life in London[29] and wrote a book on hereditary diseases published in London in 1814[30]. This was based on a lifetime of careful clinical and empirical observations. Of particular importance, Adams distinguished between what would now be considered the pedigree patterns of autosomal recessive and autosomal dominant disorders. He emphasized that the distinction was important because by confusing them we may 'excite an unnecessary apprehension in the rising generation'. He then proceeded to show that congenital disorders (present at birth) are more often *familial* (affecting siblings) than *hereditary* (affecting parent and offspring). The former tend to be more serious, resulting in death in early life:

> *congenital* diseases are more commonly familial, than hereditary; some of them being mortal, cannot indeed be transmitted, of which connate hydrocephalus or watery head is one among other instances (Ref. 30, page 14).

But he observed that in some other congenital disorders which are compatible with survival (such as congenital cataract and deaf mutism), the offspring are not affected. He recognized that inherited diseases often follow a similar course within a family and therefore where there is an early age of onset:

> those of the children who have passed that age without any of the symptoms may be considered as free from the constitutional disposition (Ref. 30, page 21).

Although Adams makes a clear distinction between what we would now consider the pedigree patterns of dominant and recessive modes of inheritance, he makes no mention of the mode of inheritance in which normal females transmit a condition which only affects males, which was of course the case in Meryon's families. This pattern of inheritance had been appreciated since the days of the Talmud. Jews excused from circumcision the sons of all the sisters of a mother who had a son with the 'bleeding disease' (haemophilia). The sons of the father's siblings were not so excused. This mode of inheritance was clearly recognized by the nineteenth century[31]. For example, John C. Otto (1774–1844) described[32] the transmission of haemophilia in 1803 as:

> males only are subject to this strange affection and that all of them are not liable to it.... Although the females are exempt, they are still capable of transmitting it to their male children (Ref. 32, page 3).

Otto therefore noted that the bleeding tendency was transmitted by healthy females but did not necessarily affect *all* males in a family, as Meryon seems to have implied in his families with muscle disease. Otto had been an apprentice to the prominent American physician, Benjamin Rush, and was himself now a senior physician at the Philadelphia Hospital. His work on the disease was well known at the time and his paper was reprinted in the *Medical and Physical Journal* in England in 1808[31]. This particular mode of inheritance was later noted in other families with the disease and these were reviewed by Nasse in 1820, who formalized this mode of inheritance[33]. Thus, as an educated and well read medical man, Meryon might perhaps have been expected to have noted the similarity between the mode of inheritance in his families with that in haemophilia, but he apparently failed to do so.

In 1879 Gowers[34] also emphasized that the muscle disease had a strong predilection for males and, when familial, was inherited through the mother. He concluded, as we shall see (Chapter 6), that this mode of inheritance was the same as haemophilia. The cytological basis of X-linkage, however, was not recognized until the early 1900s.

Finally, Meryon cannot be expected to have known of Francis Galton's important contributions on human inheritance because his earliest publication on the subject was not until 1865[35], the same year Mendel first presented his own findings and a year after Meryon's book, *Practical and Pathological Researches* on *the Various Forms of Paralysis*[20], was published.

In summary, it seems that at the time Meryon published his works on granular degeneration of the voluntary muscle, ideas about heredity were in general very confused. In commenting on Darwin's writings in *The Variation of Animals and Plants Under Domestication* published in 1868, Olby's conclusions are particularly relevant:

> Clearly he [Darwin] was writing at a time when ideas about heredity were, by contrast with modern knowledge, very confused... an amalgam of scattered empirical data, adherence to the inheritance of acquired characters, the hereditary effect of use and disuse of organs, and an understandable 'failure' to distinguish between diseases due to infection and those which we know to be genetically determined. Nor should he be considered exceptional in holding such views (Ref. 36, page 412).

Why has Meryon's contribution to muscular dystrophy been largely neglected?

It has been suggested that the reason for Mendel's findings not being recognized for over 35 years is because they were published in an obscure journal (*Transactions of the Natural History Society of Brünn*) which was not widely read. However, this seems unlikely because the journal was at the time sent to no less than 120 learned societies, academies, and libraries[37]. But could one reason for Meryon's observations being largely neglected be because they were published in the *Transactions of the Royal Medical and Chirurgical Society of London*, which may not have been widely known at the time?

The Society was founded at a meeting of physicians and surgeons on Wednesday 22 May 1805 at the Freemason's Tavern in London[38]. One of its expressed aims was 'for the purpose of conversation on professional subjects, for the reception of communications, and for the formation of a library', and to form 'a responsible centre for the reception of important communications.'

The founding members included, among others, several eminent surgeons (John Abernethy, Astley Cooper, and Sir William Blizard) and physicians (Gilbert Blane, Sir W. Farquhar, Bt), as well as those with a special interest in children's diseases (John Clarke) and what would now be called clinical chemistry (Alexander Marcet). With the exceptions of Sir W. Farquhar and John Clarke, all were, or in the case of Alexander Marcet soon became, Fellows of the Royal Society. Thus, from its inception the Society attracted many of those eminent at the time in medicine and surgery.

Eventually, the Society acquired permanent accommodation at 53 Berners Street (Figure 3.5), where it resided for 54 years, from 1835 to 1889. In 1834 the Society was granted a Royal Charter by King William IV, and so became the Royal Medical and Chirurgical Society of London. At the turn of the century it had become the oldest, largest, and most important of the various London medical societies which in 1907 amalgamated to form the now Royal Society of Medicine[39].

Even in the first 50 years of its existence, the Society had established itself as a much-respected organization with a high reputation. At the time of Meryon's presentation to the Society there were over 1700 members, with several eminent scientists from abroad having been elected to Honorary Fellowship, including Liebig, the German chemist, Rokitansky, the Viennese pathologist, Panizza, the Italian anatomist, and Magendie, the French physiologist. Honorary Fellowship had also been bestowed on a number of British dignitaries, including Robert Brown of the Linnean Society, Edwin Chadwick, Michael Faraday, and Sir William Herschel, the astronomer. The quality of the presentations at the Society's meetings can be gauged by those who had contributed by this time. These included Robert Liston, Charles Bell, Thomas Hodgkin, Sir Benjamin Brodie, Richard Bright, James Paget, Bence Jones, Alfred Garrod (father of Archibald Garrod), and Spencer Wells.

The Society attached great importance to its library (Meryon became the librarian in 1861), and from 1814 began to purchase foreign books to such an

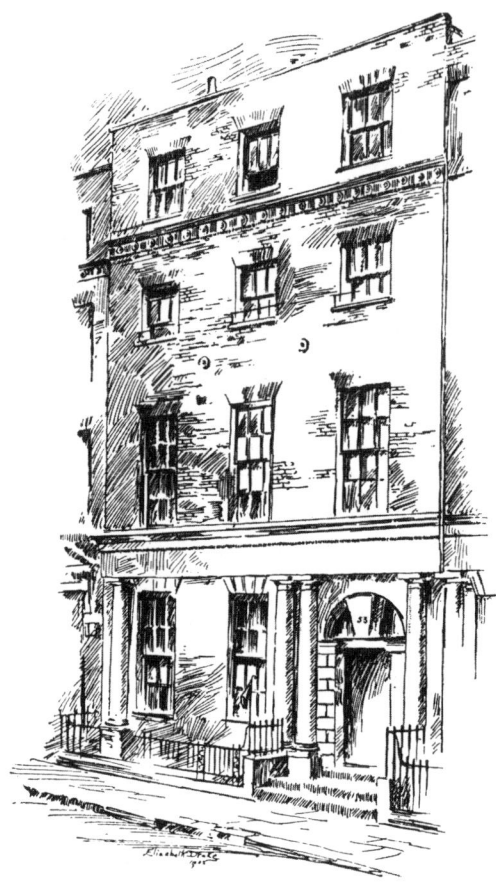

Fig. 3.5 The Royal Medical & Chirurgical Society at 53 Berners Street. (Reproduced by kind permission of the Royal Society of Medicine.)

extent that, in 1845, of 432 volumes added to the library in that year only 57 were in English. Even by 1815 the library was considered 'more comprehensive and valuable than any other collection of medical books in the country'. By the middle of the century there were over 17,000 volumes and by 1879 the number had increased to 31,000. Members were very much encouraged to use the library and its facilities.

The Society also attached great importance to the quality and originality of its communications. A special committee was set up to select papers for publication in its *Transactions* 'without undue respect of person'. In fact, only around 50% of papers presented at meetings were accepted for publication. The committee avoided anything that bordered on the non-scientific. The minutes of 1842, for example, report that in July, 'Dunn's paper on a case of

Tubercular Meningitis was ordered for publication *on condition that the author consent to omit his phrenological observations.*' On 22 November in the same year 'a paper was read on a case of Amputation of the Thigh during Mesmeric Coma by two authors, neither of them Fellows of the Society. It was not published, nor even submitted for publication; there is no abstract of it in the Minutes; and the Minute saying that it was read was excepted from confirmation.' Clearly the Society was sensitive to preserving its status. Furthermore, the aim of the Society was the presentation of original material which had not been published elsewhere, including foreign journals. Thus, in 1847 a minute states: 'That in consequence of some remarks made respecting the want of originality in parts of the papers of Dr. Johnson and Mr. Simon, a note be added as a postscript to the above papers, by the Editor, pointing-out the recent investigations which have been made in renal pathology, more especially in Germany, and which appear to have a bearing more or less direct on the contents of the above papers…'. Later in the year, however, the Council felt that it would not be expedient of the Society to 'depart from the spirit of the Advertisement inserted at the commencement of the Volume, either in corroborating statements or supplying deficiencies in any of the papers contained in the Volume'. Nevertheless the note remained recorded.

Because of the high reputation of the *Transactions*, several important foreign journals made requests for exchanges. In 1846, for example, the Institute of France requested certain back numbers they lacked, and an exchange was established with the *Comptes Rendus de l'Academie des Sciences*. It is reasonable to assume that French investigators of the time, including Duchenne, would therefore have had ready access to Meryon's 1852 publication.

Yet despite the standing of the Society and its *Transactions,* Meryon's contribution appears to have been largely neglected. It appears for the first time only in the fourth edition of Garrison & Morton's *Medical Bibliography*, published in 1983[40].

The explanation is perhaps that Meryon's contribution was published in a single relatively short (11 pages) article and only enlarged into a short chapter (15 pages) of a book not published until some 12 years later. On the other hand, Duchenne's main contributions on muscular dystrophy were published in several very extensive papers (totalling 124 pages) in a single year. The latter was perhaps also a better publicist of his findings, and of course made several important contributions to other diseases as well.

Certainly volume 35 of the *Transactions*, which contained Meryon's contribution, might well have been expected to have attracted attention later because it also included William Senhouse Kirkes' now classic description of embolism resulting from intracardiac thrombus formation[41], and which is included in Major's *Classic Descriptions of Disease*[42].

Meryon's other contributions

Meryon's book on various forms of paralysis[20] covers a great deal more than granular degeneration of voluntary muscles. It consists of six lengthy sections, the first of which deals in some detail with the structure of the nervous system. The material is largely based on a review of the work of Bell, Magendie, Brown-Séquard, Matteucci, Pflüger, Claude Bernard, and Meryon's friend, Lockhart Clarke. Again, as in his *The Constitution of Man*[4], he demonstrates his extensive reading and wide knowledge of the subject. The remaining sections deal with paralysis due to 'affections' of the spinal cord and brain (mainly inflammation, tuberculosis, neoplasms, and apoplexy), paralysis from blood poisoning (in which he includes lathyrism, plumbism, diphtheria, and syphilis), paralysis from 'reflex action' (miscellaneous conditions associated with pregnancy, teething, etc.), and, finally, progressive forms of paralysis (which includes paralysis of the insane, progressive ataxia, and granular degeneration of voluntary muscles). Clearly this classification reflected the level of knowledge at the time concerning the supposed aetiology of many of these diseases. For example, it would have been difficult to prove the syphilitic nature of many clinical problems because the Wassermann test only became available at the beginning of the next century.

The text is based on details of cases reported in the literature as well as those under his own care. At one point (page 131) he refers to a case he saw at the Hôtel Dieu in 1829, presumably while he was studying at the École de Médecine in Paris before he went to London University. In addition, on several occasions he refers to Duchenne in regard to the diagnosis of paralysis and the use of faradism.

As in his *The Constitution of Man*[4], the text is very well referenced and contributes an interesting picture of neurological practice at the time.

A few years later, Meryon became interested in the sympathetic nervous system. In June 1870 he read a paper on the subject at a meeting of the Royal Medical and Chirurgical Society[43] which was followed by a series of articles in the *Lancet* under the title 'On the functions of the sympathetic system of nerves, as a physiological basis for a rational system of therapeutics'[44]. In 1872 these articles were extended and incorporated into a book[45]. The first part is concerned with the anatomy and particularly the physiology of the sympathetic nervous system, and draws heavily on the work of Claude Bernard (1813–1878), the celebrated French physiologist. The main thrust of the book is the second part, where the author argues for the physiology of the system to form a basis for therapy:

> Seeing, therefore, that most pathological conditions are but modifications of physiological actions, and the effects of derangement of the operations of the vaso-motor

nerves, on which the healthy functions of all organs depend, it appears to me that on the knowledge and due appreciation of such aids, we may found a rational and scientific system of therapeutics (Ref. 45, page 65).

At this time, however, nothing was known of neurotransmission in the sympathetic and parasympathetic nervous systems. This was shown to be chemically mediated only some 50 years later by Henry Dale (1875–1968) and Otto Loewi (1873–1961), who shared the Nobel Prize for their work in 1936. Despite the limited knowledge available at the time, Meryon's book is of interest because it forecasts the potential for manipulating the autonomic nervous system in therapy, and thus provides a useful reference in any history of the subject. Since they are not relevant to his work in neurology, the three remaining books by Meryon merit only brief mention. In 1861 he published a *History of Medicine*[46]. It seems this was planned as a somewhat ambitious undertaking. The first volume, of some 483 pages, covers the period from the Classical Greek to the sixteenth century. Unfortunately, a second volume never appeared. But, as with his other work, it clearly reveals the very wide reading and evident scholarship of the author. In 1868 Meryon published a report of a family in which two brothers had microencephaly[47] and in 1876 he wrote a play in five acts, written mostly in verse, entitled *The Huguenot*[48]. Finally, the collected *Epigrams, Epitaphs, Personal Anecdotes*[49] of Meryon were published for private circulation around the time of his death. According to the printer, these were reproduced 'just as they were written in Dr Meryon's Common Place Book, without rearrangement, or attempt to discover the author's name where it has not been given.' This selection shows he had a nice sense of humour and little time for pomposity. But perhaps he himself might best be remembered from his family motto *Si non hodie, quando?* (If not today, when?) which, in the circumstances of Edward Meryon's neglect in the history of muscular dystrophy, would seem particularly relevant.

References

1. McCord, N. *British History 1815–1860*. Oxford: Oxford University Press, 1991.
2. Woodward, L. L. *The Age of Reform 1815–1870*, 2nd edn. Oxford: Oxford University Press, 1993.
3. Darwin, C. *On the Origin of Species by Means of Natural Selection, or The Preservation of Favoured Races in the Struggle for Life*. London: John Murray, 1859.
4. Meryon, E. *The Physical and Intellectual Constitution of Man Considered*. London: Smith, Elder & Co., 1836.
5. Lamarck, J. B. P. A. de M., de. *Philosophie Zoologique*. Paris: Baillière, 1809.
6. Jones, F. W. *Habit and Heritage*. London: Kegan Paul, Trench & Trubner, 1943.
7. Nordenskiöld, E. *The History of Biology—A Survey*. Leonard B. Eyre, tr. New York: Tudor Publishing Co., 1946; 308. (Originally published as *Biologins Historia*, 1920–24. Stockholm: Björck & Börjesson.)

8. Blumenbach, J. F. *De Generis Humani Varietate Nativa*. Göttingen: Vandenhoeck, 1775. (In the 3rd edition, of 1795, he described the five races of man.)
9. Freedman, B. J. Caucasian. *British Medical Journal*, 1984; **288**: 696–8.
10. Emery, A.E.H., Emery, M.L.H. Edward Meryon (1807–1880) and Charles Darwin (1809–1882). *On the Origin of Species. Journal of Medical Biography*, 2009; **17**: 199–201.
11. Council of the University of London. Second Statement by The Council of The University of London, Explanatory of the Plan of Instruction. 2nd edn. London: John Taylor, 1828.
12. Bennett, J. R. *Lecture Introductory to the Course of General Anatomy*; delivered in the University of London, on Wednesday, October 6, 1830. London: John Taylor, 1830.
13. University of London. *The London University Calendar for the Year MDCCCXXXI*. London: John Taylor, 1831.
14. Gull, W. W. *A Collection of the Published Writings of William Withey Gull: Medical Papers*. In: T. D. Acland (ed.) London: New Sydenham Society, 1894.
15. Meryon, E. On fatty degeneration of the voluntary muscles. [Report of the Royal Medical & Chirurgical Society, Dec. 9, 1851.] *Lancet*, 1851; **ii**: 588–9.
16. Meryon, E. On granular and fatty degeneration of the voluntary muscles. *Medico-Chirurgical Transactions*, 1852; **35**: 73–84.
17. Turner, G. L'E. *God Bless the Microscope: A History of the Royal Microscopical Society over 150 Years*. Oxford: Royal Microscopical Society, 1989.
18. Lister, J. J. On some properties in achromatic object-glasses applicable to the improvement of the microscope. *Philosophical Transactions of the Royal Society*, 1830; **130**: 187–200.
19. Bracegirdle, B. The development of biological preparative techniques for light microscopy, 1839–1989. *Journal of Microscopy*, 1989; **155**: 307–318.
20. Meryon, E. *Practical and Pathological Researches on the Various Forms of Paralysis*. London: John Churchill & Sons, 1864: 200–15. (Part previously summarized in the *British Medical Journal*, 1863; **i**: 474–8, 502–4; **ii**: 28–9, 83–6, 204–5, 449–51, 687–9).
21. Meryon, E. Case of granular degeneration of the voluntary muscles. *British Medical Journal*, 1870; **ii**: 32–3.
22. Meryon, E. On granular degeneration of the voluntary muscles. [Report of the Royal Medical & Chirurgical Society, Feb. 27, 1866.] *Lancet*, 1866; **i**: 258–60.
23. Stubbe, H. *History of Genetics*, 2nd edn. English translation, 1972. Cambridge, Mass. & London: MIT, 1965.
24. Darwin, C. *The Variation of Animals and Plants under Domestication*. London: John Murray, 1868.
25. Glass, H. B. Maupertuis, pioneer of genetics and evolution. In: B. Glass *et al.* (eds). *Forerunners of Darwin 1745–1859*. Baltimore: John Hopkins University Press, 1959: 51–83.
26. Emery, A. E. H. Portraits in medical genetics—Pierre Louis Moreau de Maupertuis (1698–1759). *Journal of Medical Genetics*, 1988; **25**: 561–4.
27. de Maupertuis, P. L. M. *Oeuvres de M. de Maupertuis*. Nouvelle édition, corrigée et augmentée. 4 vols. Lyon: J-M. Bruyset, 1756.

28. Sandler, I. Pierre Louis Moreau de Maupertuis—a precursor of Mendel? *Journal of the History of Biology*, 1983; **16**: 101–36.
29. Emery, A. E. H. Portraits in medical genetics—Joseph Adams (1756–1818). *Journal of Medical Genetics*, 1989; **26**: 116–18.
30. Adams, J. *A Treatise on the Supposed Hereditary Properties of Diseases*. London: Calow, 1814.
31. Rushton, A. R. *Genetics and Medicine in the United States 1800 to 1922*. Baltimore: Johns Hopkins University Press, 1994.
32. Otto, J. C. An account of an haemorrhagic disposition existing in certain families. *Medical Repository*, 1803; **6**: 1–4.
33. Nasse, C. F. Von einer erblichen Neigung zu tödlichen Blutungen. *Arch. Med. Erfahrung Geb. Praktischen Med. Staatsarzneikunde.* [*Horn's Archives.*] Berlin: G. Reimer, 1820: 385–434.
34. Gowers, W. R. *Pseudo-hypertrophic Muscular Paralysis—a Clinical Lecture*. London: J. & A. Churchill, 1879.
35. Galton, F. Hereditary talent and character. *Macmillan's Magazine*, 1865; **12**: 157–66; 318–27.
36. Olby, R. C. Constitutional and hereditary disorders. In: W. F. Bynum & R. Porter (eds). *Companion Encyclopedia of the History of Medicine*. London: Routledge, Vol. l. 1993: 412–37.
37. Gasking, E. B. Why was Mendel's work ignored? *Journal of the History of Ideas*, 1959; **20**: 60–84.
38. Moore, N. and Paget, S. *The Royal Medical and Chirurgical Society of London Centenary 1805–1905*. Aberdeen: Aberdeen University Press, 1905.
39. Eden, T. W. The Royal Society of Medicine. In: D'A. Power (ed.) *British Medical Societies*. London: Medical Press & Circular, 1939: 267–76.
40. Morton, L. T. *A Medical Bibliography* (Garrison & Morton), 4th edn. London: Gowers, 1983.
41. Kirkes, W. S. On some of the principal effects resulting from the detachment of fibrinous deposits from the interior of the heart and their mixture with the circulating blood. *Medico-Chirurgical Transactions*, 1852; **35**: 281–324.
42. Major, R. H. *Classic Descriptions of Disease*, 2nd edn. Springfield, Illinois: Charles C. Thomas, 1939: 502–7.
43. Meryon, E. On the function of the sympathetic system of nerves. [Report of Royal Medical & Chirurgical Society meeting of June 14,1870.] *British Medical Journal*, 1870; **ii**: 99.
44. Meryon, E. On the functions of the sympathetic system of nerves, as a physiological basis for a rational system of therapeutics. *Lancet*, 1871; **ii**: 570–2, 601–2, 631–4, 704–6, 744–5.
45. Meryon, E. *On the Functions of the Sympathetic System of Nerves, as a Physiological Basis for a Rational System of Therapeutics*. London: J. & A. Churchill, 1872.
46. Meryon, E. *The History of Medicine Comprising a Narrative of its Progress from the Earliest Ages to the Present Time and of the Delusions Incidental to its Advance from Empiricism to the Dignity of a Science*. Vol. I. London: Longman, Green, Longman, and Roberts, 1861.

47. Meryon, E. An account of some cases of arrest of development. *Transactions of the Ethnological Society*, 1868; **7**: 162–4.
48. Meryon, E. *The Huguenot*. London: E. Wilson, 1876.
49. Meryon, E. *Epigrams, Epitaphs, Personal Anecdotes,* &tc. [For private circulation. Printed just as they were written in Dr. Meryon's Common Place Book.] London, 188?

Chapter 4

The life of Edward Meryon (1807–1880)

Edward Meryon was descended from French Protestant stock, known as Huguenots, who arrived in England from France in the seventeenth century. Louis XIV had issued four edicts in 1680–1681 in an attempt to suppress Protestantism, the edict of 17 June 1681 being the final act which resulted in a huge wave of Huguenot refugees. England had provided asylum to those escaping religious persecution since the mid-sixteenth century, and when this new influx of refugees arrived, Charles II made them welcome with a proclamation granting free letters of denization (naturalization) to any who might seek refuge here. Rye, being the nearest port to the French coast, attracted many of these refugees, who were homeless, completely impoverished, and, however eager to work, dependent on charity until they could become self-supporting. Most incoming refugees travelled on to London where a Huguenot community was established and where charitable donations were given to the most needy for such basics as clothing, shoes, and, in one case, even to a locksmith, '£5 to get tools for his trade'[1].

The 1681 Relief Rolls of the French Protestant Church at Threadneedle Street, London, list a Louis Marignan (Merignan), his wife and two children, from Marennes, a small port in the Charente-Maritime district of France famous for its magnificent oysters. His occupation was given as *marinier*, or seaman, and they are recorded as having received a total of £3-2s-6d in charitable grants[1]. In another Huguenot Society publication, a Louis Merignan, his wife Hester and son Louis were listed as being denized (granted naturalization) in March 1682[2]. These entries for Louis Marignan/Merignan thus appear to be the earliest record we have of the family, who eventually settled in Rye and from whom Edward Meryon was descended. Rye, being an active port at the time, may have offered special opportunities for someone with a seaman's background and experience. Certainly, from this first Louis Marignan, who had arrived as an impoverished refugee, the family eventually became an established, prosperous, and influential part of the community (Figure 4.1).

The Huguenots were generally well received by the inhabitants of Rye and, with the approval of the vicar, the Reverend William Williams, they were

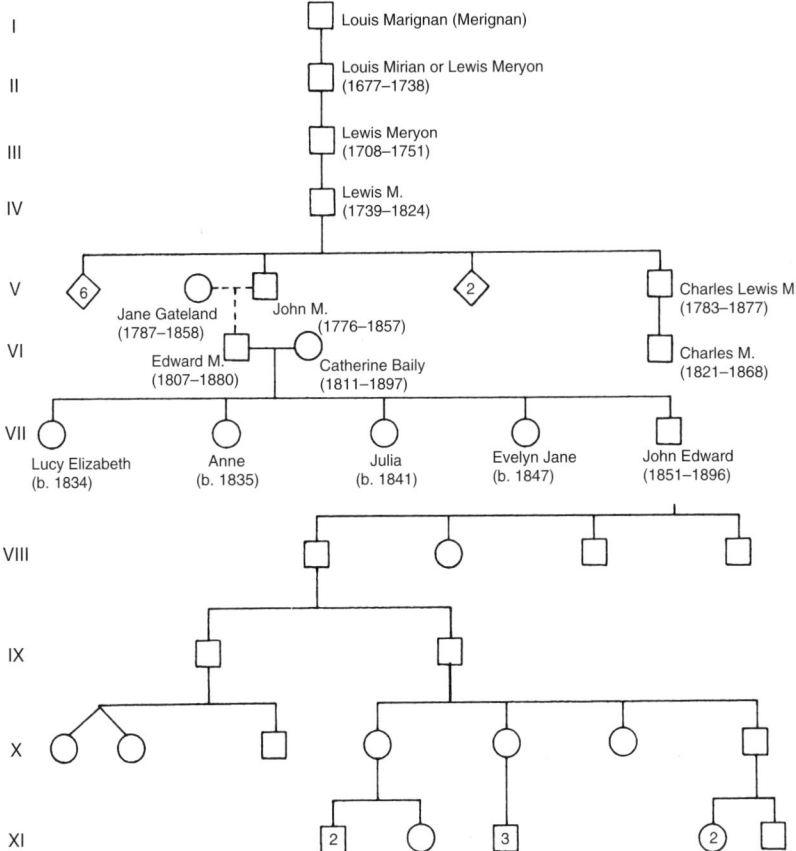

Fig. 4.1 An abbreviated Meryon family tree. Square, male; circle, female; diamond with number, number of males/females.

allowed the use of St Mary's Church for their services between the hours of 8–10 am and 12–2 pm each Sunday. The following testimony was issued on behalf of the Huguenot refugees by the towns-people:

> These are to certifie all whom it may concerne that the French Protestants that are settled inhabitants of this towne of Rye, are a sober, harmless, innocent people, such as serve God constantly and uniformly according to the usage and custome of the Church of England. And further that we believe them to be falsely aspersed for Papists and disaffected persons, no such thing appeareing unto us by the conversations of any of them. This we do freely and truely certifie for and of them. In witness whereof we have hereunto sett our hands, the 18th day of April, 1682.
> [Signed] Wm Williams, vicar; Tho Tournay; Francis Lightfoot, Coll M^tie's Customes;… Lewis Gillard, Jurat, [et al.] (Ref. 3, pages 201–2).

The records show that the family name went though a number of changes (Marignan, Merignan, Merignian, Mirinion, Merinian, Merian, Morian,

Mirian, Meryion) before finally achieving its present form, Meryon. As with other Huguenot families, a favourite Christian name has been retained, and 'Lewis' appears in every generation down to Edward Meryon's great-grandson, Peter Louis Meryon, born in 1920.

The earliest Meryons to settle in Rye were not wealthy; Louis Mirian (Lewis Meryon), son of the first known member of the family, had two of his sons, Lewis (1708–1751) and John (1716–1778), accepted by the Sanders School, a charity school established in 1720 by James Sanders (or Saunders) for the education of the poor of Rye[4]. In this school the pupils were taught 'to read in English, and write, and cast up accounts,… and the art of navigation.' (Ref. 5, page 38). By 1765, the Meryon family had obviously progressed from their humble beginnings. Lewis Meryon (1739/40–1824), who was to become Edward Meryon's grandfather, married Anne Haddock, of a fairly flourishing local family, and together they established themselves as one of the town's most industrious families. Lewis was appointed foreman for the construction of the new harbour in 1774. By 1798 he was a Freeman of the town and a landowner. He was also a merchant of corn, coal, fir timber, as well as being a brewer/maltster and Agent to the Sun Fire Office. His wife, Anne, was a stationer and bookseller in the High Street. Lewis not only owned the brewery on the Strand, but also the George Hotel, the King's Head Public House, the London Trader, and the Red Lion inns. In 1818, when the new cattle market opened in Rye, he added a large ballroom to the George Hotel in order to accommodate the farmers who then came to dine in Rye for the first time[6].

Charles Lewis Meryon (1783–1877)

Lewis Meryon and his wife, Anne, had 10 known children, the most famous of whom was Charles Lewis Meryon, MD, FRCP (1783–1877) (Figure 4.2).

He was educated at Merchant Taylor's School, London, and went on to study medicine at St John's College, Oxford and St Thomas' Hospital, London. Here, he was a pupil of Mr Henry Cline, through whose recommendation he was employed to accompany the eccentric and strong-willed Lady Hester Stanhope in the capacity of medical attendant on a voyage to Sicily and the Middle East. In fact, he is perhaps best known for this association, which lasted several decades[7,8]. He embarked with Lady Hester early in 1810 and spent 7 years travelling with her. The most arduous of his duties was to play the part of patient listener while Lady Hester indulged in her inordinate love of talking. These sessions often lasted 8, 10, or even 12 hours! Having seen her finally settled on Mount Lebanon, he returned to England to take his medical degree at Oxford in November 1817. After a year or two, at Lady Hester's request, he again returned to Syria for a short period. But he returned to England, to be admitted a Fellow of the Royal College of Physicians on 25 June 1821, and

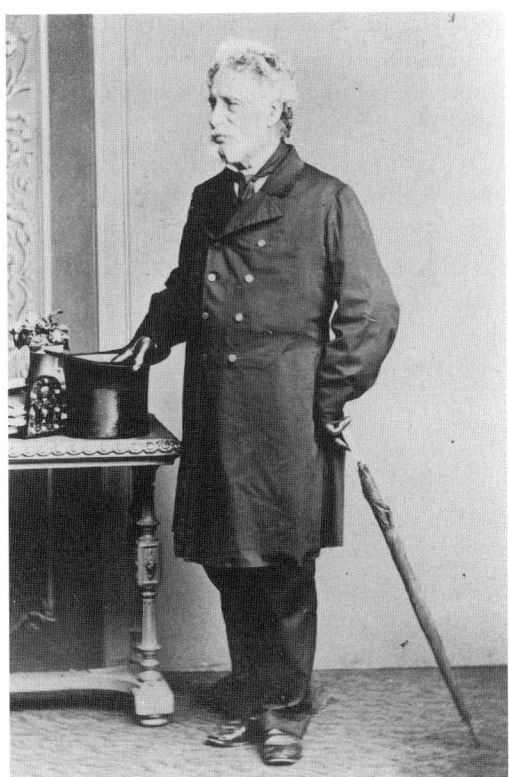

Fig. 4.2 Charles Lewis Meryon, MD, FRCP (1783–1877); Edward Meryon's paternal uncle. (Reproduced by permission of the Royal College of Physicians.)

soon afterward became domestic physician to Sir Gilbert Heathcote. Around this time he had an affair with a French dancer, Pierre-Narcisse Chaspoux, and a son was born in Paris in November 1821, called Charles Meryon, who later became a world-famous etcher (see Figure 5.1).

In 1826 his position with Sir Gilbert terminated and in 1827 he set off again for Mount Lebanon, this time with a wife and family. On the way their ship was boarded by Greek pirates and all but Dr Meryon were robbed of their money and valuables. For some reason Dr Meryon was allowed to retain his possessions except for a trifling sum and a few articles of clothing which he was invited to 'give' to the pirate crew. After this experience Mrs Meryon was reluctant to continue the journey, but after 3 years in Leghorn (Livorno), they proceeded on to Syria, arriving in late 1830. This visit lasted only until April of 1831, when relations with the fierce-tempered Lady Hester became strained. The doctor and his family departed, spending four and a half months in Cyprus on their way home. Lady Hester made one final request for the doctor to visit her, and in July 1837, he and his family landed in Beirut, departing finally on 6 August 1838. Following many years of patient tolerance of Lady Hester's compulsive talking, eccentricities, and even her 'violent and overbearing temper'[9], Dr Meryon published two three-volume memoirs of her travels and experiences[10,11].

It is likely, upon considering the circumstances of Edward Meryon's early life, that this colourful and adventurous, but clearly talented, physician may have helped and influenced his young nephew, Edward, in his schooling, university studies, and even in his medical practice, through introductions to respected members of London society.

John Meryon (1776–1857)

John Meryon, brother of Dr Charles Lewis Meryon, was the father of Edward Meryon, and an active participant in the public and political life of Rye.

Nothing is known of his early years, or his schooling, and the records for the Sanders School do not list him as a pupil. The Peacock School in Rye was an endowed grammar school established in 1636 by Thomas Peacocke, Jurat (town councillor), as a free school 'for the better Educating and Breeding of Youth there in good Literature' (Ref. 5, page 38). Instruction was given in grammar, as well as in Latin and Greek. From the contents of later documents written by John Meryon, it can be surmised that he received such instruction, perhaps at the grammar school. Unfortunately, no records now exist of those who attended the school.

John Meryon became a Freeman of Rye by birthright (i.e. his father being a Freeman) in 1798, and a Harbour Commissioner from around 1800 to the 1840s. This was a very active port and many of the townspeople depended on shipping for their livelihood. It was a significant outlet for local products, especially wool from Romney Marsh and hops from the Weald. Corn was exported in large quantities to London and Devon, and other exports included cured herrings, timber, and ironworks products. Imports included coal from the north-east of England and dairy products (cheese, butter), bacon, and livestock feeds. There was a great deal of dissension over the measures to be taken to improve the harbour and prevent silting up; the landowners and the merchants and ship owners of the town had conflicting motives, and the decisions of the Harbour Commissioners often provoked the wrath of the residents. In 1816, in fact, the exasperated town people actually took up pickaxes and shovels and breached a sluice, allowing the tide to come in and destroy it completely. The history of this long-standing conflict is recorded by John Meryon in *An Account of the Origin and Formation of the Harbour of the Ancient Town of Rye; of the Causes of its Present Decay and of the Means Whereby it may be*

Restored to its Pristine Depth and Capacity, so as to Become a Considerable Tide-Harbour, and a Useful Harbour of Refuge[12]. In this work, of 90 pages, he relates the history of the harbour from earliest times, with references to various scholarly sources (some in Greek!), and summarizes:

> The writer of these pages is now far removed from the arena of conflicting interest. Inhabiting a distant colony, descended into the vale of years, once the owner, but now no longer, of a little property in his native town of Rye, he can look and reflect dispassionately on the measures which others, whose judgment and passions are still warped by local feelings or party views…. He has learned to regard with indulgence the narrow minded selfishness of country gentlemen, who can see nothing beyond the fence of their own acres, and who are blind to the advantages of converting a small trading town into a capacious mart to which vessels of all nations might resort, and bring prosperity and wealth to the surrounding country (Ref. 12, pages 89–90).

It is evident where the sympathies of John Meryon lay. He is, however, most widely known for the part he played in the reform movement that swept through the country, including Rye, and locally for a famous altercation over the election of Mayor of the Town. With the aid of his brother, Dr Charles Lewis Meryon, and his brother-in-law, William Holloway, an 'alternative' election was held in 1825. John was made Mayor, and held the office for 6 weeks before being forced to hand power back to the legal Mayor on 29 November (Ref. 13, pages 118–19).

John Meryon was thus a colourful character in Rye. He inherited several businesses and properties from his father, Lewis, one being the brewery he managed with his brother-in-law, Meryon & Holloway (none too successfully—over their 18 years of management the prosperous firm declined into bankruptcy), ran an inn and a public house, and was a livery stable-keeper. For a time he lived at the George Hotel, another inheritance from his father, but by 1851, as shown in the Rye Census, he was living with his sister and brother-in-law at 24 High Street (now a guest house, the Holloway House), where he died on 22 March 1857, aged 80. He apparently never married.

Edward Meryon (1807–1880)

Although his actual date of birth is unknown, Edward Meryon (Frontispiece) was baptised in Rye on 10 December 1807. His mother was Jane Gateland (or Gatland) (1787–1858) (see Figure 4.1). She was about age 20 when Edward was born, and an interesting entry in the Parish Poor Book under 'Disbursements' lists a 'Mrs' Gateland, March 20, 1807, receiving £6.10s. This was a substantial sum, considering that an entry for December 1808, lists £2.11s. in payment for the upkeep of another child for 1 year[14]. It seems that Edward Meryon began life under less than favourable circumstances. John Meryon and Jane Gateland

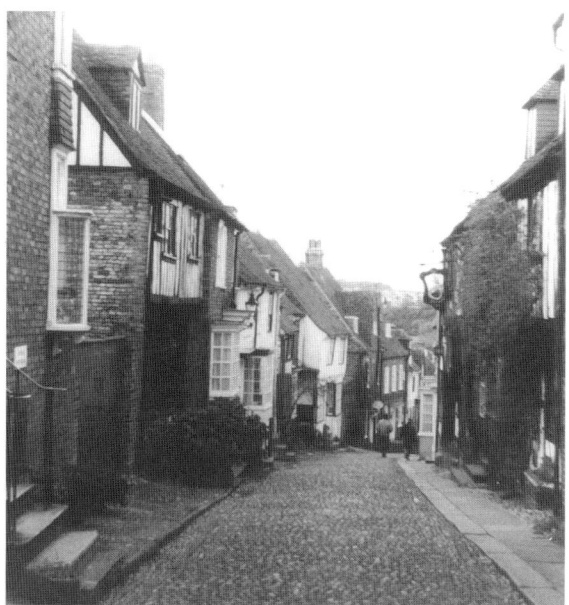

Fig. 4.3 Mermaid Street, Rye, as it is today. (Author's photograph, 1994.)

never married, but it is likely that John Meryon contributed to the upkeep and education of his son during his early years. John Meryon, who died in March 1857 aged 80, stated in his 1844 will that he left his entire estate to his 'reputed son Edward Gateland by Jane Gateland of Rye…now commonly known as Edward Meryon', although his effects were valued at under £100 by the Probate Court. John Meryon and Jane Gateland are buried next to one another in St Mary's Churchyard, Rye.

Edward's mother was listed as a 'milliner and dressmaker' living on Church Street[15], one of eight women so listed at the time. The 1841 Rye Census lists her as living alone in Mermaid Street (Figure 4.3), and in 1851 as 'unmarried', occupation, dressmaker. She died and was buried on 22 May 1858, age 71. Her parents were John Gateland and Mary Harvey Gateland, and her grandparents were Elizabeth and Isaac Gateland (a parish clerk in Rye), but little else is known of her, except that her father died when she was only 4, and she had two older sisters, Charlotte and Mary.

It is perhaps because of these circumstances that Edward Meryon chose to be silent about his early years. He lists his year of birth as 1809, and never mentions his education before his enrolment as a medical student in 1829 at the University of London, now University College. However, one trace of his schooling has been discovered. We have mentioned earlier that his uncle, Charles Lewis Meryon went to Merchant Taylors' School. Acting on the assumption that a well placed uncle might take an interest in the education of his nephews, we checked the available references to pupil enrolment at the school. In one, Robinson's *Register of the Scholars Admitted into Merchant Taylor's School*[16], there is a listing for an *Edward William Meryon*, who entered the school in October 1821. He is listed along with two of his cousins, who also entered the school in the same year: Charles Pix Meryon (1814–1879) and Meryon Holloway (1812–1828), son of William and Sarah Holloway. This information clarifies one question, but unfortunately raises several others. Charles Pix Meryon is recorded as a pupil of Merchant Taylors' from 1821–1825, and in another source[17], is listed as the son of Charles Lewis Meryon. Since he was actually the son of Thomas and Harriet Meryon, this is a peculiar error; however, his father, Thomas, died in 1820, so perhaps the school entered C. L. Meryon as his father in error. But in neither the Hart reference[17] nor the actual enrolment books checked by the school clerk, does Edward Meryon appear again. There is no additional information concerning how long he was a pupil, or who sponsored him. It seems likely, however, that Dr Charles Meryon may have played a part in the enrolment of his three nephews in his old school: he had returned from his second trip to Syria in 1820, and was still in England in June 1821, when he attained his FRCP.

According to research done by Edward Meryon's grandson, Dr Charles Evelyn Meryon (1891–1970), Edward Meryon was 'educated at Rouen, studied medicine in Paris before coming to London'. If, as seems likely, Charles Lewis Meryon was involved in Edward's education, perhaps after a term at Merchant Taylors' School in 1821, he took his nephew to France to enrol him in Rouen for the remainder of his schooling. After all, it was in November 1821 that Charles Lewis Meryon had a child born in Paris to Narcisse Chaspoux, and there might well have been journeys to France during this time. After his school years, Edward may have thought of following the profession of his uncle, and enrolled to study medicine in Paris.

Meryon states in his biographical details in later directories that he studied medicine at L'École de Médecine in Paris, although we have not as yet been able to find any record of this. This may well have been *before* he commenced medical studies in London, because, in a footnote in his book *Practical and Pathological Researches on the Various Form of Paralysis*, he states 'I also remember a case which occurred in the Hôtel Dieu, in 1829, of a woman with amaurosis....' (Ref. 18, page 131). This confirms that he spent some time there before beginning his studies in London in October of that year.

He registered as a medical student on 1 October 1829 at University College London, and gave his home address as Rye, and a London address of 6 Grafton Street East. He was nominated for entry as a student by Alexander Baring, first

Baron Ashburton (1774–1848), one of the Proprietors (as the shareholders in the new university were called). His accomplishments in his first year at the university reveal Meryon's academic ability: he was awarded a gold medal and first certificate in anatomy taught by the colourful and controversial Professor Pattison, a certificate of honour in Charles Bell's physiology course, and certificates of honour in midwifery and practical anatomy. He became embroiled in the controversy surrounding Pattison, who was accused by the students of being incompetent both as an anatomist and as a teacher (when he did turn up to lecture, he often did so in hunting pink). The lecture theatre was in constant chaos, and the students held a demonstration, which led eventually to Pattison's dismissal[19]. Meryon was apparently among those unhappy with Pattison, in spite of being awarded the gold medal in his anatomy class, for he signed a petition asking for Pattison's dismissal, and a letter from Meryon exists in the University College Archives:

> My Lords and Gentlemen
> Having heard from Mr Peart [a fellow student] that Professor Pattison has accused me of having entered his private Rooms in an insulting manner, may I request an impartial hearing by which I may be allowed to exculpate myself from so gross a charge.
> I have the honour to be
> My Lords & Gentlemen
> Your most obedient Servant
> Edwd Meryon[20]

Meryon became a member of the Royal College of Surgeons on 25 March 1831, and a Licentiate of the Society of Apothecaries on 5 May. It was customary at this time to acquire the dual qualifications to 'practise generally', that is, to practise both medicine and surgery (Ref. 21, page 17). The distinctions between physicians, surgeons, and general practitioners were becoming blurred during the period of medical reform in the first half of the nineteenth century, and this blurring allowed opportunities for advancement among all ranks of the profession[22]. From what we see of Edward Meryon's subsequent professional achievement, it is clear that he took advantage of such opportunities to acquire further qualifications and establish himself as a highly respected physician.

In the *London Times* in February 1833, an announcement was made of the marriage at Falkingham, Lincolnshire, of Mr E. Meryon, Surgeon, of Trinity Terrace, Southwark to Catherine, daughter of John Baily, Esq. of Falkingham. John Baily was an innkeeper in Falkingham, as was his son, John (Jnr), proprietor of the Greyhound Inn. How Meryon met Catherine is not certain. It may have been through her brother, James, who was probably in partnership in a wine merchant company in London with the family of Newman Smith at

20/21 Queen Street, Cheapside. Newman Smith was a friend and mentor of Edward Meryon, whose first book, published early in 1836[23] was in fact dedicated to him (see Chapter 3).

At the time of his marriage, Meryon would have been trying to establish himself as a medical practitioner. He lived on Trinity Terrace, in Southwark, and is listed in London directories of this period as 'surgeon'. Establishing oneself in practice required connections that led to patients and income, a process achieved only slowly. It was during this relatively leisurely period at the beginning of his career that Meryon developed his interests in anthropology, comparative anatomy, and geology, and was able to write his *Physical and Intellectual Constitution of Man Considered* (see Chapter 3).

By this time Meryon and his wife had two daughters, Lucy Elizabeth, born 1 February 1834, and Anne, baptised in September 1835, and soon the family moved from Trinity Terrace to 4 Bolton Street, Piccadilly.

Around 1837, Meryon must have entered into a partnership with another surgeon, Thomas Wood, for the classified listings in the London directories show Wood & Meryon, Surgeons, at the Bolton Street address. Thomas Wood had been listed as a surgeon at this address for several years previously. The benefits of buying into a partnership, or even outright purchase, for a new medical man, were many. Conditions of work in a prosperous partnership were better than those in a single practice. A buyer who moved into an established practice had ready introductions to patients, and did not have to wait for his income to build up. It removed the pressure of having to be constantly available to patients. In fact, many single practitioners feared that if they left time for a holiday they would lose patients to their competitors. It was also a way of buying a place, literally and figuratively, in the community. The established partner introduced the new man to his patients, in itself a form of recommendation, and a possible way of preventing a dissatisfied patient from perhaps changing to another practice. By 1839 Wood had left the scene, and Meryon was the sole practitioner at Bolton Street.

University College London did not offer degrees until 1839, and Meryon took the examinations and was awarded the degree of Bachelor of Medicine in 1841, the same year in which his third daughter, Julia, was born. A year later he applied for, and was offered, the lectureship in comparative anatomy at St Thomas' Hospital Medical School. One of the governors on the board approving this appointment was Newman Smith, a 'very active and influential governor'[24]. In August 1843 Meryon requested to be excused from teaching the course the following year 'in consequence of the state of his health'[25], and for the next 2 years St Thomas' appointed another lecturer. In 1845, Meryon again applied for the chair in comparative anatomy at St Thomas', and taught there from May 1846 until July 1854, when he again regretfully tendered his resignation. He was replaced by T. H. Huxley (who in 1860 defended vigorously Darwin's *Origin of Species* against Bishop Wilberforce at the famous debate in Oxford); after a year, however, Huxley too resigned 'unwillingly' on the grounds of his engagements, and health. During Meryon's tenure, Meryon encouraged the medical school to enlarge its collection of zoological preparations, and offered to provide a list of animals required. In addition, he offered to 'set [Newman Smith, presently at Brighton] to work to procure as many specimens as he can get...'[26].

Meryon must have spent some time studying following his 1843 resignation from St Thomas', because in December 1844 he took the examinations and was awarded the MD degree. Submission of a thesis was not mandatory, and London University have no records of a thesis by Meryon. He may have felt his energies could be better spent in enlarging his practice and observing cases of particular interest to him, pursuing his interests in anthropology and history, and becoming a member of a gentleman's club, The Athenaeum.

In the 1845 medical directory he lists himself as 'Candidate, Athenaeum Club', though he was actually nominated and finally became a Member in 1850, supported, among others, by his medical colleagues Richard Bright and Richard Partridge, as well as Charles Landseer, the Keeper of the Royal Academy and brother of Sir Edwin, the famous painter. Club membership would bring invaluable social and professional contacts, though Meryon was already involved in a number of societies through his interests in anthropology, geology, and history. From 1845 onwards, he lists membership in the Ethnological Society of London, to whom he delivered a paper, published in their *Transactions* of 1868[27], the Royal Institution (founded to promote scientific progress and which at this time was perhaps more respected than the Royal Society itself), where he in turn proposed another 20 candidates for membership; in 1846 he was elected a Fellow of the Royal Medical and Chirurgical Society of London (Figure 4.4) and in 1857 he became a Fellow of the Geological Society. He took an active part in these societies, serving as council member and vice president of both the Geological and the Medical and Chirurgical Societies, as well as librarian of the latter.

His fourth daughter, Evelyn Jane, was born in 1847. Perhaps his growing family required a larger house, for in that year the Meryons moved to 14 Clarges Street (Figure 4.5), not far from his Bolton Street home. It was certainly not the grandest house on Clarges Street; the tax rolls show it to be assessed at a lower rate than its neighbours. It had been the home of William Mitford, the historian, from 1810 to 1822, and occupied by a solicitor, Thomas Walford, for a year before the Meryons bought it.

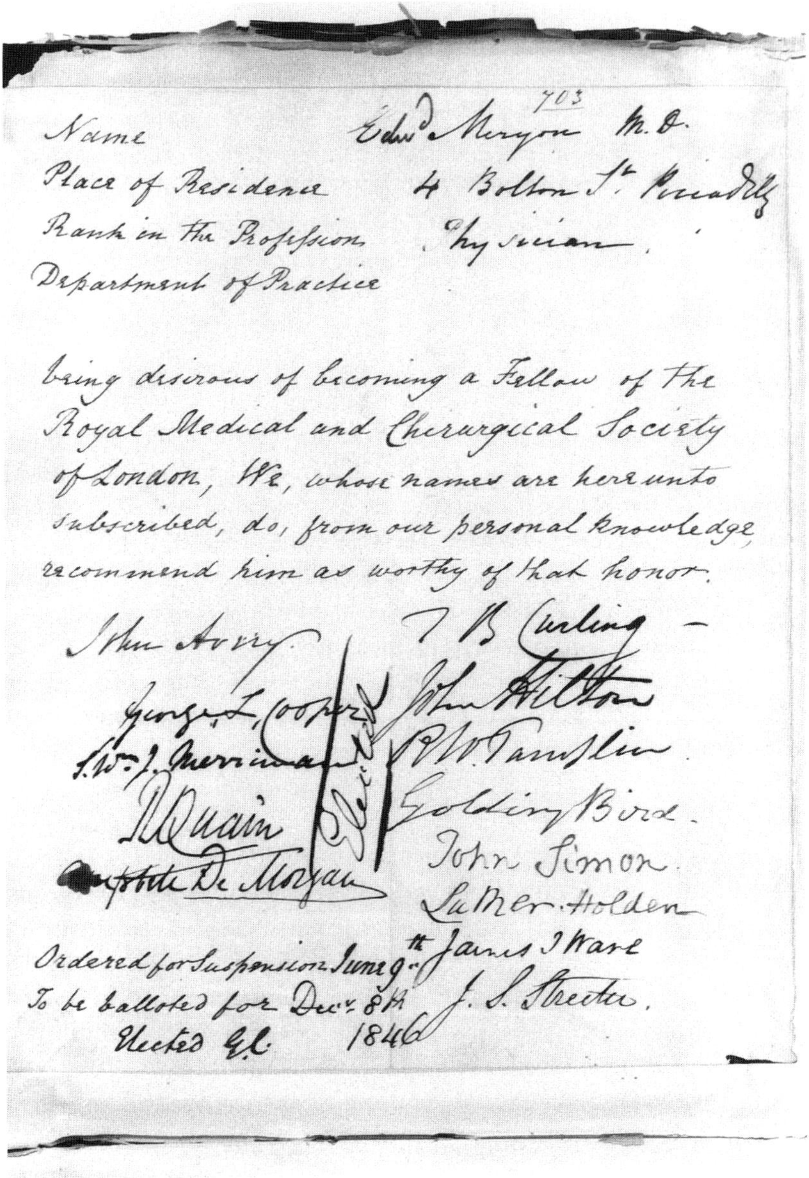

Fig. 4.4 Edward Meryon's election to Fellowship, the Royal Medical and Chirurgical Society, 1846. (Reproduced by kind permission of the Royal Society of Medicine.)

In 1851 his son, John Edward, was born, from whom several Meryons alive today are descended, including Iona Clare Meryon (XI$_8$ in Figure 4.1), born in 1984, who recently graduated in medicine, carrying on Edward Meryon's (her great-great-great grandfather) interest in medical science.

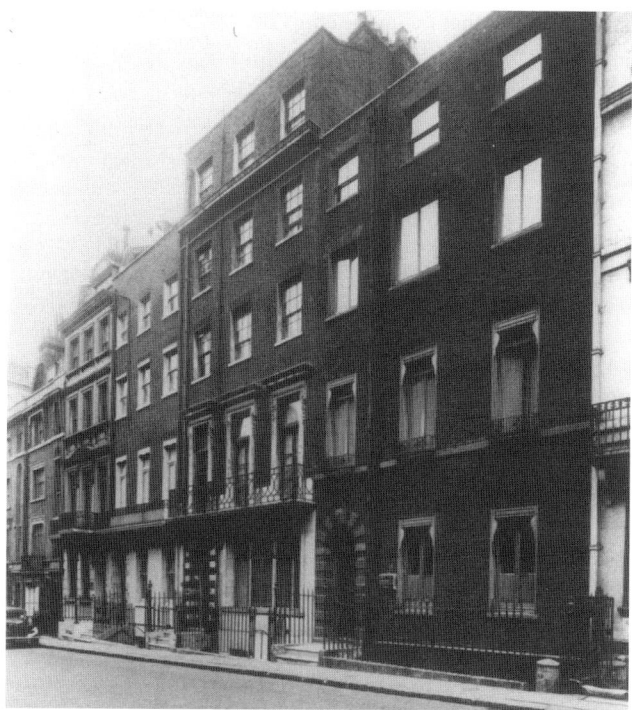

Fig. 4.5 Edward Meryon's residence from 1847 to 1880 at 14 Clarges Street, Piccadilly (house on the right hand side). The building was destroyed in the Second World War and a new building on the site now bears a plaque to Meryon's former home. (Reproduced by kind permission of the Greater London Photograph Library.)

Meryon took the examination for Licentiate of the Royal College of Physicians in April, 1851. He went from being an LRCP to FRCP in 1859. The College had no Members until the 1858 Medical Act, which also granted the College Council power to nominate 'distinguished licentiates... to the fellowship'[28], and, as Meryon appeared in the 1859 College *List* as a Fellow, not a Member, it seems likely that he was nominated in this way. Meryon's academic and medical accreditation was thus complete, and his status as a respected member of the medical community was assured.

Meryon's interest in nervous and muscle diseases and his numerous publications have been discussed in the preceding chapter. He was certainly a prolific writer and active participant in the various societies to which he belonged. It was perhaps for his social standing as much as his medical qualifications that around 1868 he was appointed physician to the relatively recently established London Infirmary for Epilepsy and Paralysis, later to become the Maida Vale Hospital for Nervous Diseases. The hospital was founded in 1866 through the initiative of Julius Althaus (1833–1900), a German who came from a strongly

Protestant family, his father being the equivalent of a rural dean in the Anglican Church. He studied medicine at Göttingen and Heidelberg, receiving his MD from Berlin. He was attracted to the study of nervous diseases and studied as a postgraduate under Charcot at the Salpêtrière before settling in London. The appointment of Meryon as physician was probably a shrewd move on the part of Althaus, for, as Feiling has written:

> with himself as a foreigner and comparative stranger to London, assisted by quite junior and undistinguished colleagues, the medical staff lacked professional prestige. Edward Meryon, although not really distinguished in medicine, was clearly a well-known figure in London society at the time....The author of books on the history of medicine and on the functions of the sympathetic system of nerves, he was a man of wide learning and of many friends whom he delighted to entertain at the Athenaeum Club (Ref. 29, pages 4–5).

Like most who have written on the history of paralysis and nervous diseases, it is obvious that Feiling too was unaware of the significance of Meryon's original contributions on, for example, muscle disease.

In 1869 the wives of the physicians were requested to form a committee, each inviting the cooperation of three friends, and as house visitors, to supervise the general domestic arrangements of the establishment. The hospital grew and in 1872 moved to new premises, a house on Portland Terrace on the north side of Regent's Park, and a year later changed its name to the Hospital for Diseases of the Nervous System to avoid confusion with the similarly named National Hospital in Queen Square. The lay members of the management committee were exceedingly lax about attendance at meetings, and the hospital was in effect governed by its medical staff, Althaus in particular, with Althaus and Meryon often chairing the meetings. The hospital suffered numerous financial crises, and appeals for funds were made to defray expenses, especially after the 1875 explosion of a barge on a nearby canal which damaged the hospital building. Mrs Meryon (Figure 4.6) was actually called in to assist in the housekeeping. It is clear that Althaus and Meryon, the two stalwarts, and their wives were the most 'devoted servants of the young hospital' (Ref. 29, page 8).

During his years with the infirmary, Meryon continued to write, and find time to undertake the duties of a vice president of the Royal Medical and Chirurgical Society and a Council member of the Royal College of Physicians. He had become a distinguished and respected member of the London medical community (Figure 4.7).

Among Meryon's publications, perhaps the most unusual is the play mentioned earlier (Chapter 3), partly in verse form, entitled *The Huguenot*[30], which is now to be found in the UK only in the library of his club, the Athenaeum

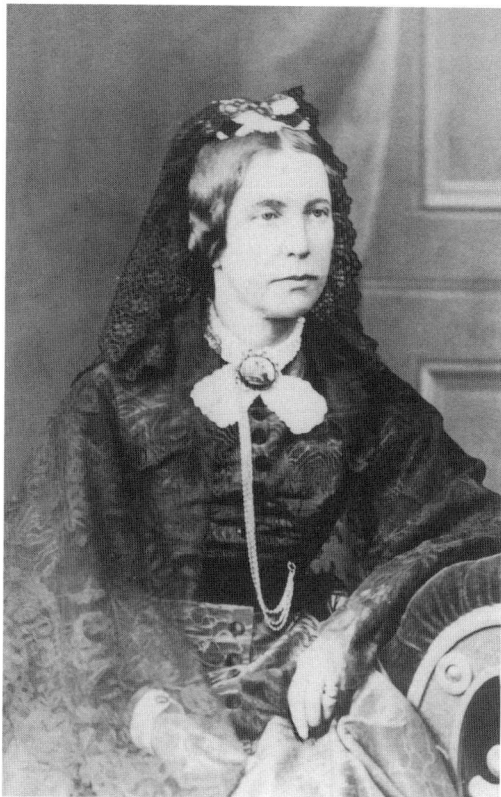

Fig. 4.6 Catherine Meryon (née Baily) (1811–1897), c. 1861. (Reproduced by kind permission of Mr. David Easton.)

(inscribed 'for private distribution' with a handwritten dedication to 'The Athenaeum Club from the Author'). The work is a highly dramatic historical romance between the Catholic Marguérite de Lanoy and Gaspar Lomagne, her childhood love and a Huguenot, which takes place in France in 1572 at the time of the St Bartholomew's day massacre.

Meryon's ill-health forced him to resign from his position as physician to the Hospital in 1879. It is known that at this time Meryon's two eldest daughters, Lucy Elizabeth and Anne, were both married (the great-grandson of Lucy is David Easton, born in 1930, who has been of exceptional help to the authors in their research on the Meryon family), and that Meryon's son, John Edward, had chosen a career in the Royal Navy and married Isobella Chalmers, a descendant of the famous Scottish theologian, Thomas Chalmers. They had four children, the first a son, Edward David Meryon, born in 1880. Evelyn, Meryon's youngest daughter, who suffered from a severe visual impairment, remained at home, unmarried.

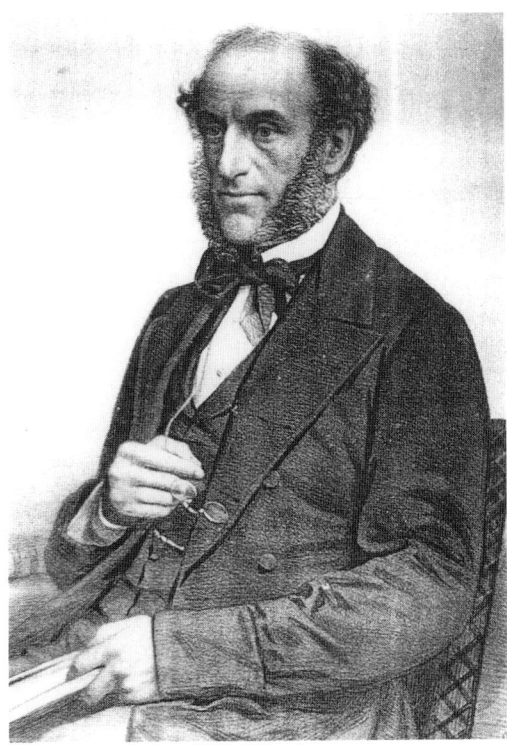

Fig. 4.7 Edward Meryon. (Engraving by J. R. Black of London, c. 1862.) (Reproduced by kind permission of Mr. David Easton.)

Edward Meryon (Figure 4.8) died suddenly, at home, on Monday, 8 November 1880[31], according to the death certificate of 'Gout, many years, Heart disease, several months'. His obituaries[32,33] clearly demonstrate he was a much liked and respected gentleman, held in esteem by both colleagues and friends.

> By the sudden death, on the 8th inst., of Dr Edward Meryon, at his residence, Clarges-street, Mayfair, the profession has sustained the loss of an accomplished and practical physician, and those who knew him a trusty and sincere friend. In the practice of his profession he not only brought his great professional experience to bear thoughtfully and conscientiously in every case in which he was consulted, but his kind and friendly sympathy was ever called into exercise as an auxiliary to his skill. He was single-minded, liberal, and accomplished, and his well-stored mind rendered his society at once entertaining and instructive.... In the memory of a large number of old acquaintances, especially many members of the Athenaeum Club, he will long live as the type of a good, noble, and true-hearted gentleman'.[32]

He was buried at Brompton Cemetery, London (Figure 4.9). He had had a happy and fulfilling life as a London physician and family man, but perhaps without ever realizing the important contributions he had made to muscular dystrophy.

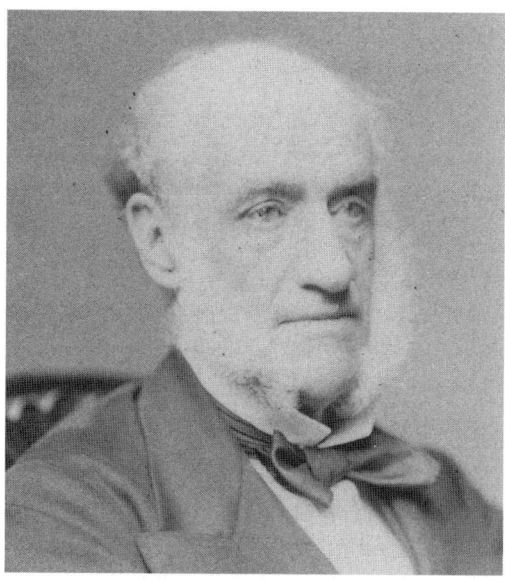

Fig. 4.8 Edward Meryon in later years, c. 1880. (From *Epigrams, Epitaphs, Personal Anecdotes, &tc.*, London: for private circulation [188?].)

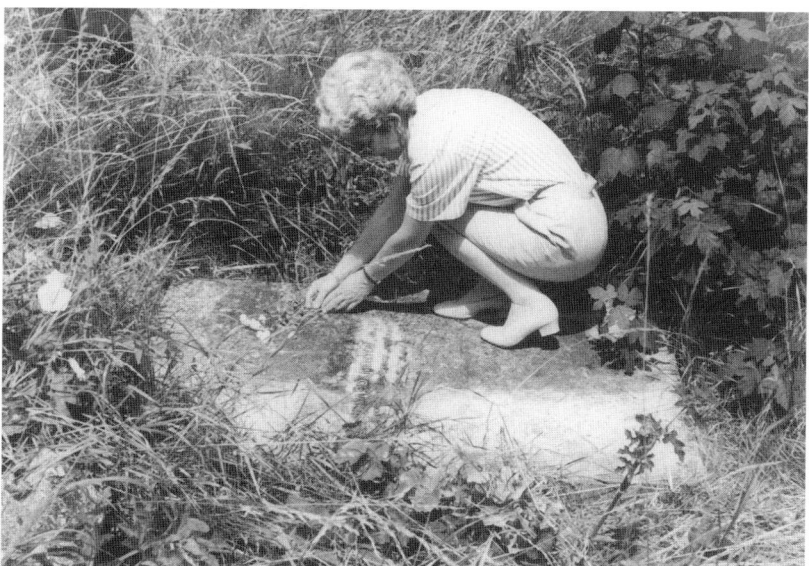

Fig. 4.9 Rediscovery in 1993 of Edward Meryon's long neglected grave in Brompton Cemetery, London, being cleaned by one of the authors. The inscription simply reads 'In memory of Edward Meryon, MD who died November 8th 1880 aged 73 years'.

References

1. Hands, A. P., Scouloudi, I. *French Protestant Refugees Relieved through the Threadneedle Street Church, London 1681–1687*. Vol. 49. Quarto Series of Publications. London: Huguenot Society, 1971: 135.
2. Shaw, W. A. *Letters of Denization and Acts of Naturalisation for Aliens in England & Ireland 1603–1700*. Vol. 18. Quarto Series of Publications. London: Huguenot Society, 1911.
3. Cooper, W. D. Protestant refugees in Sussex. *Sussex Archaeological Collections*, 1861; **13**: 180–208.
4. Rye Records. *Lists of Scholars attending Sanders' School 1722–1828*. Lewes: East Sussex Record Office, 1722–1828. [Ref. no. 114/10].
5. Clark, Kenneth. *Rye—A Short History*. Rye: Anthony Neville, 1991.
6. Fabes, A., Gibson, E. *The Meryon Story*. Rye: Privately published, 1985.
7. Haslip, J. *Lady Hester Stanhope: A Biography*. Harmondsworth: Penguin, 1934, 1945.
8. Gibb, L. *Lady Hester: Queen of the East*. London: Faber, 2005.
9. Bishop, T. H. Charles Lewis Meryon (1783–1877): physician and biographer of Lady Hester Stanhope. *Medical Bookman and Historian*, 1948; **2**: 412–14.
10. Meryon, C. L. *Memoirs of the Lady Hester Stanhope, as related by herself in Conversations with her Physician*. 3 vols. London: Henry Colburn, 1845.
11. Meryon, C. L. *Travels of Lady Hester Stanhope, Forming the Completion of her Memoirs*. 3 vols. London: Henry Colburn, 1846.
12. Meryon, John. *An Account of the Origin and Formation of the Harbour of the Ancient Town of Rye*. [Rye Manuscripts. Rye Harbour. Lewes: East Sussex Record Office, 1845].
13. Vidler, L. A. *A New History of Rye*. Hove: Combridges, 1934.
14. Rye. *Parish Poor Book*. Lewes: East Sussex Record Office, 1803–1811. [Ref. no. PAR 467/30/13.]
15. Pigot & Co. *Pigot's London Directory*. London: Pigot & Co., 1839. (Includes provincial listings.)
16. Robinson, Rev. C. J. *A Register of the Scholars Admitted into Merchant Taylors' School, from A.D. 1562 to 1874*. Vol. 1–2. Lewes: Farncombe & Co., 1882–1883.
17. Hart, Mrs. E. P. (ed.) *Merchant Taylors' School Register, 1561–1934*. Vol. 1–2. London: Merchant Taylors' Company, 1936.
18. Meryon, E. *Practical and Pathological Researches on the Various Forms of Paralysis*. London: John Churchill & Sons, 1864.
19. Pattison, F. L. M. *Granville Sharp Pattison, Anatomist and Antagonist 1791–1851*. Edinburgh: Canongate Publishing Ltd, 1987: 149–73.
20. Meryon, E. Letter. University College London Library. Manuscripts and Rare Books. [College Collection Correspondence: No. 2052, Meryon]: 1830.
21. Peterson, M. J. *The Medical Profession in Mid-Victorian London*. Berkeley: University of California Press, 1978.
22. Loudon, I. *Medical Care and the General Practitioner 1750–1850*. Oxford: Clarendon Press, 1986: 189–90.
23. Meryon, E. *The Physical and Intellectual Constitution of Man Considered*. London: Smith, Elder & Co., 1836.

24. Parsons, F. G. *The History of St. Thomas's Hospital.* Vols 1–3. London: Methuen & Co. Ltd., 1932–36; Vol. 3: 90.
25. St. Thomas's Hospital Mss. *Minute Book. Medical & Surgical School, St. Thomas's, 1842–1845.* London. [Medical Library Archives, Ref. 30.i .3, 30 August 1843.]
26. St. Thomas's Hospital Mss. Medical Officers & Lecturer's Committee. St. Thomas's Medical & Surgical School, Minutes of Meetings, 1849–1854. London. [Medical Library Archives, Ref. 30.i .9, 12 December 1849.]
27. Meryon, E. An account of some cases of arrest of development. *Transactions of the Ethnological Society*, 1868; **7**: 162–4.
28. Cooke, A. M. *A History of the Royal College of Physicians of London.* Oxford: Oxford University Press for the Royal College of Physicians, 1972; Vol. 3, p. 808.
29. Feiling, A. *A History of the Maida Vale Hospital for Nervous Diseases.* London: Butterworth & Co., 1958.
30. Meryon, E. *The Huguenot.* London: Effingham Wilson, 1876.
31. Obituary. Edward Meryon MD. *Times*, November 10, 1880.
32. Obituary. Edward Meryon, MD, FRCP. *Lancet*, 1880; **ii**: 833.
33. Obituary, Meryon, Edward. In: Brown, G. H. comp. *Lives of the Fellows of the Royal College of Physicians, 1826–1925.* London: Royal College of Physicians, 1955. [*Munk's Roll, IV.* p. 113.]

Chapter 5

Duchenne de Boulogne (1806–1875)

By almost any criteria one wishes to take, Duchenne must count among the great in neurology. He played a singularly important role in the history of muscular dystrophy and, according to Sir Arthur Keith, he was 'one of the most remarkable figures which has ever appeared on the medical stage'[1]. An excellent multi-authored and beautifully illustrated book on the life and work of Duchenne was published in Paris in 1999 by the *École nationale supérieure des beaux-arts*.

Duchenne's life

Guillaume Benjamin Amand Duchenne, or Duchenne de Boulogne as he signed himself in order not to be confused with Duchesne, a fashionable society physician in Paris at the time, was born in the town of Boulogne-sur-Mer on 17 September 1806. This was some 7 years after the French Revolution. France was now in its ascendancy and Claude Clodion, for instance, had just started the Arc de Triomphe in Paris. But Boulogne, a busy fishing town situated on the north coast of France, being distant from Paris, was spared some of the excesses of the Capital.

Until Napoleon's abdication in 1814, French privateers operated from most of the French Channel ports, including Boulogne, and played an important role in the war against England. Duchenne's father was a renowned privateer of the time and later became supervisor of the port. For this he was awarded the Légion d'Honneur by Napoleon himself in 1804. No doubt his son's character was influenced by this background: basically that of a fisherman—strong, independent, clumsy in speech, yet kind and generous. In later years the arrival on the wards of Paris hospitals of this rather taciturn little man from the provinces must have been surprising to the establishment. He never became part of Paris Society.

He was one of four brothers, and from the age of 10 was educated at the Collège de Monseigneur Haffreingue where he showed a particular predilection for the natural sciences. In 1825, at the age of 19, he received his 'Bachelier ès Lettres'. His father then expected him to go to Naval School and was very disappointed when his son expressed a wish to study medicine, especially since his other sons had also chosen careers other than the sea. However, despite some reluctance, the captain agreed and Duchenne left for Paris at the end of 1825. He had only been in Paris a few weeks when his father died of a cerebral haemorrhage. Having returned to Boulogne to comfort his mother and family, he returned to Paris in March 1826 to begin his studies. Laënnec (the inventor of the stethoscope) died in August, but other teachers in Paris at the time included Joseph Récamier (1774–1852), who first recognized the process of metastasis, Guillaume Dupuytren (1777–1835), a famous surgeon whose name is still associated with contractures of the fingers, and Jean Alibert (1768–1837), a physician who first described mycosis fungoides, as well as various other skin disorders. There was also the beginning of a new generation of celebrities which included the experimental physiologists François Magendie (1783–1855) and later Claude Bernard (1813–1878), and the renowned pathologist Jean Cruveilhier (1791–1874).

The French Revolution had swept away the traditional system of recruitment and the old restrictions on entry into the medical profession. Protestants and Jews were no longer excluded[2]. We have already seen that Edward Meryon studied at the École de Médecine around this time (Figure 5.1). Could their paths therefore have crossed? This is an intriguing possibility but our research on this point has so far been unhelpful.

The Faculty of Medicine in Paris had been established in the mid-thirteenth century[3], some years after the renowned school at Montpellier. Over the years, Paris established its pre-eminence as a centre for clinical teaching, though it was only in the wake of Claude Bernard and Pasteur that biological and laboratory disciplines began to be considered important in the medical curriculum. For example, in his clinical lectures at the Hôtel-Dieu in 1857, Professor Armand Trousseau (1801–1867) could say to his students:

> The small amount of time that you dedicate to medicine makes it very difficult for you to study auxiliary sciences. You must have sufficient notion of chemistry and physics to be able to understand the application of these sciences to medicine. But I should profoundly deplore the time that you might lose in order to acquire a more extended knowledge of chemistry… So, gentlemen, let us have a little less science and a little more art.

In Duchenne's time the doctorate in medicine or surgery involved 4 years of study which included anatomy, physiology, pathology and nosology, materia medica, chemistry, and pharmacy. There were no less than 23 professors in the faculty at the time. We may assume therefore that Duchenne received a good grounding in the basics, with an especially good training in clinical medicine which was to prove particularly important to him in the future. There were written and oral tests in Latin and a terminal thesis was required which had to be in French or Latin[4].

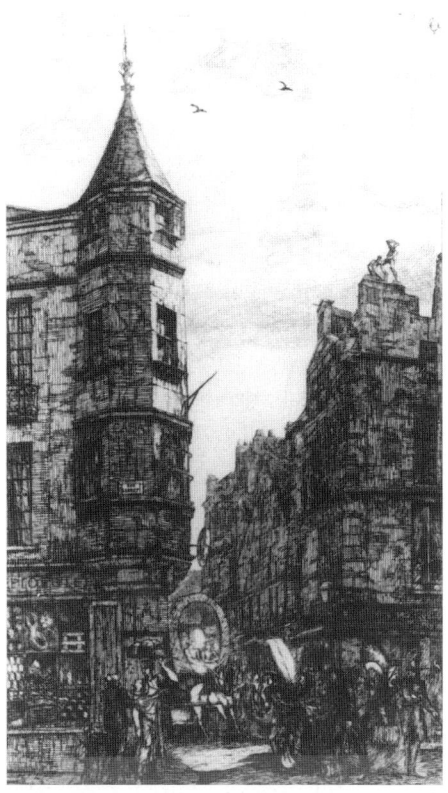

Fig. 5.1 Rue de L'Ecole de Médecine, 1861 (showing the Tourelle, the house in which Charlotte Corday assassinated Jean-Paul Marat). (Etching by Charles Meryon.)

After an undistinguished career as a student, Duchenne graduated in 1831 with a thesis, *Essays on Burns*, of 34 pages, probably inspired by Dupuytren, He then returned to Boulogne with the sole ambition of becoming a 'médecin de famille'. In December he married a young lady of the same town, a Mlle Barbe Boutroy. According to Guilly[5], in his comprehensive biography of Duchenne, it was a love match, and in January 1833 a son was born, christened Guillaume Maxime Emile Duchenne. But 2 weeks after giving birth, the young mother died of puerperal sepsis. Duchenne had attended his wife's confinement and his mother-in-law unfairly reproached him for her death. In his distraught state of mind Duchenne allowed her to take over the upbringing of his young son, a decision which he later very much regretted. The future seemed quite hopeless. He became severely depressed and ignored his patients and his practice. He was often seen idling about the harbour. At home he consoled himself by reading and playing Bach and Beethoven on his violin. But after some time he gradually began to recover and his patients, mainly poor fishermen and their families, began to return to his practice.

Then, in 1835 a chance event occurred which changed his life. He had occasion to treat, by electropuncture, one of his patients with neuralgia, and the question arose as to why the electric current produced a localized contraction of muscle fibres.

> l'ouverture brusque du courant produisait au point de la piqûre, une contraction isolée, circonscrite, limitée à un seul faisceau musculaire (Ref. 5, page 11).

He found this intriguing and became obsessed with the effects of electrical stimulation. This was the beginning of his interest in the application of electricity to medicine. He found there was no need to puncture the skin to stimulate muscles; after all, this was painful and there was a very real risk of infection. He found he could use two metallic electrodes (which he called 'rhéophores') applied to the surface of skin which had been dampened. Subsequently he built his own apparatus (faradic induction coil and batteries) for the electrical stimulation of muscles and nerves[5–7]. His new studies so excited him that in 1842, at the age of 36, he left Boulogne for Paris where there were greater opportunities for him to pursue his work on *l'électrisation localisée* (Figure 5.2). But there may also have been other reasons for his return to Paris. There is a suggestion that there may have been some sort of neurological disease in his own family. In the archives of the library of Boulogne-sur-Mer, Cuthbertson[8] has located an anonymous letter of 24 April

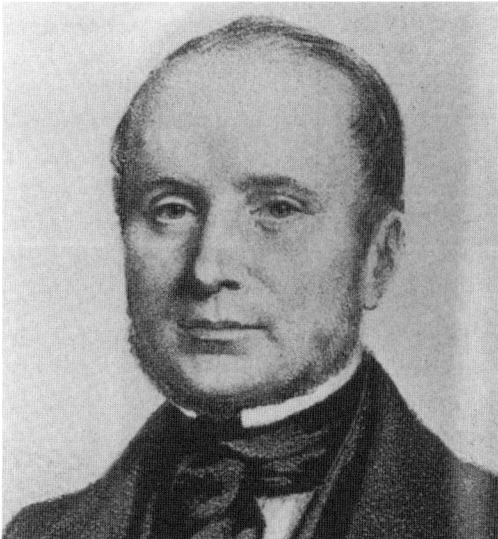

Fig. 5.2 Duchenne around the time he began his research into muscle disease. (Reproduced with permission from *The Founders of Neurology*, edited by Webb Haymaker, 1953. Courtesy of Charles C. Thomas, Publishers, Springfield, Illinois.)

1889 in which the writer apparently provides evidence of this possibility. As Cuthbertson comments:

> such a family history could certainly have provided an impetus to push an introverted and melancholy young man into a lifetime study of neurological disease.

A third reason may have been disillusionment with Boulogne following a disastrous second marriage in 1839 to his cousin, a widow, Honorine Lardé. Whatever the reason, his return to Paris went unnoticed. He was, as Cuthbertson says, 'an unknown provincial doctor, with little grace and less money'. From such an inauspicious start so began a career which was to have a major influence on neurology. His home at 21 Boulevard des Italiens (now occupied by the offices of *Le Monde* newspaper) was to include a room for seeing patients, a workshop for making instruments, a study, and a darkroom for photography. In this way it became the fulcrum for his work.

La Salpêtrière

Although he was never attached to any one department, and was therefore free to trace and follow up his patients wherever he wished, he spent much time at the Hôtel Dieu and, most fruitfully, at the Salpêtrière (Figure 5.3). It was here

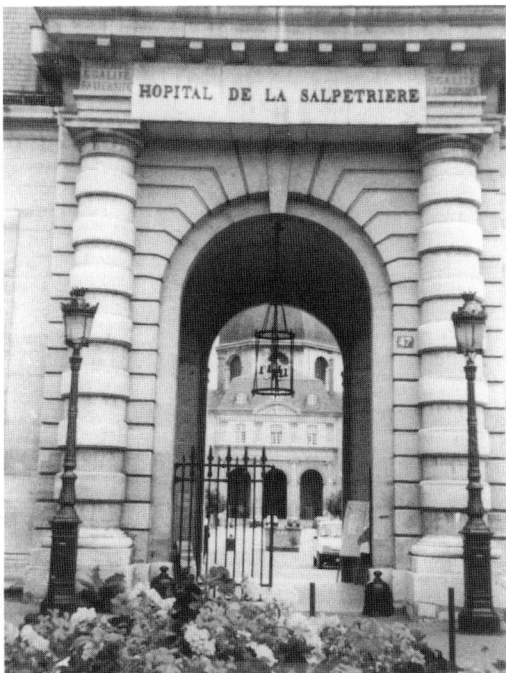

Fig. 5.3 The entrance to the Hôpital de la Salpêtrière as it is today. (Author's photograph,1994.)

that later Jean-Martin Charcot (1825–1893) was to become a close friend and was much influenced by Duchenne. Charcot was also to make enormous contributions to neurology, for example in delineating amyotrophic lateral sclerosis, and various other conditions with which his name is still associated: Charcot–Marie–Tooth disease, Charcot's joint, Charcot's triad[9,10]. Charcot's initial interest in neurological diseases in fact stemmed from Duchenne's influence. Duchenne discussed with Charcot his ideas and the results of his research and taught him photography. In return, Charcot taught Duchenne histology and the importance of pathological anatomy[11]. Like Charles Bell before them, these men also opposed animal experiments and their contributions to neurology came exclusively from studying patients.

However, at the beginning, Duchenne's time in Paris was difficult. Many did not accept his ideas. There were frequent arguments with associates, often centred on questions of priority. Others regarded him more good-humouredly as a harmless crank. But he persevered and continued to work hard, making copious and detailed notes on all the patients he saw, often applying his electrical methods in treatment (Figure 5.4).

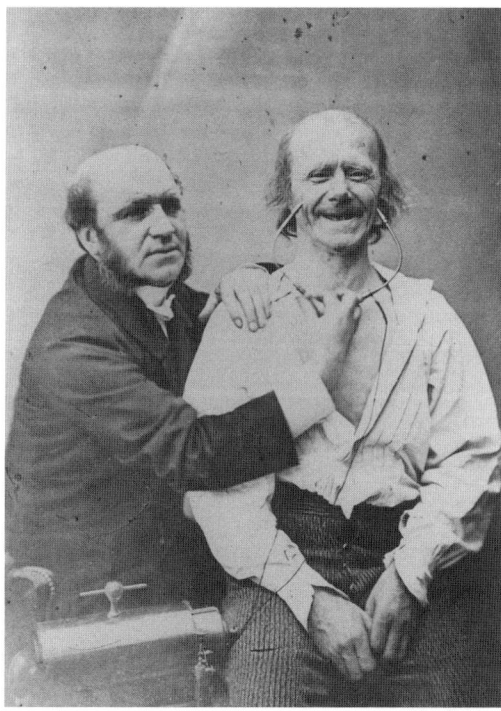

Fig. 5.4 'An electro-physiological experiment' from Duchenne's *Mécanisme de la Physionomie Humaine*.

By 1851 his work was gradually being recognized and the Académie de Médecine awarded him the Itard Prize for a paper entitled *Fonctions des muscles de la face démontrées par l' localisée*. In the same year his mother-in-law died and his son, Emile, came to live with him in Paris. But in the intervening years Emile's feelings about his father had been coloured by his embittered grandmother, and after a few months the two separated. Emile went off to study medicine and some years later, in 1864, published his thesis on a subject doubtless influenced by his father, namely, *La Paralysie Atrophique Graisseuse de l'Enfance*. In it he credits his father with having first described 'paralysie hypertrophique' and throughout refers frequently to his father's work[12].

From the early 1850s onwards, however, Duchenne's work began to attract increasing attention, largely through his numerous publications. In 1855 the first edition of his *De l'Électrisation Localisée*[13] appeared, the second edition of which 6 years later would contain important details of a case of muscular dystrophy. In the following year he became a Chevalier de la Légion d'Honneur.

The year 1862 saw the publication of his classic work, *Méchanisme de la Physionomie Humaine*, concerning the facial expression of emotion[14], and the return of his son, Emile, (now also a doctor), with whom a close and loving relationship developed at last. Duchenne was now comfortably established (Figure 5.5), enjoying his practice and his two grand-daughters. He was always

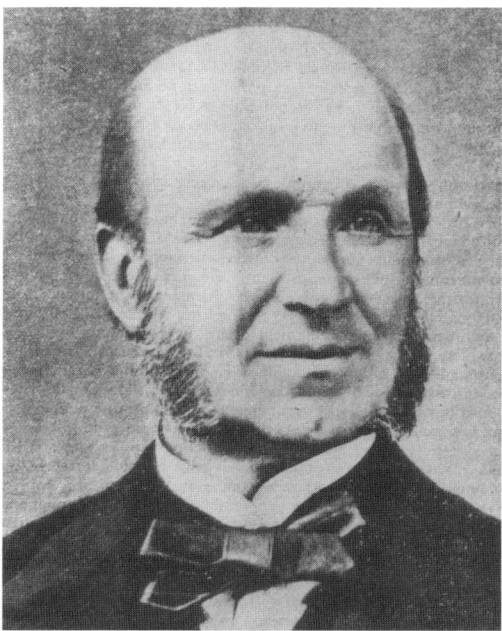

Fig. 5.5 Duchenne in middle age. (Kindly provided by Professor Fernando Tomé, Paris.)

hospitable and a generous host. He would often give dinner parties for his medical colleagues (Nélaton, Broca, Charcot, Potain, and Vulpian). After the meal, the idea was to discuss muscle pathology from lantern slides. But Duchenne always asked if he might first show a few magic lantern slides to amuse his little grand-daughters. And so, before his distinguished guests could discuss their latest findings in muscle histology, they had to view 'The tale of Bluebeard' or 'The adventures of "Riquet à la Houppe"'! He was often teased for his absent-mindedness. He turned up in evening dress for a formal dinner party given by Baron Haussmann, the distinguished planner of the city of Paris, a week late! On another occasion, as a joke his daughter-in-law served grilled croutons and asked how her father-in-law enjoyed the beefsteak, to which the old doctor replied 'Your steak was excellent, my dear—it was just right, for I don't like my meat over-cooked'.

In 1870 the Franco-Prussian War began, and during the subsequent siege of Paris Duchenne became involved in treating the wounded and sick. In December his wife died, and a month later his son was reported to have died of typhoid. But Cuthbertson[8] has located correspondence of the time which suggests that Emile may have been mentally ill, was institutionalized, and may have died in a mental hospital. All this contributed to Duchenne's profound depression, in which he remained until his death in 1875.

During his declining years Duchenne was cared for by his daughter-in-law. Around this time he visited England, Austria, and Spain, and although he was much fêted and honoured, he remained depressed. He had published over 90 articles and books during his lifetime, but in his remaining years many took advantage of his work. His secretary was alleged to have stolen some of his papers to give to ambitious young colleagues. Duchenne seemed indifferent to all this.

He suffered a cerebral haemorrhage in August 1875 and Potain and Charcot never left him during the last weeks of his illness, taking it in turns to sleep by his bed. He died on 17 September 1875 on his sixty-ninth birthday. An appreciation appeared in the *Medical Times & Gazette* on October 2nd and on October 30th the Paris correspondent of the *Lancet*, commenting on Duchenne's life and work, wrote that, despite many adverse circumstances:

> his reputation has come out clear and bright as an honest, hard-working, acute, and ingenious observer, an original discoverer, a skilful professional man, and a kind-hearted, benevolent gentleman.

He had been elected a corresponding member of various academies and universities throughout Europe, but he never became a member of the

Académie de Médecine de Paris or the Institut de France. When pressed to become a member of the latter, Duchenne replied characteristically:

> Non, ma seule ambition est de revivre dans mes ouvrages. Il en est qui ont les honneurs aujourd'hui; plus tard, ils seront oubliés et mes livres vivront (Ref. 5, page 220).

He was without a doubt a man who had happily, and with success, dedicated his life entirely to medical science.

Paralysie hypertrophique de l'enfance

Unlike Meryon, when Duchenne began his work on muscle disease in Paris this was not inspired by a general interest in the subject among colleagues. On the contrary, at the beginning there was, as we have seen, little interest in his work and he was often ridiculed. Furthermore, the Salpêtrière at the time, though to prove a very valuable source of clinical material, was a huge rambling collection of old buildings housing a vast number of chronically sick and incurable patients, usually poor and vagrant. Yet against this unprepossessing background, Duchenne made almost all his major contributions.

In the second edition of his *L'Électrisation Localisée*, published in 1861[15], he describes the case of a young boy he first saw in 1858, then 9 years of age, with what Duchenne refers to as *Paralysie hypertrophique de l'enfance* (Figure 5.6). The following year, in an album of clinical photographs to accompany his book[16], Duchenne published a photograph he took himself of this same patient (Figure 5.7).

The clinical features of the case were as follows. Not until around 18 months of age did the child attempt to stand without support. When he was seen by Duchenne he walked only with great difficulty and soon tired, and if he fell he was unable to get up again. He was also developing an equinovarus deformity, the cause of which Duchenne, in his later publication[17], rightly attributes to muscle imbalance. Duchenne was especially impressed by the enlargement of certain muscles, particularly the sacrospinalis and gastrocnemius muscles, despite the fact that the lower limbs were obviously weak. The upper limbs appeared much less affected, which accounts for Duchenne's use at this time of the alternative term *paraplégie* for this disorder. Because the boy also had some intellectual impairment, Duchenne wondered if the cause might therefore be cerebral (*paralysie hypertrophique de l'enfance de cause cérébrale*). The clinical details of this case are much less detailed than those given by Meryon, whose work is not mentioned, and at this stage, Duchenne provided no histological findings. However, this case clearly intrigued Duchenne because over the next few years he studied a number of similar cases, details of which were published

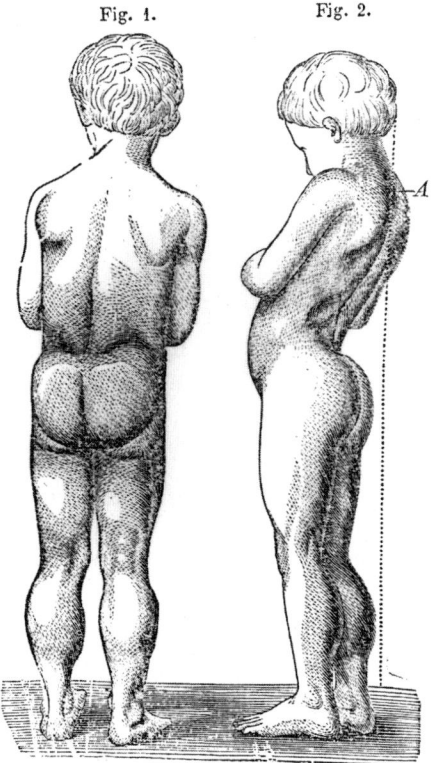

Fig. 5.6 Duchenne's case number 68, published in 1861[15]. Note the lordosis and enlarged calves.

in an extensive series of articles in 1868[17]. It is largely on the basis of this that his name became widely associated with the condition. Later, in 1883 these and various of his other publications were translated, edited, and condensed for the New Sydenham Society by Poore[18].

In the 1868 publications[17] Duchenne reviewed his original case in considerable detail, plus 12 further cases, two of whom were young girls. He notes that his observations on the condition in 1861 had attracted more attention in Germany than in France and that between 1861 and 1867 details of no less than 15 cases had been published in Germany (Table 5.1). Duchenne reviewed the findings in these cases as well, but he failed to include Oppenheimer's study[19] of six cases, published in 1855. He does, however, refer to Meryon's work, though, as we shall see, he misinterprets Meryon's findings and here also gives the date of Meryon's publication as 1866 whereas it was originally published in 1852 (though much later in the text (page 429) he quotes the correct date).

PARALYSIE HYPERTROPHIQUE DE L'ENFANCE | 83

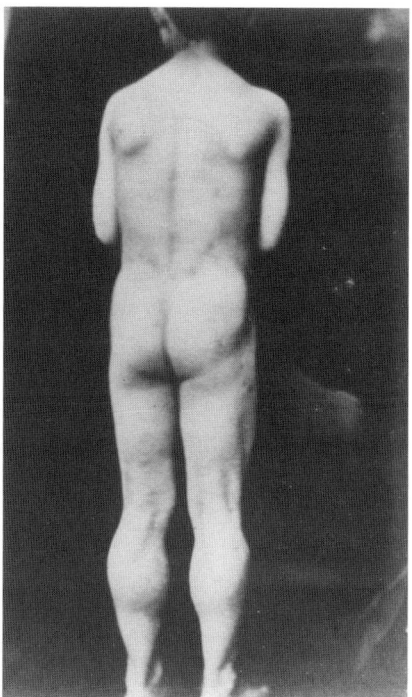

Fig. 5.7 Duchenne's own photograph of his patient with *Paralysie hypertrophique* (Figure 13 in Ref. 16).

From his studies Duchenne recognized several stages in the progress of the disease, though there was some overlap between them. The first stage was characterized by progressive weakness of the lower extremities and lumbar muscles, beginning usually in early childhood (though at age 10 in one of his female cases). This weakness resulted in a tendency to fall, an inability to rise without help, and difficulty in climbing stairs. He noted the lordotic waddling gait in these children and, like Bell before him, he was struck by the peculiar way of getting up from the floor or a chair:

> Le penchait-on un peu en avant, il ne se redressait qu'en s'aidant de ses mains accrochées à un meuble ou appuyées sur ces cuisses (Ref. 17, page 20).

At a later stage there appeared a gradual increase in size of some of the affected muscles, particularly the gastrocnemius muscles, and the progress of the disease appeared to arrest for a period, perhaps for 2–3 years. In the final stage the weakness progressed and involved the upper extremities. By adolescence ambulation was lost altogether and death occurred later (in his own cases the cause is given as pneumonia in one and phthisis in two others). He also records

Table 5.1 Cases in the German literature reviewed by Duchenne[17]*

Case numbers	Year	Author(s)	Reference
1	1862	Spielmann, C. A.	Gazette Médicale de Strasbourg, 5: 85
2	1862	Kaulich, J.	Vierteljahrschrift für die Praktische Heilkunde (Prag), 1: 113 (Old Series v. 73)
3	1863	Berend, H. W.	Berliner Allgemeine Medizinische Centralzeitung, 9
4	1866	Eulenberg, A. & Cohnheim, J.	Verhandlungen der Berliner Medicinischen Gesellschaft, 1: 191–205
5 & 6 (brothers)	1867	Wernich, A.	Deutsches Archiv für Klinische Medicin, 2: 232–43
7	1865	von Stofella, E. R.	Medizinische Jahrbücher (Wien), 9: 85–98
8	1865	Griesinger, W.	Archiv der Heilkunde, 6: 1–13
9–12 (same family)	1866	Heller, A.	Deutsches Archiv für Klinische Medicin, 1: 616–29
13–15 (same family)	1867	Seidel, M.	Die Atrophia musculorum lipomatosa (sogenannte Muskelhypertrophie) Jena. 1867 (book review). In: Centralblatt für die Medicinischen Wissenschaften (Berlin), 5(42, 28 Sept): 666–9

*References have been verified as completely as possible and, where necessary, corrected by the authors.

that, although one case (no. 11, a girl) was highly intelligent, another was mentally retarded and she had reduced intellect (*intelligence obtuse*). By now, however, he had abandoned the idea that the disease had a cerebral cause, because in many of his cases there was no intellectual deficit.

It seemed to Duchenne that, based on these clinical features, an appropriate name for the condition might be *paralysie musculaire pseudo-hypertrophique* or pseudohypertrophic muscular paralysis. However, based on his pathological findings he thought it could also be termed *paralysie myo-sclérosique*.

Muscle pathology

It is perhaps Duchenne's contribution to muscle pathology which established his association with the disease as much as his clinical findings.

Although Meryon had previously described in some detail the microscopic findings in muscle, his observations had been limited to material obtained at autopsy, the so-called diagnosis of Morgagni.

Duchenne, however, was keen to study muscle from living patients but objected to open biopsy on the grounds that it exposed the patient to the risks of anaesthesia and problems of wound healing, which in his opinion were unjustified when this was being carried out purely for scientific reasons:

> Est-il juste d'exposer des malades à de pareils dangers, pour atteindre un résultat purement scientifique qui ne peut leur être d'aucune utilité? Nous ne le pensons pas (Ref. 17, page 203).

—a sentiment just as valuable nowadays!

Duchenne therefore proceeded to design a muscle biopsy needle or punch (*emporte-pièce histologique*) to obtain specimens in life. His instrument apparently caused no serious problems and seemingly little pain. He emphasized that the punch had to be introduced at right angles to the direction of the muscle to ensure an adequate specimen was obtained, and that it had to be very carefully cleaned after use and stored in alcohol. But this was no prescience of the relation between micro-organisms and wound infection, which would not be reported by Robert Koch for another decade or so. It was to eliminate any material after use which might produce artefact and to prevent the instrument from rusting! These measures nevertheless account for his never having problems with wound healing.

This was a forerunner of subsequent biopsy needles, a technique which is now widely used for obtaining tissue for diagnosis in muscular dystrophy. Some authorities, such as Dubowitz[20], believe Duchenne was the first to introduce this technique, but this is not so. Griesinger[21], for example, some years previously attempted to obtain muscle tissue from his patient (Figure 5.8) using a biopsy needle designed by Middeldorpff, a surgeon in Breslau at the time. Duchenne first tried this instrument himself, but found it unsatisfactory for several reasons. He therefore designed his own, with which he had much greater success.

Duchenne used the technique on several of his patients, and in some cases from different muscles, and at different times in the same case. He then compared his histological findings with those of others and concluded (Ref. 17, pages 309–17) that the most striking and, in his opinion, fundamental abnormality was hyperplasia of the fibrous connective tissue *(myo-sclérosique)*, and that the increase in such tissue was related to the increase in the size of certain muscles. Interestingly, however, and to his complete surprise, he found no apparent increase in fibrous connective tissue in a biopsy specimen from one of the young girls he studied (case 13). Later, fatty tissue predominated. The muscle fibres themselves were often smaller in diameter (though this was variable) and cross-striations were faint; sometimes they were not visible at all and

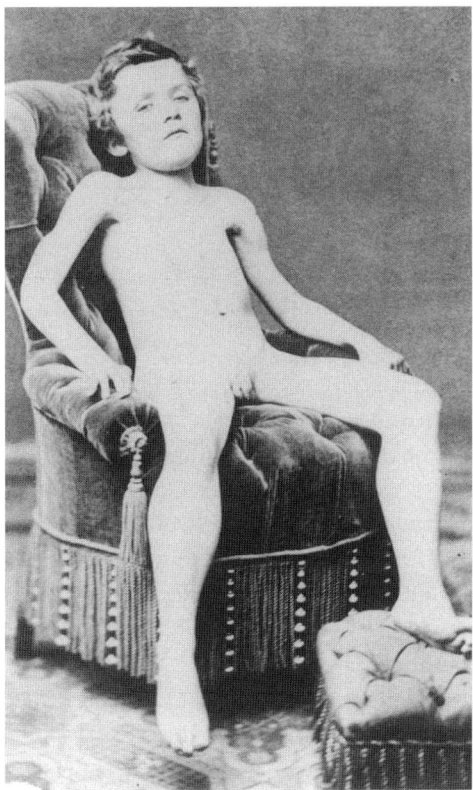

Fig. 5.8 The patient studied by Griesinger[21]. Note the enlarged calves.

had been lost completely. He does *not* consider that the sarcolemma might itself be defective, as Meryon did, but only ponders on its relationship with the increase in fibrous connective tissue ('Le tissu fibroïde interstitiel de la paralysie pseudo-hypertrophique est-il composé pas des sarcolèmes vides (ou) est-il le produit de la dégénérescence fibroïde?').

The illustrations accompanying these discussions are works of art in themselves (Figure 5.9).

Duchenne's views on aetiology and pathogenesis

Duchenne considered that this was essentially a disease of childhood with a predilection for boys. But though he was aware that familial cases had previously been reported by Meryon and later in Germany, none of his own cases apparently had a family history of the disease. With regard to the possibility of a neurogenic basis, he refers to a German case reported in 1866 which came to autopsy. The spinal cord was examined by Julius Cohnheim (1839–1884), a

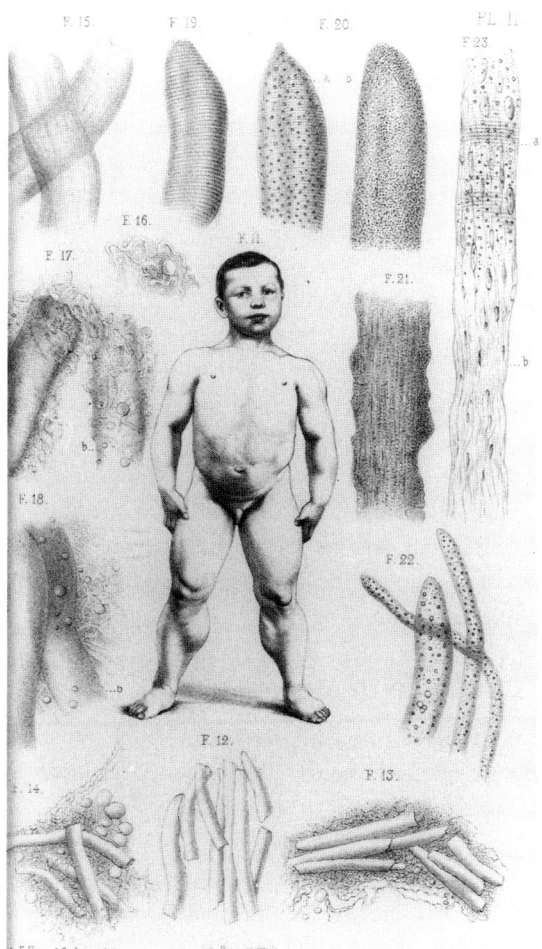

Fig. 5.9 An illustration from Duchenne's 1868 publication[17].

pathologist and pupil of Virchow and whose name is still remembered in myology for the apparent grouping of muscle fibrils within each muscle fibre, so-called Cohnheim's areas. No apparent abnormality was found in the cord. Nevertheless, Duchenne cautions that, despite the acknowledged eminence of the pathologist, there was a need to confirm this finding. It would not be until 1871 when, in collaboration with Charcot, Duchenne himself was able to examine microscopically a spinal cord from a patient and to confirm that it was normal.

It will be remembered that Meryon had considered the possibility of there being a neurogenic basis for the disease in 1852 and found the spinal cord to be normal in one of the cases he studied at the time. Later, in 1864, as we have seen, he went further and compared the microscopic findings in the cord of a patient with a normal healthy individual and found no difference. Duchenne makes no reference to these earlier studies of Meryon which, in the circumstances, proved particularly relevant with regard to the cause of the disorder.

In discussing the cause of the disease, Duchenne excludes any external cause but thinks that it may be related to a vasomotor disturbance affecting the capillary circulation of the muscle—a view held by some until comparatively recently (reviewed in Ref. 22).

He considered the proliferation of the fibrous connective tissue to be particularly relevant to pathogenesis. Interestingly, this idea was revived nearly a hundred years later[23]. Furthermore, though we now know the primary defect is a deficiency of dystrophin, a cytoskeletal protein, it has now been suggested that this could in some way lead to increased mast cell function (a major factor in fibrosis) and therefore be important in the pathogenesis of the disease[24]. Duchenne himself, however, was at a loss to explain how this increase in connective tissue could occur, and had to conclude, as we would have done ourselves until 1987, 'la pathogénie de la paralysie pseudo-hypertrophique est très obscure; elle doit être réservée.'

Duchenne's attitude to Meryon's work

Duchenne refers on several occasions to Meryon's publication of 1852[25], which he dismisses because he believed that the disease Meryon described was *progressive muscular atrophy*:

> Mais l'observateur distingué, M. Edw. Meryon, qui en a exposé la relation, les ayant évidemment confondus avec l'atrophie musculaire progressive, je dois me réserver d'en discuter le diagnostic différentiel, avant de les ranger ici parmi les cas de paralysie pseudo-hypertrophique précédents (Ref. 17, page 25).

Duchenne goes to great pains to emphasize the differences between *paralysie pseudo-hypertrophique* and two other conditions which cause weakness in childhood: *atrophie musculaire graisseuse progressive de l'enfance* (progressive muscular atrophy of childhood or spinal muscular atrophy) and *paralysie atrophique graisseuse de l'enfance* (atrophic paralysis of childhood or, as we now know it, acute poliomyelitis).

The distinguishing features were mainly clinical but Duchenne also laid emphasis on differences in muscle histology:

> la dégénérescence granuleuse ou graisseuse de leurs fibres musculaires et la substitution graisseuse de leur tissu interstitiel, il devient impossible de confondre avec elle la paralysie pseudo-hypertrophique dans laquelle la lésion anatomique des muscles est bien différente (Ref. 17, page 554).

But perhaps of greater significance is his use of the phrase *dégénérescence granuleuse ou graisseuse* (granular or fatty degeneration) in describing the histology in muscular atrophy because Meryon had referred to the muscle disorder he studied as '*granular and fatty degeneration of muscle*'[25]. Furthermore, Duchenne describes the muscle histological findings reported by Meryon as 'transformation granuleuse ou graisseuse' (Ref. 17, page 432). This confusion over terminology may possibly explain Duchenne's assessment and dismissal of Meryon's work. This could have subsequently influenced others and may therefore have been a factor in Meryon's work being largely ignored and Duchenne given precedence.

But could this have been the result of a genuine misunderstanding by Duchenne? Meryon's findings were in fact summarized in detail in a French journal at the time and this would have been available to Duchenne[26], but which adds to the confusion by concluding '*La dégénérescence graisseuse serait donc dans cette théorie une des formes de l'atrophie*'! Incidentally, Meryon's findings were also reported in a German journal[27].

Even in England this misconception was perpetuated. William Roberts (1830–1899) of Manchester, for example, who later became professor of medicine, a Fellow of the Royal Society and was knighted[28], wrote an influential book in 1858 on wasting palsy[29]. It is quite clear from the text that he too believed Meryon had described cases of progressive muscular atrophy, or *Cruveilhier's atrophy*, and in his analysis Roberts includes Meryon's cases with others who clearly had this disease.

But though it seems to the present authors that this was most likely to have been the result of genuine misunderstanding, there are suggestions in both Poore (Ref. 18, page xiv) and in Duchenne's obituaries[30,31] that Duchenne was not averse to disputes over priorities.

In his 1864 book[32], Meryon is clearly aware of Duchenne's interpretation and refutes it: he states quite clearly that the disorder described by Duchenne as *atrophie musculaire progressive* is not what he described (page 200), and later goes on:

> M. Duchenne has referred my first case to a category of diseases which he has denominated '*Paralysie atrophique graisseuse de l'enfance*', and which he defines as nervous in character, resulting from some antecedent febrile affection, and terminating either in rapid recovery or degeneration of the affected muscles into fat. I would beg to point out, however, that the cases which I have described have not presented a symptom of nervous disturbance, neither have they followed any febrile affection, nor have they resulted in the structural lesion which he has indicated. They have, in fact, nothing in common with the so-called '*Paralysie atrophique graisseuse de l'enfance*', except the failing of muscular power (Ref. 32, page 204).

It seems that at the time it was difficult for many to accept that muscle weakness could occur in the absence of a defect in the nerve supply to the muscle.

A few years later Gowers, in his major study of the disease[33], states quite clearly that Duchenne:

> at first denied that Meryon's cases were of the same nature as his own, but most other writers on the disease have recognized their identity, and it seems to me undoubted (Ref. 33, page 2).

An assessment of Duchenne's contribution

There is little doubt that the clinical picture presented by Duchenne, if somewhat repetitious and long-winded, is far more detailed than that given by Meryon. But in the 1860s others had also given very detailed descriptions of the disease and for a time it was, for example, referred to as Duchenne–Griesinger disease after Wilhelm Griesinger (1817–1868), professor of psychiatry and neurology at the University of Berlin[34], who described the disease in considerable detail in 1865[21]. However, Duchenne was not able to satisfy himself that the spinal cord was normal in the disease, he failed to note the breakdown of the sarcolemma, which we now know is important in pathogenesis, and did not emphasize the familial nature of the disease, all aspects of the disease which Meryon addressed and emphasized in the cases he studied. However, Meryon made few other original contributions to medical neurology, whereas Duchenne is remembered for a variety of significant contributions to the field. He introduced the use of electricity in diagnosis and treatment and the study of the effects of electrical stimulation of muscle in health and disease. More specifically, he was the first to describe the conditions of progressive muscular atrophy (Duchenne–Aran disease), progressive bulbar palsy (Duchenne's paralysis), the effects of partial brachial plexus palsy (Duchenne–Erb palsy), and, though he was certainly not the first to describe tabes dorsalis, he gave one of the earliest detailed accounts of the condition which was once therefore referred to as Duchenne's disease. Duchenne made major advances in the techniques of examining the nervous system, both at the bedside and in the laboratory. He was throughout his entire professional life a hard-working and dedicated investigator.

Meryon, on the other hand, was more in the mould of the English physician who, having made an inspired and thoughtful study of a disease, allowed his other professional and family interests thereafter to occupy his attention. In both their professional and private lives, the two men were very different yet both made profoundly important contributions to our understanding of the disease.

References

1. Keith, A. *Menders of the Maimed.* London: H. Frowde, 1919: 91.
2. Ramsey, M. *Professional and Popular Medicine in France 1770–1830; The Social World of Medical Practice.* Cambridge: Cambridge University Press, 1988.
3. Binet, L., Vallery-Radot, P. *La Faculté de Médecine de Paris—Cinq Siècles d'Art et d'Histoire.* Paris: Masson et Cie, 1952.
4. Coury, C. The teaching of medicine in France from the beginning of the seventeenth century. In: C. D. O'Malley (ed.) *The History of Medical Education.* Los Angeles: University of California Press, 1970: 121–72.
5. Guilly, P. *Duchenne de Boulogne.* Paris: Baillière et Fils, 1936.
6. Kaplan, E. B. Duchenne de Boulogne and the physiologie des mouvements. In: S. R. Kagan, (ed.) *Victor Robinson Memorial Volume Essays on History of Medicine in Honor of Victor Robinson.* New York: Froben Press, 1948: 177–92.
7. Jokl, E. Guillaume Benjamin Amand Duchenne de Boulogne et la physiologie des mouvements. *Episteme*, 1967; **1**: 273–83.
8. Cuthbertson, R. A. *Duchenne de Boulogne; his Life, his Times and the Significance of his Work with Special Reference to his Study of Mechanism of Human Facial Expression* (Thesis). University of Melbourne, Melbourne, Australia, 1977. (See also: Cuthbertson, R. A. *The Mechanism of Human Facial Expression.* New York: Cambridge University Press, 1990: 226–7.)
9. Ekbom, K. The man behind the syndrome: Jean-Martin Charcot. *Journal of the History of Neuroscience*, 1992; **1**: 39–45.
10. Hierons, R. Charcot and his visits to Britain. *British Medical Journal*, 1993; **307**: 1589–91.
11. Capildeo, R. Charcot in the 80's. In: F. C. Rose & W. F. Bynum (eds). *Historical Aspects of the Neurosciences.* New York: Raven Press, 1982: 383–96.
12. Duchenne (de Boulogne) fils. De la paralysie atrophique graisseuse de l'enfance. *Archives Générales de Médecine*, 1864; **2**(6th Ser., tome 4): 28–50; 184–209; 441–55.
13. Duchenne, G. B. A. *De L'Électrisation Localisée et de son Application à la Physiologie, à la Pathologie et à la Thérapeutique.* Paris: J.-B. Baillière et Fils, 1855.
14. Duchenne, G. B. A. *Mécanisme de la Physionomie Humaine.* Paris: Vve. J. Renouard, 1862. (Now edited and translated by R. A. Cuthbertson in *The Mechanism of Human Facial Expression.*New York: Cambridge University Press, 1990.)
15. Duchenne, G. B. A. Case 68: paraplégie cérébrale, congénitale, hypertrophique. In: *L'Électrisation Localisée et de son Application à la Pathologie et à la Thérapeutique*, 2nd edn. Paris: J.-B. Baillière et Fils, 1861: 354–6.
16. Duchenne, G. B. A. *Album de Photographies Pathologiques.* Paris: J.-B. Baillière et Fils, 1862.
17. Duchenne, G. B. A. Recherches sur la paralysie musculaire pseudo-hypertrophique ou paralysie myo-sclérosique. *Archives Générales de Médecine*, 1868; **11**: 5–25, 179–209, 305–21, 421–43, 552–88.
18. Poore, G. V. *Selections from the Clinical Works of Dr. Duchenne de Boulogne.* London: The New Sydenham Society, 1883: 186.
19. Oppenheimer, G. *Ueber progressive fettige Muskel-Atrophie.* Heidelberg: Habilitationschrift, 1855. Reviewed in: *Canstatt's Jahresbericht über die Fortschritte der Gesammten Medicin in allen Ländern*, 1855; **3**: 74–87.

20. Dubowitz, V. History of muscle disease. In: F. C. Rose and W. F. Bynum (eds). *Historical Aspects of the Neurosciences*. New York: Raven Press, 1982: 213–22.
21. Griesinger, W. Ueber Muskelhypertrophie. *Archiv der Heilkunde*, 1865; **6**: 1–13.
22. Emery, A. E. H. *Duchenne Muscular Dystrophy*, 1st edn. Oxford: Oxford University Press, 1987: 130–31.
23. Golarz, M. N., Bourne, G. H. The histochemistry of muscular dystrophy. In: G. H. Bourne and M. N. Golarz (eds). *Muscular Dystrophy in Man and Animals*. New York: Hafner Publishing Company, 1963: 90–157.
24. Gorospe, J. R. M., Tharp, M.D, Hinckley, J., Kornegay, J. N., Hoffman, E. P. A role for mast cells in the progression of Duchenne muscular dystrophy? Correlations in dystrophin deficient humans, dogs and mice. *Journal of the Neurological Sciences*, 1994; **122**: 44–56.
25. Meryon, E. Granular and fatty degeneration of the voluntary muscles. *Medico-Chirurgical Transactions*, 1852; **35**: 73–84.
26. Meryon, E. Dégénérescence graisseuse des muscles volontaires. *Gazette des Hôpitaux*, 1854; **6**: 506.
27. Meryon, E. Ueber die Fettdegeneration der thierischen Gewebe. *Schmidt's Jahrbücher der in- und ausländischen Gesammten Medicin*, 1854; **82**: 362–3.
28. Brockbank, W. *The Honorary Medical Staff of the Manchester Royal Infirmary 1830–1948*. Manchester: Manchester University Press, 1965: 43–6.
29. Roberts, W. *An Essay on Wasting Palsy (Cruveilhier's Atrophy)*. London: J. Churchill, 1858.
30. Obituary. Duchenne. *Medical Times & Gazette*, 1875; **2**: 398–9.
31. Obituary. Duchenne. *Lancet*, 1875; **ii**: 645.
32. Meryon, E. *Practical and Pathological Researches on the Various Forms of Paralysis*. London: J. Churchill & Sons, 1864.
33. Gowers, W. R. *Pseudo-hypertrophic Muscular Paralysis—a Clinical Lecture*. London: J. & A. Churchill, 1879.
34. Goldstein, J. Psychiatry. In: W. F. Bynum and R. Porter (eds). *Companion Encyclopedia of the History of Medicine*, Vol. 2. London: Routledge, 1993: 1350–72.

Chapter 6

Refining the clinical picture

Up to the mid-nineteenth century there had been very little interest among physicians in muscle disease per se, no doubt because most of their attention understandably focused on 'fevers' or, as we now know, infectious diseases (Chapter 3). But in the 1860s there had obviously been some interest because by 1868 Duchenne was able to review nine reports of *muscle paralysis* in the German literature. Then, 10 years later Gowers identified no less than 81 reports from both European and American journals. How can we account for this dramatic rise in interest?

Increasing interest in muscle disease

Duchenne's publications in the late 1860s and early 1870s no doubt played a very important role in increasing interest in muscle diseases. There was also a greater interest in medical nosology in general. After the 1880s the germ theory offered an explanation for many diseases and this recognition then resulted in others, which were not infectious, being given more attention. But the impact of the germ theory on nosology should not be overstated. Most of the diseases in which an infectious agent turned out to be the cause already had reasonably specific clinical and pathological identities, even if their aetiology had previously been unclear[1]. Nevertheless, clarification of the origins of such diseases threw into greater prominence others for which the causative agent was still a mystery. In the case of muscle disease an interest was no doubt also fuelled by improvements in techniques for the microscopical study of tissues (Chapter 3).

Whatever the cause for this increase in interest, the next few years were to witness several studies of large numbers of patients. In this way the phenotype became more and more refined and the *spectrum* of abnormalities which can occur in the disease became clearer. These studies also heralded the concept of clinical and genetic heterogeneity within this group of diseases and eventually led to attempts at classification. One investigator at this period who played a crucial role was the English physician William Richard Gowers.

William Richard Gowers (1845–1915)

By any standards Gowers was one of the most outstanding neurologists of his time. Much of what we know of his life and work is due to Macdonald Critchley's detailed and excellent biography of the man, to which source the present authors are greatly indebted[2]. Apart from his study of muscular dystrophy he made a number of major contributions to other branches of neurology. Like many before him in this history, his origins were humble. His father was a boot- and shoe-maker or cobbler and William was born in his father's little shop in Hackney, East London on 20 March 1845. When he was 11 years old his father died, and he and his mother went to live in Headington near Oxford to be with her family. Here he gained a place at Christ Church College School which provided him with an excellent education. In 1860, at the age of 15, he left school and the following year became apprenticed to a local practitioner, Dr Thomas Simpson of Coggeshall in Essex. In this way his lifelong interest in medicine began. It was also at this time that he became acquainted with a family in the village with four boys afflicted with a strange disorder of locomotion, with wasting of some muscles and enlargement of others. This encounter was later to stimulate his interest in muscular dystrophy.

Even at this period of his life he spent much of his leisure time studying and improving his knowledge of languages, mathematics, and chemistry. His only recreational activities appear to have been chess and botany. Then in 1863 he moved with his mother to London and entered University College Hospital as a medical student where Meryon, some 35 years previously, had also been a student. At the time, there was a certain bias toward neurology at University College and this no doubt influenced Gowers.

After qualifying in 1867 and taking the Membership of the Royal College of Surgeons (MRCS), he worked as an assistant to one of the most distinguished doctors of the time, Sir William Jenner, court physician and President of the Royal College of Physicians. This appointment was no doubt due to Gowers' obvious ability and was to be a great help in furthering his future career. Two years later, in 1869, he passed the MB degree of London with first class honours, having already secured gold medals in botany, physiology, anatomy, and materia medica, and silver medals in pathological anatomy and practical physiology and histology. To add to this he was awarded a gold medal for his MD degree the following year. With such qualifications and with such support his future seemed assured right from the beginning.

In 1870, at age 25, he was appointed medical registrar at the National Hospital for the Paralysed and Epileptic in Queen Square (eventually in 1948 to assume its present title: National Hospital for Nervous Diseases), which had opened 10 years previously with two physicians, J. S. Ramskill and C. E. Brown-Séquard[3]. Two years afterward he became honorary assistant physician. Later he was also to be appointed professor of medicine and physician to University College Hospital, though at the age of 43 he resigned from these positions to devote more of his time to writing and to his work at the National Hospital. At the age of 30 Gowers married a Miss Baines and set up house at 50 Queen Anne Street where he remained and practised until his retirement.

During his lifetime he received a number of honours for his work, including being elected a Fellow of the Royal Society at the age of 42 and knighted 10 years later on the occasion of Queen Victoria's Diamond Jubilee. Honorary Fellowships were also bestowed on him by a number of prestigious foreign associations and societies. In 1893, the Royal Medical and Chirurgical Society awarded him the Marshall Ball Prize for the best original work in English on the anatomy, physiology, or pathology of the nervous system (Figure 6.1).

Although a great deal has been written about Gowers' contributions to medicine and to neurology in particular, not a great deal has been published about his personal life. His clinical work and writing took up most of his time. However, he was an enthusiast for shorthand, which he taught himself and encouraged his staff to do the same. He made shorthand notes on all his cases and in 1894 founded and became the first president of the Society of Medical Phonographers. He also had a very keen interest in botany and became an authority on mosses, though he never became a Fellow of the Linnean Society,

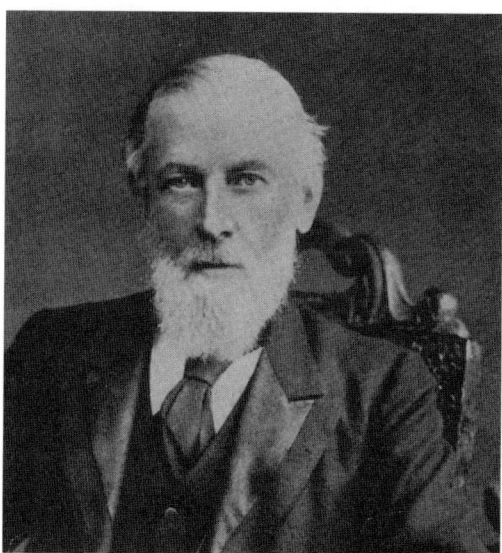

Fig. 6.1 Sir William Gowers (1845–1915). (Reproduced by kind permission of Dr. Macdonald Critchley.)

the Society of natural history and taxonomy. He was also an accomplished etcher and engraver and actually exhibited at the Royal Academy during one year. Although music apparently had little appeal to him personally, he made certain that his children became accomplished instrumentalists. He concerned himself with the acoustics of music, initiating correspondence on the subject of an improved scientific designation of musical notes in the *Musical News*. Thus his interests and hobbies were those that would appeal to someone with an interest in detail and of an obsessive, perhaps somewhat introspective, personality.

From his mid-twenties and for around 10 years he suffered recurrent attacks of abdominal pain. This he attributed to 'perityphlitis' (appendicitis) which seems eventually to have settled down with conservative treatment. Perhaps this had a functional origin. According to Macdonald Critchley:

> Gowers was not a man with a wide circle of professional friends and correspondents. He was reserved and apparently difficult to know. Warmness and conviviality were foreign to him and he remained among his colleagues a lonely and unapproachable figure, admired but not understood.

Although a member of the Savile Club and the Athenaeum he played little part in their activities and preferred his own company to that of others. Yet beneath this rather forbidding exterior, his colleagues found him genial and loyal, and to his junior staff he was very supportive and encouraging. Interestingly, his few close friends were drawn mainly from outside the medical profession and included the eminent geologist Thomas Bonney, the composer Walford Davies, and the writer Rudyard Kipling.

He was never very robust and the last few years of his life were dogged by ill-health. In 1894 he suffered a 'breakdown' and to recover went on a cruise to South Africa. But he never completely recovered and at 62 he was forced to retire from practice. In 1914 both he and his wife developed pneumonia, to which Lady Gowers succumbed. He rallied, but his condition gradually deteriorated and he died on 4 May 1915. Although he contributed so much to neurology, he never had a fashionable and lucrative practice; he was never wealthy and left little when he died.

Gowers' contribution to medicine and neurology

Gowers was essentially a careful clinical observer and an excellent teacher. His diagnostic accuracy was legendary and his aphorisms were widely quoted. For example:

> decisive hesitation is far wiser than hesitating decision.
> Cultivate the habit of viewing a chronic case fresh from time to time.

> Certain symptoms are very frequent in a given disease... but their absence does not prove that the disease does not exist.

He also introduced several new terms into medicine which are now widely used, including *abiotrophy*, *knee jerk*, and *fibrositis*. The term *abiotrophy* referred to decay or degeneration and he considered the dystrophies as representing muscular abiotrophies.

He was the *first* to describe 'musicogenic' epilepsy and the 'nasal smile' in myasthenia gravis, as well as the syndromes widely associated with the names of Foster Kennedy and Kinnier Wilson. Yet, though Gowers' name is associated with the peculiar manner of rising from a seated position in those with pelvic girdle weakness, as we have seen, this had actually been described previously by Bell and Duchenne. Eponymous associations sometimes seem to be a lucky chance, and, rather ironically, Gowers eschewed the use of eponyms himself.

He had an inventive mind and the devices he constructed or invented included a haemoglobinometer, a haemocytometer, a 'safety' hypodermic syringe, a portable reading lamp to take on long railway journeys, a telephone switchboard in his home, and an improved Duchenne dynamometer.

He made special studies of ophthalmoscopy and epilepsy, and wrote a *Manual of Diseases of the Nervous System*[4] which became a standard work for many years. He wrote over 330 articles and books during his lifetime, almost all as the single author. These are listed in Critchley's biography[2]. But here we are particularly concerned with his contributions to muscular dystrophy.

Pseudohypertrophic muscular paralysis

In his lifetime Gowers published several articles as well as a book on muscular dystrophy. His first article on the subject appeared as early as 1874 and was based on a lecture presented at the Royal Medical and Chirurgical Society[5]. It was co-authored with J. Lockhart Clarke (1817–1880) who by this time was well known for his researches on the spinal cord and for having introduced the method of mounting microscopic sections in Canada balsam. He was born in London, the son of a woollen draper who died when Clarke was 7 years of age. For reasons which are not entirely clear his mother then took her seven children to France for their education. It was probably familiarity with the language and culture that helped him a great deal when later in his professional life he met and collaborated with Duchenne. His life and work have been detailed elsewhere[6].

Clarke became a close and long-standing friend of Meryon. When he visited Paris in 1867 he was asked to see one of Duchenne's cases (details of which

Duchenne published the following year—case no. 12 at the Hôpital Sainte-Eugénie[7]), and on his return to London he discussed Duchenne's findings at a meeting of the Pathological Society[8]. However, like many others at the time, he misinterpreted the nature of the disease described by Meryon. Could this be in part due to Duchenne's influence? Later, in 1871 he was sent muscle specimens by Duchenne for his opinion. Thus it seems more than likely that, through his association with Meryon and his familiarity with Duchenne's work, it was Lockhart Clarke who encouraged Gowers' interest in the subject of muscle disease.

Gowers' paper with Clarke[5] is essentially a lengthy and detailed account of an affected boy who died at the age of 14. Interestingly, the Achilles tendons were divided at age 9 in the belief that this would keep him walking. In fact, the operation was used for this purpose until comparatively recently but is now no longer recommended. When the case came to autopsy, muscle histology revealed some variation in fibre size, loss of cross-striations, and a predominance of fat and connective tissue, findings which confirmed earlier studies. The spinal cord was fixed and studied by Lockhart Clarke. But though there is much detail of various apparent abnormalities (probably the result of spinal deformity and post-mortem artefactual changes), there is no clear statement on the possibility of the anterior horn cells being affected. This information had to wait until it was addressed in Gowers' monograph published 5 years later.

In 1879 Gowers gave a series of lectures at the National Hospital for the Paralysed and Epileptic on 'pseudo-hypertrophic muscular paralysis' (a literal translation of Duchenne's term for the disorder). These lectures subsequently appeared in *Lancet* in July of the same year[9], and were later published in his now famous monograph on the subject[10]. This was based on data from 220 cases which included 24 he had seen himself (including the four brothers from Coggeshall he first saw as an apprentice), 20 seen by colleagues, and 176 from 81 published reports in the literature. In this comprehensive and detailed study, Gowers attempted to give as complete a picture of the disease as possible, including the clinical features, pathology, prognosis, and possible treatment. As with all of Gowers' writings, clarity, thoughtfulness, and good prose are evident, qualities which he himself always prized in others. For example, the graphic description on the first page (which has since been reproduced many times by writers on the subject) reads:

> The disease is one of the most interesting, and at the same time most sad, of all those with which we have to deal: interesting on account of its peculiar features and mysterious nature; sad on account of our powerlessness to influence its course, except in a very slight degree, and on account of the conditions in which it occurs. It is a disease of early life and of early growth. Manifesting itself commonly at the transition from infancy to childhood, it develops with the child's development, grows with his

growth—so that every increase in stature means an increase in weakness, and each year takes him a step further on the road to a helpless infirmity, and in most cases to an early and inevitable death (Ref. 10, page 1).

It is useful to summarize his conclusions regarding the clinical presentation because they have hardly been improved upon since.

- Onset is usually before age 6, standing is lost around age 10–12, and death usually occurs between 14 and 18
- Muscle enlargement (pseudohypertrophy) most often affects the calf muscles but may involve other muscles as well (e.g. the vasti, glutei, sacrospinalis, deltoids, buccinators, etc.). The tongue may also be enlarged
- Muscle wasting (at least at the beginning) is *selective* (e.g. the sternocostal part more than the clavicular part of the pectoralis major) and the proximal muscles are affected more than the distal muscles (the small muscles of the hands are scarcely ever affected)
- Weakness of the knee and hip extensors results in what is nowadays referred to as Gowers' manoeuvre or Gowers' sign (Figure 6.2), which he describes in this way:

> In getting up they first put the hands on the ground (1), then stretch out the legs behind them far apart, and, the chief weight of the trunk resting on the hands, by keeping the toes on the ground and pushing the body backwards, they manage to get the knees extended, so that the trunk is supported by the hands and feet, all placed as widely apart as possible (2). Next the hands are moved alternately along the ground backwards, so as to bring a larger portion of the weight of the trunk over the legs. Then one hand is placed upon the knee (3), and a push with this and with the other hand on the ground is sufficient to enable the extensors of the hip to bring the trunk into the upright posture (Ref. 10, page 36).

Gowers at first thought the action of putting the hands on the knees, then grasping the thighs higher and higher ('climbing up his thigh') so as to extend the hips and push up the trunk was pathognomonic of the disease. He later realized, however, that this could be seen in other diseases where the same muscle groups were affected.

- A waddling gait occurs and results from weakness of the gluteus medius. This weakness causes the pelvis to tilt down toward the unsupported side when the child raises a leg from the ground, to compensate for which the body is inclined toward the supporting leg, an action which, when repeated, results in a broad-based waddling gait
- Lordosis occurs as a result of weakness of the hip extensors, which causes the pelvis to tilt forward with the development of a compensatory lumbar lordosis

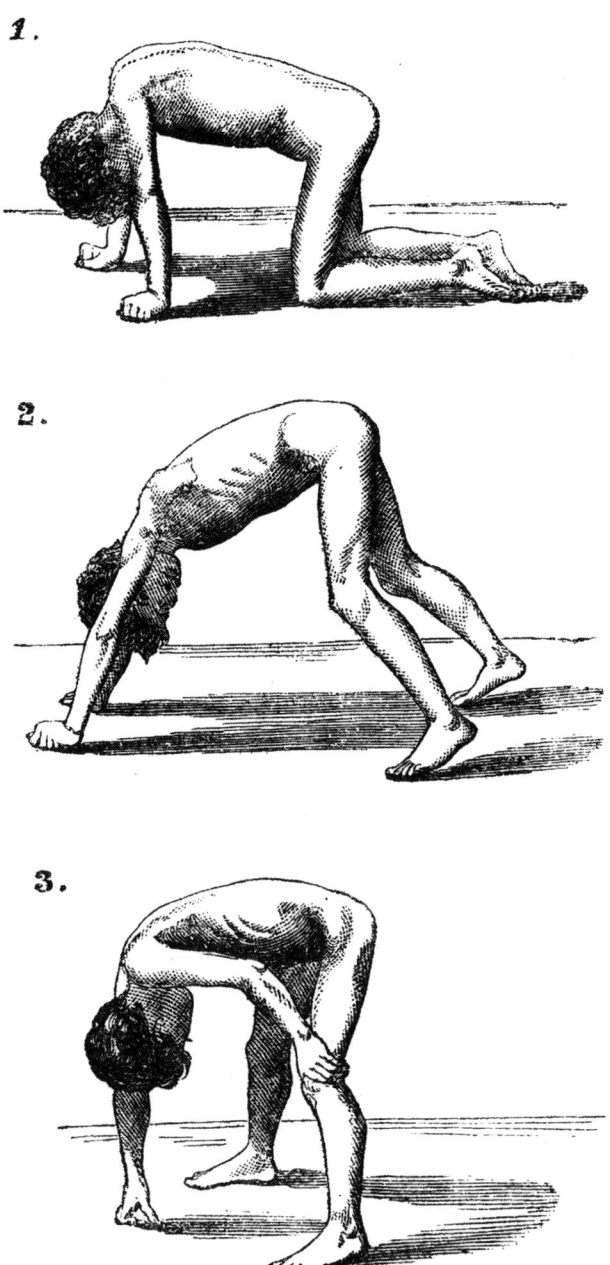

Fig. 6.2 Gowers' manoeuvre or sign. (From W. R. Gowers' *Pseudo-hypertrophic Muscular Paralysis*, 1879.)

- Contractures and deformities develop later in the course of the disease as a result of muscle imbalance and habitual posture (e.g. talipes and contractures of the knees, hips, and elbows, and lateral curvature of the spine or scoliosis)
- The heart may also become affected ('in the same way as the voluntary muscles, but recorded evidence scarcely at present establishes the fact.') (Ref. 10, page 29)

Gowers, however, failed to recognize that mental handicap can be part of the clinical picture (Ref. 10, page 38). We now know that this can occur, to varying degrees, in a significant proportion of boys with the disease.

Gowers appreciated that most cases die from an intercurrent respiratory infection as a result of 'weakness and wasting of the thoracic muscles, for instance, [which] gradually lessen the respiratory power'. For cases that would now be clearly categorized as Duchenne muscular dystrophy and if two cases who died accidentally in early childhood are excluded, then the age at death in Gowers' series is little different from our own up to 1983 (Table 6.1). It would seem that if there had been any improvement in survival this had been slight, though a large survey in Japan in 1987 suggested that hospitalized patients survived longer[12], and this is now borne out in recent years where assisted respiration is offered.

Gowers' views on muscle histology were not novel, but with Lockhart Clarke he did examine the spinal cord in a case that came to autopsy, which they had described previously[5], but now stressed that the anterior horn cells were in fact normal, in contrast to the situation in progressive muscular atrophy. His most interesting observations, however, focus on the predilection for the male sex and its familial nature.

Of the total of 220 cases he reviewed, 190 (86%) were males and, interestingly, he notes that in many cases in girls the onset was somewhat later and the progression slower. We shall return to this point later (Chapter 9).

Table 6.1 Age at death and year at death recorded in 73 affected boys in our own series over the 50-year period 1934–1983 (Ref. 11, page 40) compared with data from Gowers[10]

	1934–1963	1964–1973	1974–1983	Gowers
Number	13	32	28	25
Mean	16.27	16.63	16.83	15.36
s.d.	4.09	2.6	2.53	2.46

Furthermore, of the 220 cases, 102 were apparently isolated, while in the remainder other family members were believed to be affected. This relatively high proportion of familial cases was no doubt the result of bias in the selection of cases. However, his observations on the familial cases are particularly important:

> the disease is almost never to be heard of on the side of the father; when antecedent cases have occurred, they have almost invariably been on the side of the mother (Ref. 10, page 23).

and later, in some families:

> a woman's children by different husbands were affected… [and in one family] a son of a woman by one husband and two sons by another, were all affected, and the mother's brother was also the subject of the disease (Ref. 10, page 24).

Parental consanguinity, he stresses, was not important, the only significant factor being inheritance *through the mother*. Gowers concluded that this predilection for males and maternal inheritance was in fact the same as in haemophilia.

> The character of limitation to males and unilateral inheritance from the ovum only, the mother not being affected, but the mother's brothers suffering, is seen also in some cases of haemophilia, and perhaps in no other diseases (Ref. 10, page 49).

He could not pursue the matter of inheritance further at this time because the cytological basis of X-linkage would not be known for at least another 30 years[13].

However, by 1908 it is obvious that over the intervening period Gowers had given much thought to the hereditary basis of a number of neurological diseases. At a meeting of the Royal Society of Medicine in that year[14], he attempted to classify such disorders and categorized pseudohypertrophic muscular paralysis as a *heredity abiotrophy*. Most interestingly, he reported the details of the follow up of a family in which the disease had been transmitted through two maternal lineages over several generations (the affected boys in one branch of this family had been reported previously by Meryon {Family P}). William Bateson also attended this meeting and would no doubt have been very interested in Gowers' observation, particularly since Bateson was especially concerned with explaining hereditary disease in terms of the newly re-discovered Mendelian principles of heredity. The following year saw the publication of Bateson's book on the subject in which he discusses sex-limited descent, using the examples of haemophilia, colour blindness, and pseudohypertrophic muscular paralysis (Ref. 15, pages 222–5). He comments, somewhat prophetically in the light of future developments:

> In Gowers' disease we have perhaps also to deal with more than one condition, and the evidence suggests that the recessiveness in females is not universal (Ref. 15, page 225).

Treatment

With regard to treatment, Gowers wrote:

> The treatment of the disease has to be directed rather against the effects of the morbid process than against the morbid process itself, which, whatever be its nature, is certainly to a large extent beyond our influence (Ref. 10, page 52).

This has remained essentially true ever since. His discussion of various remedies in use at the time adds little. But he does emphasize the need for passive exercises to prevent contractures, the possible use of 'mechanical appliances' to help prolong ambulation, and spinal jackets in the hope of impeding the development of spinal deformity. All these measures have since become accepted practice and his reference to what we now know as physiotherapy seems to have been the first time that this was clearly recommended in the care of patients with muscular dystrophy.

Clinical heterogeneity

A close study of the details of some of the cases published up to and including Gowers indicates that some may have been affected by forms of muscular dystrophy somewhat similar to, but now known to be different from, Duchenne disease. For example, the onset of the disease was somewhat later and the subsequent progression slower in some cases, suggesting that they had what we would now refer to as *Becker muscular dystrophy* (for example, family T in Meryon[16]; and cases 23, 35, and 36 in Gowers[10]).

It is also now recognized that occasionally female *carriers* may actually show some signs of the disease, ranging from significantly enlarged calves to marked muscle weakness, so-called *manifesting carriers*. Significantly enlarged calves in females were noted in Meryon's family 87[17] and marked muscle weakness in Gowers' cases 7 and 8[10]. These appear to be the first reports of manifesting carriers in Duchenne muscular dystrophy.

Also, affected brothers and sisters have been recorded (for example, cases 89 and 90 in Meryon[17], and the family reported separately[18]; and cases 14 and 15, whose parents were also cousins, and cases 25 and 26 in Gowers[10]), which suggests that these may have been families with the condition which came to be referred to as *severe childhood autosomal recessive muscular dystrophy*.

Thus, with hindsight it is clear that not all individuals considered up to this time to have pseudohypertrophic muscular paralysis had an identical disease. Gowers himself felt classification had serious pitfalls: 'Nature is prone to ignore our divisions and to blend that which we distinguish.'

First attempts to resolve such clinical heterogeneity and to differentiate Duchenne's pseudohypertrophic muscular paralysis from other types of muscle disease therefore had to await the work of others.

References

1. Bynum, W. F. Nosology. In: W. F. Bynum and R. Porter (eds). *Companion Encyclopedia of the History of Medicine.* Vol. 1. London & New York: Routledge, 1993: 335–56.
2. Critchley, M. *Sir William Gowers (1845–1915)—A Biographical Appreciation.* London: William Heinemann, 1949.
3. Aminoff, M. J. *Brown-Séquard, a Visionary of Science.* New York: Raven Press, 1993: 41,102.
4. Gowers, W. R. *A Manual of Diseases of the Nervous System.* 2 vols. London: J. & A. Churchill, 1886–88.
5. Clarke, J. L., Gowers, W. R. On a case of pseudo-hypertrophic muscular paralysis. *Medico-Chirurgical Transactions,* 1874; **57**: 247–60. (NS, **39**: 247–60).
6. Emery, A. E. H., Emery, M. L. H. Lockhart Clarke (1817–1880): his role in the early history of muscular dystrophy. *Neuromuscular Disorders,* 2000; **10**: 530–3.
7. Duchenne, G. B. A. Recherches sur la paralysie musculaire pseudohypertrophique ou paralysie myo-sclérosique. *Archives Générales de Médecine,* 1868; **11**: 25.
8. Clarke, J. L. Paralysis with muscular degeneration (paralysie myosclérosique), or paralysis with apparent hypertrophy (translated from the French manuscript of Dr Duchenne by Mr Lockhart Clarke, and communicated by him, in the name of the author, with remarks). *Transactions of the Pathological Society of London,* 1868; **19**: 6–15.
9. Gowers, W. R. Clinical lectures on pseudo-hypertrophic muscular paralysis. *Lancet,* 1879a; **ii**: 1–2, 37–49, 73–5, 113–16.
10. Gowers, W. R. *Pseudo-hypertrophic Muscular Paralysis—A Clinical Lecture.* London: J. & A. Churchill, 1879b.
11. Emery, A. E. H. *Duchenne Muscular Dystrophy,* 2nd edn. Oxford: Oxford University Press, 1993.
12. Mukoyama, M., Kondo, K., Hizawa, K., Nishitani, H. and the DMDR Group. Life spans of Duchenne muscular dystrophy patients in the hospital care program in Japan. *Journal of the Neurological Sciences,* 1987; **81**: 155–8.
13. McKusick, V. A. *On the X Chromosome of Man.* Washington, DC: American Institute of Biological Sciences, 1964.
14. Gowers, W. R. Heredity in diseases of the nervous system. *British Medical Journal,* 1908, **ii**: 1541–3. (See also: *British Medical Journal,* 1908; **ii**: 1467–9.)
15. Bateson, W. *Mendel's Principles of Heredity.* Cambridge: Cambridge University Press, 1909.
16. Meryon, E. On granular and fatty degeneration of the voluntary muscles. *Medico-Chirurgical Transactions,* 1852; **35**: 73–84.
17. Meryon, E. *Practical and Pathological Researches on the Various Forms of Paralysis.* London: J. Churchill, 1864.
18. Meryon, E. Case of granular degeneration of the voluntary muscles. *British Medical Journal,* 1870; **ii**: 32–3.

Chapter 7

Resolution of heterogeneity

As more and more cases of 'muscular paralysis' were studied so it became increasingly clear that there was considerable variation in the clinical picture. The question therefore arose as to whether this represented variability within a single disease entity, or represented several different diseases which mimicked that described by Meryon, Duchenne, and Gowers? In other words, was this variability merely a reflection of a spectrum of clinical manifestations within a single disease? This was a question which investigators would have to face in future in regard to many other genetic diseases. But it seems that muscular dystrophy was probably the first major group of diseases where this was recognized to be a problem and where attempts were made to resolve it.

Early studies of the problem—Leyden and Möbius

First attempts to resolve the problem of heterogeneity can be attributed to Leyden and Möbius. In 1876, Ernst von Leyden, professor of medicine at various times in Berlin, Königsberg, and Strasbourg argued that a familial form of atrophic pelvic girdle muscle disease was similar to but probably different from Duchenne's pseudohypertrophic muscular paralysis (Ref. 1, page 540). In his words, the 'hereditäre Form der progressiven Muskelatrophie' was different from 'lipomatöse Muskelhypertrophie':

> Dennoch bin ich geneigt, sie als zwei verschiedene Formen anzusprechen, sofern die letztere Krankheit durch ihre ganz typische Verbreitung und eigenthümliche Lipomatomatose einen besonderen Typus erhält (Ref. 1, page 540).

Three years later Paul Möbius, a private neurologist in Leipzig, reviewed no less than 94 reports of what he referred to as 'Pseudohypertrophia musculorum' and more or less agreed with Leyden's conclusions[2]. For some years afterwards this was referred to as the *atrophic, pelvic girdle* or *pelvifemoral type of Leyden–Möbius*. Later it was realized that cases of Leyden–Möbius disease with early onset were no different from Duchenne's disease except for the apparent absence of pseudohypertrophy. This is, however, a variable feature in Duchenne's disease in any event. However, cases of Leyden–Möbius disease with *later* onset probably did represent a different disease entity.

Although this delineation therefore proved to be somewhat artificial, it no doubt stimulated others to consider the possibility of heterogeneity. For first attempting a rational classification of these diseases, credit must be given to the German neurologist Erb, a man who in some ways was not unlike Gowers.

Wilhelm Heinrich Erb (1840–1921)

Erb was born the son of a forester on 30 November 1840 in the village of Winnweiler in the Palatinate, a region of south-west Germany[3]. He began studying medicine at the early age of 17 in Heidelberg and later in Erlangen and Munich where he graduated in 1864. He then returned to Heidelberg to work with Nikolaus Friedreich (1825–1882). The latter was already an established authority on neurological disorders and his work was extensively quoted by Leyden and Möbius. He is credited, for example, with having first described *a* particular form of hereditary ataxia now referred to as Friedreich's ataxia.

At age 25 Erb became a Privatdozent, a term reserved for a university lecturer who at the time was often not salaried. According to Max Nonne, who later became one of his students, he was meticulously punctual, and took considerable care in planning his ward rounds and, like Gowers, liked to examine each newly admitted patient himself[4].

It was through Friedreich's influence that Erb became interested in neurological disorders and their pathology, and his subsequent accomplishments, again like Gowers, were largely based on careful and detailed clinical studies. After a period of 3 years in Leipzig, he returned in 1883 to Heidelberg to succeed Friedreich as Ordinarius (professor) and it was here that his important studies of muscular disorders culminated in two major articles published in 1884, and 1891[5,6]. The second and more detailed was published in the first issue of the *Deutsche Zeitschrift für Nervenheilkunde* (*German Journal of Neurological Science*), of which he was one of the four founders (Figure 7.1).

Apart from his observations on 'dystrophia muscularis progressiva', he also studied Thomsen's disease, or autosomal dominant myotonia congenita, giving a graphic and detailed description of the disorder[7].

During his lifetime he became a much respected neurologist and worked to establish the subject as a special field in its own right and separate from psychiatry. But it would be some years before this division was generally accepted.

What of the man? Like Gowers he was a cultured gentleman and was always impeccably dressed. He was highly intelligent, rather formidable, and somewhat detached though he had many friends, including Alois Alzheimer, the psychiatrist. However, he could quickly lose his temper and was apparently given to strong language when irritated. Here he was very different from Gowers!

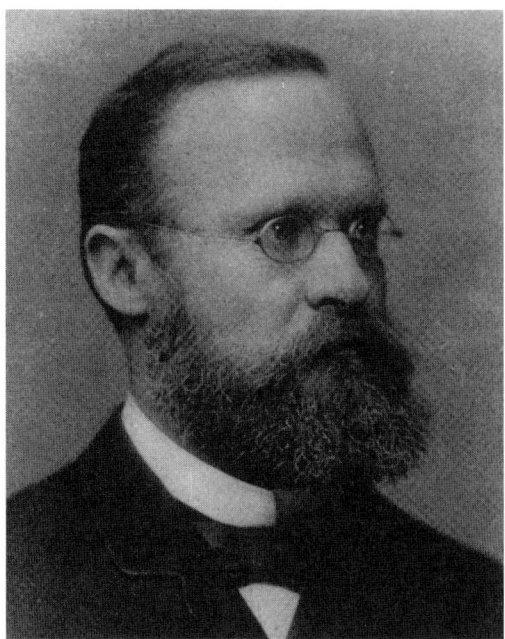

Fig. 7.1 Wilhelm Heinrich Erb (1840–1921). (Reproduced with permission from *The Founders of Neurology*, ed. by Webb Haymaker, 1953. Courtesy of Charles C. Thomas, publishers, Springfield, Illinois.)

He was a man of many ideals. Above all else he loved learning, and he was a fanatical seeker of the truth: the breach was irreparable between Erb and anyone with whom he worked if he discovered they were involved in the slightest 'corriger la vérité' (remarks by Dr H. M. Mayer in the 1990 *Festschrift*, Wilhelm-Erb-Gymnasium, Winnweiler, Germany, page 14).

He was extremely conscientious and hard-working, and produced 273 publications during his lifetime, only slightly fewer than Gowers. He was, like many neurologists of the time and later, a great bedside teacher and valued the systematic examination of the nervous system for significant signs and symptoms.

He was held in great esteem during his lifetime both in Germany and abroad. In later years he was much saddened by the deaths of two of his four sons and a third who was killed on the first day of the First World War. He died of a heart attack in October 1921, aged 81, it is said while listening to Beethoven's *Eroica*.

Erb's contributions to neurology

During his lifetime he became an enthusiastic exponent of electrodiagnosis and in fact has been considered the founder of the discipline[8].

He was the first to demonstrate increased electrical irritability of motor nerves in tetany (so-called Erb's phenomenon). He was also the first to use electrical stimulation of the brachial plexus to localize nerve root lesions. With Duchenne he described the clinical effects of such a lesion (Duchenne–Erb palsy), which Duchenne correctly attributed to birth trauma when the infant's head is pulled laterally to deliver the shoulder.

He was also among the first neurologists to use a reflex or tendon hammer and, with Westphal, discovered the diagnostic importance of the tendon knee reflex which, a few years later, Gowers referred to as the 'knee jerk' (Chapter 6). The somewhat unusual way in which Erb and Westphal reported their findings is recounted in Spillane's *Doctrine of the Nerves* (Ref. 9, page 328). Apparently, Erb submitted a paper on the subject for publication in the German *Archives of Psychiatry and Nervous Diseases* in 1875, only to learn that the editor himself, Carl Westphal, was preparing a similar paper. They therefore agreed to publish simultaneously. Erb was the first to use the term 'acute anterior poliomyelitis' which we have seen (Chapter 5) that Duchenne referred to as 'paralysie atrophique graisseuse de l'enfance'. Duchenne's use of the term 'atrophique' in this way had led to semantic confusion.

With Goldflam he also gave a detailed account of myasthenia gravis, which for some time was referred to as Erb–Goldflam disease, though actually the condition had first been described by Thomas Willis in 1672[10]. Finally, he gave accurate descriptions, along with Charcot, of chronic spastic spinal paralysis, which can be hereditary or due to environmental causes such as tabes. Like Gowers he also wrote an esteemed textbook on nervous diseases[11]. According to Viets[3], Erb was the father of neurology in Germany and was to his country what Charcot was to France and Gowers to England.

Dystrophia muscularis progressiva

Toward the end of the nineteenth century neurologists were beginning to recognize a variety of disorders in which muscle wasting and weakness were cardinal features. These included poliomyelitis, polyneuritis, syringomyelia, and syphilitic amyotrophy[12].

Erb[5,6] set out to differentiate those cases with a pathological lesion within the central (or peripheral) nervous system from those which appeared to be the result of a primary disease of muscle. He critically analysed previously published reports and presented details of his own cases. These studies were noteworthy for the very detailed and meticulous way in which Erb described the involvement of different muscle groups in different cases. It was this attention to detail which led him to conclude that 'spinalen Form der progressiven

Muskelatrophie' represented a separate group of conditions in which the pathological lesion resided in the central nervous system. This was not so in the remaining cases, which resulted from degeneration of the muscle itself. This notion was not entirely new because Meryon, for example, had also made the point some 30 years previously (Chapter 3). However, Erb marshalled a great deal more convincing clinical and pathological data to support the idea. He also saw that the use of the term 'atrophie' in the names of both groups of disorders had added to the confusion. He therefore proposed that the primary muscle disorders be referred to as 'Dystrophia muscularis progressiva' (progressive muscular dystrophy), a term which in one form or another has been used ever since. Erb also concluded that dividing cases according to whether there was or was not a family history was artificial and misleading.

He also described a 'juvenile' scapulohumeral form of progressive muscular dystrophy which he considered to be a separate condition, with onset usually early in life, affecting both sexes, and in which the shoulder girdle and the upper limb musculature was primarily involved, *but not the face*. Erb recognized that cases in which the facial muscles were involved probably represented yet another disorder, the first clear and detailed description of which is attributed to Landouzy and Dejerine.

Facioscapulohumeral muscular dystrophy of Landouzy and Dejerine

A number of early reports of 'muscular paralysis' failed to mention whether or not the facial muscles were involved. Duchenne recorded facial weakness in many of the cases he referred to as 'l'atrophie musculaire graisseuse progressive de l'enfance' which would no doubt now be designated facioscapulohumeral muscular dystrophy[13]. Such a case is most graphically illustrated in Figure 16 in Duchenne's *Album de Photographies Pathologiques*[14] (Figure 7.2).

The first detailed description of muscular dystrophy with facial weakness was, however, provided by Landouzy and Dejerine, and their names were eponymously associated with the condition until relatively recently.

Louis Théophile Joseph Landouzy (1845–1917) was born in Reims where his father was a professor in the school of medicine. He obtained his medical degree in Paris and, under the tutelage of Charcot, became interested in neurological disorders, an interest he retained throughout his life. But outside this speciality he is perhaps better remembered for his work on tuberculosis and his interest in physiotherapy[15]. In 1901 he became professor and was elected dean of the medical faculty, a position he held for the rest of his life.

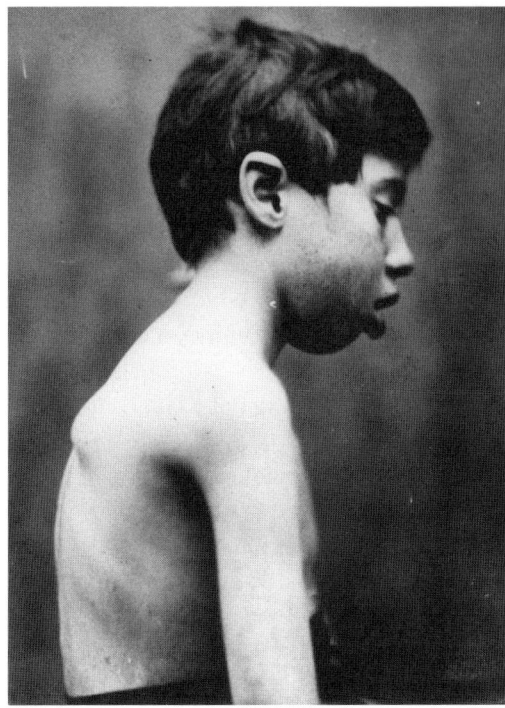

Fig. 7.2 One of Duchenne's cases illustrated in Figure 16 of his *Album de Photographies Pathologiques*[14]. Note the facial weakness and winging of the scapula.

Like many of his predecessors in neurology he was a fine teacher but his interests extended far beyond medicine. He was an accepted authority on art, a noted bibliophile, and confirmed traveller (Figure 7.3).

Joseph Jules Dejerine (1849–1917), whose name, contrary to popular belief, does not have acute accents, was born in Geneva of French parents and later moved to Paris to study medicine.

Apparently he was an able scholar but preferred the pleasures of boxing, swimming, and sailing to studying. After qualification he worked at the Salpêtrière and the Bicêtre and in 1910 became professor of clinical neurology in the Faculty of Medicine. He made many important contributions to neurology, a number of them in collaboration with his wife, Augusta Dejerine-Klumpke (1859–1927), who had previously been one of his students. She belonged to a famous San Francisco family and had studied medicine in Paris[16]. Despite a great deal of opposition, in 1887 she became the first woman to receive the title of *interne des hôpitaux*. In the following year they married, with Professor Landouzy being one of the witnesses. Her name is perhaps nowadays

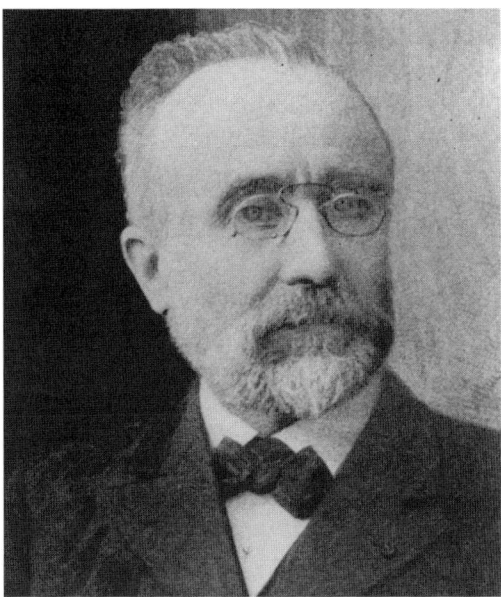

Fig. 7.3 Louis Théophile Joseph Landouzy (1845–1917). (Reproduced with permission from *The Founders of Neurology*, edited by Webb Haymaker, 1953. Courtesy of Charles C. Thomas, publishers, Springfield, Illinois.)

best known for a particular paralysis of the small muscles of the hand (Klumpke's paralysis).

With Jules Sottas, Dejerine described 'hypertrophic polyneuropathy' (Dejerine–Sottas disease). He also published works on olivopontocerebellar atrophy and the thalamic syndrome. He was one of the pioneers in the localization of brain function and with his wife published a famous text on the subject[17]. He was also interested in functional disorders, though insisting that the personality of the therapist was an important factor to be considered[18]. He died in 1917 at the age of 68, worn out by his work in a military hospital during the First World War (Figure 7.4).

His wife thereafter continued his clinical work and research, becoming president of the Société de Neurologie, of which her husband had been one of the founders, and an officer of the Légion d'Honneur. She died in 1927 at the same age as her husband.

The story of the definition of facioscapulohumeral muscular dystrophy by Landouzy and Dejerine has been recounted by Sorrel-Dejerine and Fardeau[19]. On the 20th of June 1880, a 21-year-old man was admitted to the Hôpital de la Charité in Paris with severe muscle wasting and weakness. The history was that from the age of 3, following an attack of measles, the parents had noticed

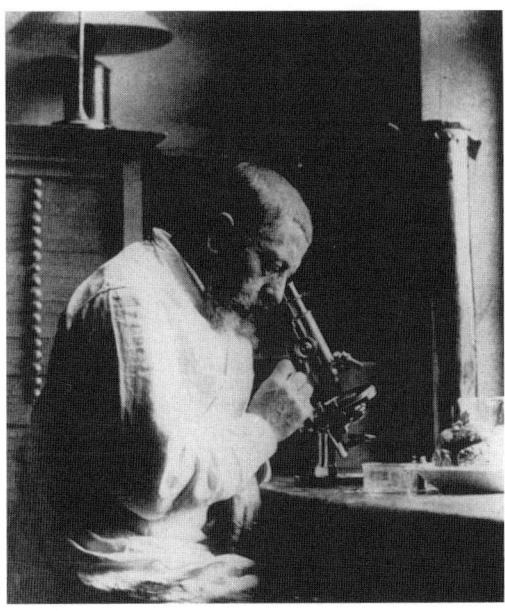

Fig. 7.4 Joseph Jules Dejerine (1849–1917). (Reproduced with permission from *The Founders of Neurology*, ed. by Webb Haymaker, 1953. Courtesy of Charles C. Thomas, publishers, Springfield, Illinois.)

a change in his facial appearance. This was apparently the only complaint until around age 17 when he developed weakness of the shoulder girdle and upper arm muscles. The weakness progressed and eventually the lower limbs became affected.

When examined, the facial appearance was noted as 'une bouche de tapir' and the facial muscles were weak, resulting in a transverse smile. There was marked weakness and wasting of the shoulders and upper arms as well as the lower limbs. There were no sensory changes and the tendon reflexes were absent. There were six brothers and two sisters in the family. A younger brother and two sisters, one of whom had died at age 20, were similarly affected, and the disease could be traced back through the father over four generations in the family.

On the 25th of October 1883, at the age of 24, the patient died of tuberculosis. At post mortem no abnormalities were found in the brain, spinal cord or peripheral nerves. Thus, although the clinical findings were similar to cases reported by Duchenne, the cause was not neurogenic as he had surmised, but myopathic. Landouzy and Dejerine presented their conclusions at l'Académie des Sciences in January 1884 where they emphasized the myopathic nature of the disorder ('myopathie sans neuropathie') and suggested the title 'myopathie atrophique progressive'[20]. They then proceeded to document details of this and other cases and to discuss the relevance of similar cases previously reported in the literature[21–23].

Their conclusions were that facial weakness (excluding the extraocular muscles, which remained unaffected) was a significant manifestation of the disorder which may be apparent from early childhood, along with involvement of the pectoral girdle and upper limb musculature at first and only later the lower extremities, slowly progressive course, absence of pseudohypertrophy, and absence of muscle fasciculations. Also, the apparent age at onset was variable and not necessarily in childhood, and the disease varied in severity in different individuals from the same family. Finally, it could be inherited over several generations. The subsequent history of this disorder has been outlined elsewhere.

From the point of view of the present discussion, the detailed studies and descriptions provided by Erb and by Landouzy and Dejerine now made it possible to attempt a classification of progressive muscular dystrophy. This was first suggested by Erb (Ref. 6, pages 259–60), who proposed the following:

1. Childhood types
   Hypertrophic form
   Atrophic form (with or without facial involvement)

2. Juvenile and adult types
   Scapulohumeral form(s).

However, he was mindful that there could be overlap between the types and therefore included a claim for 'gemischte und unbestimmte' (mixed and uncertain) forms! But since cases with facial weakness could begin in later life this classification was not entirely satisfactory. The problems of classifying these diseases would now begin increasingly to engage the interest of those working in the field of neuromuscular disorders.

References

1. Leyden, E. von. Hereditäre Formen der Progressiven Muskelatrophie; Die Lipomatöse Muskelhypertrophie. *Klinik der Rückenmarkskrankheiten.* Vol. 2. Berlin: A. Hirschwald, 1876: 525–40.
2. Möbius P. J. Ueber die hereditären Nervenkrankheiten: II. Die hereditäre oder degenerative Muskelatrophie. *Sammlung Klinischer Vorträge in verbindung mit Deutschen Klinikern, herausgegeben von Richard Volkmann (Leipzig). (Innere Medicin No. 57)* 1879; **171**: 1510–31.
3. Viets, H. R. Wilhelm Heinrich Erb (1840–1921). In: Haymaker, W. (ed.) *The Founders of Neurology.* Springfield, Ill: Charles C. Thomas, 1953: 279–82.
4. Nonne, M. Wilhelm Erb. In: Kolle, K. (ed.) *Grosse Nervenärzte.* Stuttgart: Thieme, 1956.

5. Erb, W. Ueber die 'juvenile Form' der progressiven Muskelatrophie und ihre Beziehungen zur sogenannten Pseudohypertrophie der Muskeln. *Deutsches Archiv für klinische Medicin*, 1884; **34**: 467–519.
6. Erb, W. Dystrophia muscularis progressiva: klinische und pathologisch–anatomische Studien. *Deutche Zeitschrift für Nervenheilkunde*, 1891; **1**: 13–94, 173–261.
7. Kuhn, E., Rüdel, R. Wilhelm Heinrich Erb (1840–1921). *Muscle & Nerve*, 1990; **13**: 567–9.
8. Swift, T. R. The Breathing Arm: 1993 Presidential Address, American Association of Electrodiagnostic Medicine. *Muscle & Nerve*, 1994; **17**: 125–9.
9. Spillane, J. D. *The Doctrine of the Nerves: Chapters in the History of Neurology*. Oxford: Oxford University Press, 1981: 328.
10. Hughes, J. T. *Thomas Willis 1621–1675: His Life and Work*. London: Royal Society of Medicine, 1991: 81–3.
11. Erb, W. H. *Handbuch der Krankheiten des Nervensystems*. 2 Vols. Leipzig: F. C. W. Vogel, 1876–78.
12. Walton, J. N., Nattrass, F. J. On the classification, natural history and treatment of the myopathies. *Brain*, 1954; **77**: 169–231.
13. Padberg, G. W. A. M. *Facioscapulohumeral disease*. (Doctoral dissertation), University of Leiden, 1982.
14. Duchenne, G. B. A. *Album de Photographies Pathologiques*. Paris: J. B. Baillière et Fils, 1862.
15. Alpers, B. J. Louis Théophile Joseph Landouzy (1845–1917). In: Haymaker W. (ed.) *The Founders of Neurology*. Springfield Ill: Charles C. Thomas, 1953: 317–20.
16. Zupanc, M. Madame Augusta Dejerine-Klumpke. In: Ashwal, S. (ed.) *The Founders of Child Neurology*. San Francisco: Norman Publishing, 1990: 215–21. (See also Bailey, H., Bishop, W. J. *Notable Names in Medicine and Surgery*. London: H. K. Lewis, 1959: 168–9.)
17. Dejerine, J. J., Dejerine-Klumpke, A. *Anatomie des Centres Nerveux*. 2 Vols. Paris: Rueff et Cie, 1895–1901.
18. Zabriskie, E. G. Joseph Jules Dejerine (1849–1917). In: Haymaker, W. (ed.) *The Founders of Neurology*. Springfield, Ill: Charles C. Thomas, 1953: 271–5.
19. Sorrel-Dejerine, Y., Fardeau, M. Naissance et métamorphoses de la myopathie atrophique progressive de Landouzy et Dejerine. *Revue Neurologique (Paris)*, 1982; **138**: 1041–51.
20. Landouzy, L., Dejerine, J. De la myopathie atrophique progressive (myopathie héréditaire débutant, dans l'enfance, par la face, sans altération du système nerveux). *Comptes Rendus de l'Académie des Sciences (Paris)*, 1884; **98**: 53–5.
21. Landouzy, L., Dejerine, J. De la myopathie atrophique progressive. Myopathie sans neuropathie, débutant d'ordinaire dans l'enfance, par la face. *Revue de Médicine*, 1885; **5**: 81–117, 253–366.
22. Landouzy, L., Dejerine, J. Nouvelles recherches cliniques et anatomo-pathologiques sur la myopathie atrophique progressive à propos de six observations nouvelles, dont une avec autopsie. *Revue de Médicine*, 1886; **6**: 977–1027.
23. Landouzy, L., Dejerine, J. Contribution à l'étude de la myopathie atrophique progressive (myopathie atrophique progressive, à type scapulo-huméral). *Comptes Rendus Société de Biologie (Paris)*, 1886; **3**(8 sér.): 478–81.

Chapter 8

Nosology of the dystrophies

By the end of the last century the concept of muscular dystrophy being a primary disease of muscle was finally accepted. It could be defined as a disease characterized by progressive muscle wasting and weakness, in which the muscle histology had been shown by Erb and others[1] to have certain distinctive features (such as muscle fibre degeneration and necrosis, increased amounts of connective tissue and fat, etc.), and in which there was no evidence of spinal cord or peripheral nerve involvement and no myotonia. It was also recognized that it was often hereditary. But it was also becoming evident that there was more than one type of dystrophy and the problem of classifying them was only just beginning.

The classification of diseases, or the science of *nosology*, is more than an academic exercise, though it is doubtless an intellectual challenge. We now know that hereditary diseases which are clinically similar may be genetically different, and the recognition of such heterogeneity is essential in interpreting the results of studies designed to investigate aetiology and pathogenesis. Furthermore, genetically different disorders may have different prognoses and respond differently to any proposed therapy—what is effective in one form of a disease may prove to be ineffective or even deleterious in another. It is now recognized that such heterogeneity may be the result of different alleles at the same gene locus or to different gene loci. In the latter situation the disorder may then exhibit different modes of inheritance: as an autosomal dominant, autosomal recessive, or X-linked recessive trait[2].

Up to the end of the nineteenth century so little was known about the basis of inheritance that no real headway could be made in resolving genetic heterogeneity within the muscular dystrophies. Only as Mendel's principles of heredity began to be recognized and accepted did the situation become clearer. But this did not occur immediately. Mendel's principles could be demonstrated in plants and animals but this was far more difficult in humans, where controlled matings were impossible and generation times long. The physician could only observe a pedigree and draw inferences from it. The acceptance of the relevance of Mendelian principles in human disease was a slow process and many physicians persisted in using terms such as 'heredo-familial' and the transmission of 'degenerative factors'. To many it seemed extraordinary that sex could influence the onset of a disease such as Duchenne dystrophy.

In 1907 P. C. Knapp, addressing the American Neurological Association, argued that applying Mendelian principles to human disease seemed so difficult that it might well take many years to resolve. In fact, the application of these principles in neurology began very gradually and only became generally accepted after 1920. This may therefore partly explain why there was little advance in further resolving heterogeneity in muscular dystrophy for some 30 years after Erb's seminal publications. It is also possible that much research around this time may have been interrupted by the devastating effects in Europe of the First World War. But, whatever the reason, it was not until around the late 1920s that publications began to appear which gave any detailed and significant consideration to the problem of *genetic* heterogeneity.

However, not all were in fact convinced that such heterogeneity already existed. One factor may have been that it was not always appreciated that an isolated case of a disorder in a family could still be genetic. But perhaps more importantly, it may have been that 'lumping' disorders together often had more appeal than what some, like Gowers, viewed as unjustified 'splitting'[3]. This problem is well exemplified by the early family studies of Ade T. Milhorat.

Genetic heterogeneity

Milhorat was born in 1899 in New Jersey. He graduated from Columbia University in 1924 and from Cornell University Medical College 4 years later.

While at Columbia University, Milhorat studied under Thomas Hunt Morgan (1866–1945), the renowned geneticist. Morgan's pioneering work on the fruit fly, *Drosophila*, helped to establish the chromosome theory of inheritance and the physical basis of Mendelism, an idea independently proposed by Walter Sutton and Theodor Boveri in the early 1900s[4,5]. With colleagues, including Calvin Bridges and, notably, Alfred Sturtevant, Morgan studied the phenomenon of genetic linkage or the arrangement of genes on the chromosomes. Eventually, in *Drosophila* they were able to draw the first chromosome map with the positions of several *sex-linked* characters, a term which Morgan emphasized was more appropriate than the previously used term, sex-limited. In 1933 Morgan was awarded the Nobel Prize for Physiology and Medicine[6].

When Milhorat attended Columbia University, Morgan was then at the height of his research in genetics and his enthusiasm was proverbial. Milhorat would no doubt have been impressed by Morgan and would have appreciated as much as anyone the implications of such genetic research for diseases in humans.

After internship at Columbia-Presbyterian Hospital, Milhorat was awarded a National Research Council Fellowship to study physiological chemistry for 2 years under Karl Thomas in Leipzig. It was around this time that he became increasingly interested in Gowers' writings and decided to devote himself to research into muscular dystrophy. On his return to the United States in 1932 he established a large clinic at the New York Hospital-Cornell for patients with muscular dystrophy, and through these patients and their families was formed the Muscular Dystrophy Association of America in 1950. The history of this organization, dedicated to the care of patients with muscular dystrophy and to research, and the first of its kind in the world, would make an interesting study in its own right. Milhorat also established a research laboratory at his hospital, mainly concerned at first with creatine metabolism (an important aspect of muscle breakdown). This later formed the basis of The Institute for Muscle Disease in 1959 with Milhorat as its Director, a position he retained until his retirement in 1973 (Figure 8.1). The Institute became an important focus for research into muscle disease and quickly established an international reputation in the field.

Milhorat became professor of clinical medicine at New York Hospital-Cornell in 1956 and was given emeritus status in 1968. After his retirement he became a consultant to the Muscular Dystrophy Association and continued his

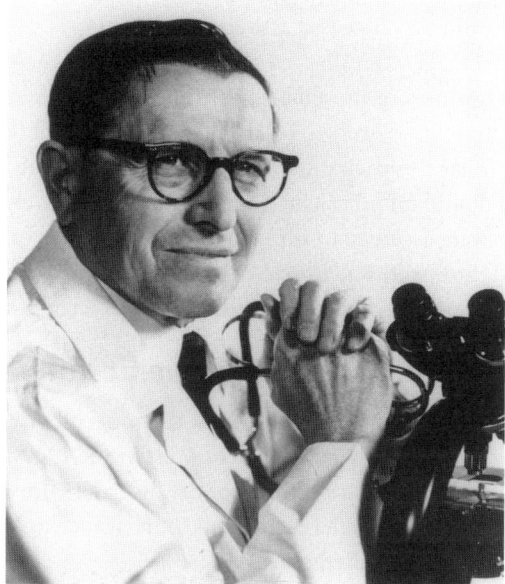

Fig. 8.1 Ade T. Milhorat. (Reproduced by kind permission of his son, Thomas H. Milhorat, MD.)

research. His wide interests included geology and medical history. He was always particularly interested in the *first* descriptions of diseases and he is also descended from French Huguenot stock, like Edward Meryon, remarkable coincidences in this history! He died in 1997 at the age of 98.

In the intervening years after his return from Germany to the United States in 1932, he had studied 85 individuals with muscular dystrophy and obtained information on further cases in affected families, making a total of 125 cases[7]. No doubt because of his earlier interest in genetics he set about studying the families of these individuals. Although others had reported on the hereditary nature of the disease, this study marked a new departure because of the scale of the studies and his attempt to classify the role of genetic factors in the disease. In summary, his findings revealed clear sex-linked recessive inheritance in 26 cases and dominant inheritance in 14. In 27 only siblings were affected. The remaining cases were all isolated and he speculated as to the reasons for this: some could be sporadic (i.e. new mutations), or be abortive in the parents or other family members (i.e. incomplete penetrance), or sex-linked recessive which only by chance affected one boy in the family, or might be due to recessive factors in some families. The latter is a particularly interesting possibility which had, for example, been proposed to explain a large inbred family in Switzerland reported by Minkowski and Sidler a few years previously[8].

Such an extensive and detailed family study of the disease was a major step forward. But the possibility that genetic differences reflected fundamental differences and should be related to associated phenotypes was not seriously considered. In fact, Milhorat lumped all the cases together to show that 'the earlier in life symptoms of muscular dystrophy develop the more rapid the progression of disability is likely to be'. He further noted that the disease tended to follow a similar course in different members of the same family and that in families with dominant inheritance the disease was relatively milder. At the time these ideas were assumed to apply to inherited diseases in general[9].

The real need, however, was to relate genetic differences to clinical differences, and in the next few years many attempted such an approach.

Nosology based on clinical and genetic differences

It was now beginning to be recognized that the muscular dystrophies were both genetically and clinically heterogeneous. From the 1940s onwards many groups contributed to the classification of the disorders. In some, emphasis was placed more on clinical differences, while others, such as Milhorat, placed more emphasis on genetic differences.

Those that have best stood the test of time have attempted to include as many relevant factors as possible. Some of the more important earlier studies of the problem include those of Julia Bell[10], Tyler and Wintrobe[11], Levison[12], Becker[13], Stevenson[14], and Lamy and de Grouchy[15]. These do not exhaust the studies being carried out around the time, but they do represent some of the more significant contributions on the problems of nosology.

Bell's often-quoted study[10] was based on an extensive survey of well over 1000 cases, but since most of the information was gained rather uncritically from reports in the literature, serious doubts have been expressed about her conclusions. However, as a guide to the earlier literature it is nevertheless a valuable publication. All the other studies were based on personally examined cases and family members, and therefore the results are more valuable. There is perhaps little to be gained from considering the details of these earlier publications which, in any event, with the exception of two[13,15] have all been critically evaluated by Walton and Nattrass[16]. But certain conclusions can be drawn from these studies.

Firstly, Lamy and de Grouchy[15], based on their very thorough and careful genetic study of 102 families, emphasized the distinctive and homogeneous nature of the dystrophy described by Duchenne, but that in a minority of families with a similar clinical picture little girls could be affected and the mode of inheritance was autosomal recessive. Stevenson[14] also distinguished what he referred to as 'autosomal limb girdle muscular dystrophy' from Duchenne dystrophy but in the former condition there was considerable variation in clinical presentation and in age at onset, many beginning in adulthood. The apparent differences in cases of autosomal recessive muscular dystrophy in these two studies no doubt reflect the different ways in which families were ascertained: whereas Lamy and de Grouchy's study was based on a *children's* hospital in Paris, Stevenson attempted complete ascertainment of *all* cases in the province of Northern Ireland. Ascertaining cases through nursing homes and hospitals could also lead to a bias by excluding milder cases of the disease[17].

Secondly, the facioscapulohumeral type of muscular dystrophy, described earlier by Landouzy and Dejerine, was confirmed as a distinct entity inherited as an autosomal dominant trait[11,12]. A study of a very large Mormon family of 1249 individuals over six generations, of whom 159 were affected, provided an ideal opportunity to assess the extent of clinical variability with the same mutant gene[18].

Finally, Becker[13], who at the time made perhaps the most extensive clinical and genetic analysis of affected individuals within a relatively well defined region (Südbaden, Germany), confirmed the distinctive identity of at least three forms of dystrophy: two pelvic girdle forms, one rapidly progressive and X-linked and one possibly more benign and autosomal recessive; and a pectoral girdle form, with facial weakness and autosomal dominant inheritance.

The emphasis was now clearly turning away from purely clinical and pathological studies of the disease. The need to consider genetic factors, as Milhorat had attempted, was now being accepted. In fact, the time would shortly come when genetic factors would not only be considered in terms of understanding the basic cause of dystrophy but also as an actual *aid to diagnosis*[19], in a way a volte-face from many of the earlier studies of the disease.

At the same time other clinically distinctive, but rarer, forms of dystrophy were beginning to be recognized. The single most important contribution on the subject, in which all these factors were carefully considered, was that of Walton and Nattrass in 1954, which proved to be a landmark in the history of muscular dystrophy[16].

The classification of Walton and Nattrass

How John Walton first became interested in muscular dystrophy is related in his autobiography[20]. He was just completing his thesis on subarachnoid haemorrhage for the MD degree of Durham University. In Britain this is a postgraduate degree and is usually necessary to specialize later on. At this time he was no doubt becoming a little concerned about his future, which is not unusual some 4 or 5 years after qualification, when serious consideration had to be given to a choice of speciality. Apparently, the professor of medicine (F. J. Nattrass) had been asked for advice by Dr Albertine Winner of the Department of Health regarding correspondence the Ministry had received concerning patients with 'muscular dystrophy' who appeared to have recovered or had at least failed to deteriorate as had been suggested by the diagnosing physician. As Walton says, Professor Nattrass

> to his everlasting credit, felt that the story was one which warranted further study and hence sought financial support through (Durham) University and from the Department of Health in order to establish a research post... (Ref. 20, page 161).

Walton was duly appointed as research assistant with the primary objective of studying those patients who had so unexpectedly recovered from what had seemed a progressive and incurable disease. On subsequent careful analysis these proved to be cases of benign congenital myopathy, dermatomyositis, or polymyositis[21]. It was also suggested that Walton should survey all the patients with muscular dystrophy in the region. Often in this history, we have seen how the encouragement and support of a senior colleague has resulted in a young assistant making a major contribution to the subject. This was certainly so in this case and throughout his life Walton has always acknowledged the support he received from Nattrass.

Frederick John Nattrass was born on 6 August 1891, the son of a Methodist minister. He was educated at King Edward's School, Birmingham, and later the Medical School of Durham University where he was an outstanding student, graduating with distinctions in no fewer than 11 subjects, and with first class honours in 1914. He later served in the Royal Army Medical Corps in the First World War and was eventually captured. After the war he returned to Newcastle where he gained the MD degree with gold medal, and subsequently became a consultant physician and finally professor of medicine with a particular interest in neurological disorders (Figure 8.2). When the Muscular Dystrophy Group of Great Britain was founded, as an independent charity on 1 May 1959, he was chosen as the first chairman and spent most of his life, even after retirement, in furthering the interests of the group. He had abiding interests in ornithology, art, and music, and for many years was a member of a Bach Choir. He died 2 weeks after his eighty-eighth birthday in 1979[22].

When Walton started his research into muscular dystrophy it is doubtful that he ever imagined how this would develop and what effects it would have on his own future and on the subject in general. John Nicholas Walton was born in 1922 in a small village in a mining region of County Durham in Northumberland, both his parents being teachers. After attending the local high school he won a scholarship to study medicine at King's College, Durham, later to become the University of Newcastle, and graduated in 1945 with first class honours with distinctions in medicine, surgery, and midwifery. Following

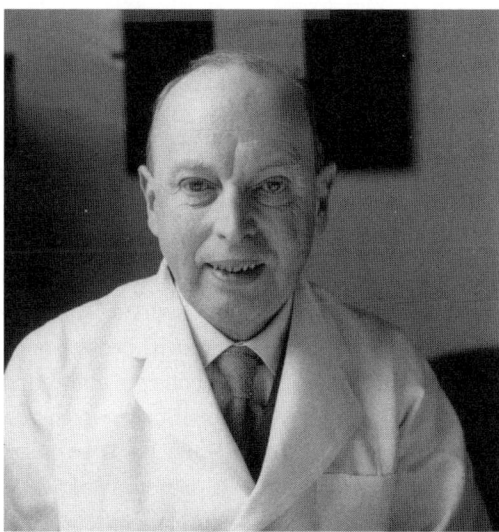

Fig. 8.2 Frederick John Nattrass. (Reproduced by kind permission of Lord Walton.)

the usual junior hospital appointments, he spent a period of National Service in the Royal Army Medical Corps, which he clearly enjoyed because later he joined the Territorial Army, eventually becoming honorary colonel of the local regiment.

He returned to Newcastle in 1949 where he was appointed medical registrar and began to hone his clinical skills in neurology, which were to prove invaluable in his later work on neuromuscular diseases. It was shortly after this that he became research assistant to Professor Nattrass. Thereafter, he began the steady climb up the academic ladder, eventually becoming professor of neurology. His department in Newcastle became internationally recognized as one of the great centres of research into neuromuscular disorders. He became chairman of the Muscular Dystrophy Group of Great Britain, a position he held for 25 years, as well as at different times being chairman of its Research Committee and its Medical and Social Services Committee. Like Ade Milhorat in the United States, John Walton did much to stimulate and support research into neuromuscular disease in his own country. In fact, a chance meeting with him in Edmonton, Canada in 1963 was largely responsible for encouraging the author (AEHE) to set up a research group of his own in Manchester with funding from the Muscular Dystrophy Group.

Over the years he and his colleagues in Newcastle have published a great many research papers on muscular dystrophy and related disorders. In the past these have been mainly concerned with clinical, pathological, and biochemical studies, but the group he founded is now also recognized internationally for its work in molecular genetics. He has written or edited nine books, and in regard to neuromuscular disorders the most relevant are his *Skeletal Muscle Pathology*[23] and *Disorders of Voluntary Muscle*[24].

Apart from his clinical and research interests, he became a highly regarded and efficient administrator. He was elected dean of medicine in Newcastle, a position he held for 10 years. Later, in 1983 he was appointed warden of Green College, Oxford. The College was founded in 1979 and named after its benefactor, Dr Cecil Green, formerly president of Texas Instruments, and is centred around the very beautiful eighteenth-century Radcliffe Observatory and associated buildings. During this period he proved himself a much liked warden and was respected by the College Fellows and students alike. Following his retirement as warden in 1989, he took up residence in Osler's Oxford house, which he and his late wife, Betty, enjoyed restoring in Osler's memory. He has been elected presidents of the World Federation of Neurology, the Royal Society of Medicine, the British Medical Association, and the General Medical Council. He was knighted in 1979 and 10 years later became a Peer with the title The Right Honourable Lord Walton of Detchant, named after the small village in Northumberland where he and his family have had a holiday cottage for many happy years. He is now 'retired' but still continues his work and interest in neuromuscular disorders and his work in broader medical and educational issues through various Select Committees of the House of Lords. He is patron, president and Advisory Board member of innumerable charities and maintains his lifelong burning interests in cricket, golf, and the fortunes of Newcastle United football team (Figure 8.3).

The Walton and Nattrass publication of 1954[16] is noteworthy in several respects. Firstly, strenuous efforts were made to ascertain every case in the population studied (Northumberland and Durham). Secondly, all patients and their available family members were interviewed in detail and examined personally. Thirdly, all were subsequently admitted to hospital for electromyography and muscle biopsy to confirm the diagnosis and for independent assessment by Professor Nattrass.

In total there were 84 'pure' cases of muscular dystrophy, which included 48 cases of the Duchenne type. In one of these cases (family D6, with five other affected males in two generations), onset was at age 26, he became confined to a wheelchair when aged 30, and was still alive at age 44. In two other families the clinical picture was similar. For this reason the authors rejected Stevenson's idea that the disease was always restricted to 'young boys'. It now seems very likely that these were cases of the more benign Becker type of X-linked muscular dystrophy. Walton failed to accept that such a benign form existed as

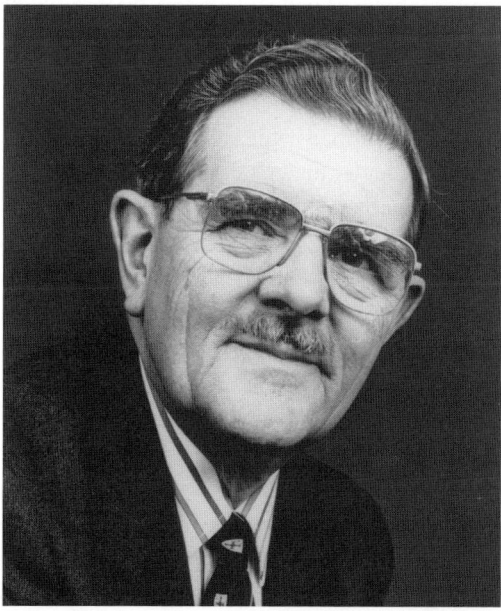

Fig. 8.3 John Nicholas Walton. (The Right Honourable, Lord Walton of Detchant.)

a separate disease entity even as late as 1963 (Ref. 25, page 271), though admittedly at this time he was not alone in this regard.

There were also three sporadic cases of girls with a disorder which clinically and in its rate of progression was somewhat similar to that in affected boys. Walton and Nattrass could offer no clear explanation for these cases.

In their survey there were four families with autosomal dominant facioscapulohumeral muscular dystrophy. Among the 18 affected, three were relatives who believed themselves to be unaffected until examined. The occurrence of such very mild (*abortive*) cases was to be repeatedly emphasized by Walton in future and became an important consideration in genetic counselling.

There were also 18 cases of what the authors referred to as 'limb girdle muscular dystrophy'. According to Walton and Nattrass, the diagnostic features of this group included expression in males or females, onset usually after the second decade, predominant involvement of the proximal limb girdle musculature, relatively slow progression, and, rarely, muscle pseudohypertrophy. However, the authors comment:

> the natural history of the disease in these cases of limb girdle myopathy shows much more variation than in the other groups; whereas the course is sometimes as insidious as in the average facioscapulohumeral case... in other cases weakness increases more rapidly... (Ref. 16, page 207–8).

We now know that a limb girdle group so defined is itself very heterogeneous. They considered it to be usually inherited as an autosomal recessive trait.

Finally, there were two cases of myopathy predominantly affecting the *distal* limb musculature (distal myopathy), and a single case with ptosis and impaired ocular movements (ocular myopathy).

Although the authors' study had helped to classify the clinical features in these five types of dystrophy, a better understanding of their inheritance was crucial. Walton therefore set about a detailed genetic analysis[26–28]. These studies are interesting because they include the first attempts to locate the responsible genes by searching for linkage to known genetic markers[26]. The markers used included colour blindness, various blood groups, and the ability to taste PTC (phenylthiocarbamide). This was an imaginative and so far unexplored approach in muscular dystrophy. Unfortunately, however, none of these markers proved to be linked to any of the forms of dystrophy. Later, Duchenne muscular dystrophy and the Xg blood group would both be shown to be on the short arm of the X chromosome, but this blood group was not discovered until 1962[29].

Walton recognized that isolated cases of Duchenne muscular dystrophy might be due to new mutations and determined the mutation rate using Haldane's formula[30], as had Stevenson previously[14]. Walton arrived at a figure of 43×10^{-6}, a somewhat low figure we now know, probably because, despite all his effort, not all cases in the population had been ascertained.

Of particular interest was a large family with nine affected males in four generations and with an affected *female* who was apparently as badly affected as the males[27]. Walton speculated as to how a female could be affected in this way and wondered if this could be due to her having some X chromosomal abnormality. In fact, she proved to have no 'drumsticks' in her polymorphonuclear leukocytes (i.e. male type) and Walton therefore suggested[28] she had Turner's syndrome (ovarian agenesis). These females, we now know, usually only have a single X chromosome (like normal males); if the disease were on the X chromosome it would explain why this girl was affected. This was the first such case reported in the world's literature. Later, other X-linked recessive diseases would also be reported in XO Turner's syndrome.

This was in 1956–1957, around the time Tjio and Levan published their famous paper in which they described a greatly improved method for studying human chromosomes, which previously had not been possible[31]. It would be another 3 years, however, before Turner's syndrome was shown to be associated with 45 chromosomes and an XO sex chromosome constitution[32]. Walton's ideas about his case were therefore in this respect ahead of their time.

The obvious maternal inheritance in Duchenne muscular dystrophy, first reported by Meryon, and the fact that mothers occasionally had had affected sons by different husbands, and now with this female case with Turner's syndrome, all led to the conclusion that Duchenne muscular dystrophy was most likely X-linked[33]. At the time, not all were entirely convinced.

In human genetics the mode of inheritance of a disorder had usually to be inferred from the pedigree pattern, but for various reasons this was far from satisfactory and could be misleading. For example, in a family with only one boy affected with a particular disorder, this might be an autosomal dominant with sex limitation and a new mutation or non-penetrant in one parent, an autosomal recessive with sex limitation, or an X-linked recessive. In an effort to better establish the mode of inheritance in human disorders, statistical methods, referred to as *segregation analysis*, were being developed, most notably by Fisher, Weinberg, Haldane, and Hogben. Segregation analysis was applied for the first time to muscular dystrophy in 1959 by Morton and colleagues, who also introduced the method of *discriminant analysis* to help resolve genetic heterogeneity in this group of disorders.

Discriminant and segregation analysis

Newton Morton's contribution to muscular dystrophy was not unlike that of one or two others in this history. He made an important and significant contribution and then never returned to the subject again.

He was born in New Jersey in 1929. From early on he had an interest in the more mathematical aspects of genetics and for this reason went to the University of Hawaii to study the population genetics of the fruit fly, *Drosophila*, where there was already a flourishing interest in the subject. However, he became increasingly interested in the mathematical problems of human genetics and for a time worked at the Atomic Bomb Casualty Commission in Hiroshima. He then returned to the United States, to Madison, Wisconsin, where he completed his PhD in 1955. The subject of his dissertation was *Sequential Tests for the Detection of Linkage*. Morton did not discover the so-called lod (*logarithm of the odds*) statistic. This was apparently developed by Wald for quality control of bombs during the war and was not published because of censorship until after the war[34]. But Morton certainly pioneered its use in human genetics and almost all studies of gene mapping of human diseases are now based on this methodology.

While continuing his postdoctoral studies in Wisconsin, he was searching for a problem to which he could apply his mathematical skills to analysing human pedigree data. A fortunate meeting occurred with the neurologist Henry Peters, who had a large clinic for patients with muscular dystrophy in Wisconsin. Also at this time Morton's colleague, C. S. Chung, was just finishing his PhD on mathematical genetics but wanted to remain in Wisconsin because his fiancée had just been hospitalized with tuberculosis. This concatenation of events led to a very successful collaboration between the three in the computer analysis of patients and families with muscular dystrophy. Morton later became professor in the department of genetics and in the School of Public Health in Hawaii. From 1988 he was professor and director of the Cancer Research Campaign Research Group in Genetic Epidemiology in Southampton, England, and now continues in retirement as professor of human genetics (Figure 8.4).

The two papers that Morton and Chung published in 1959 addressed two problems: the delineation of types of muscular dystrophy and their genetics. They first applied the method of *discriminant analysis* to a large body of data[35] to clarify distinctions between different groups. This type of analysis was not new. R. A. Fisher (1890–1962), a renowned geneticist and statistician, had first devised the method in 1936 for differentiating groups using multiple measurements in each group and for this purpose had devised discriminant functions[36,37]. However, Fisher's interest at the time was the application of the method for differentiating two species of iris plants according to their petal length, petal width, sepal length, and sepal width. Before Morton's work this approach had never been applied to any large body of medical data and

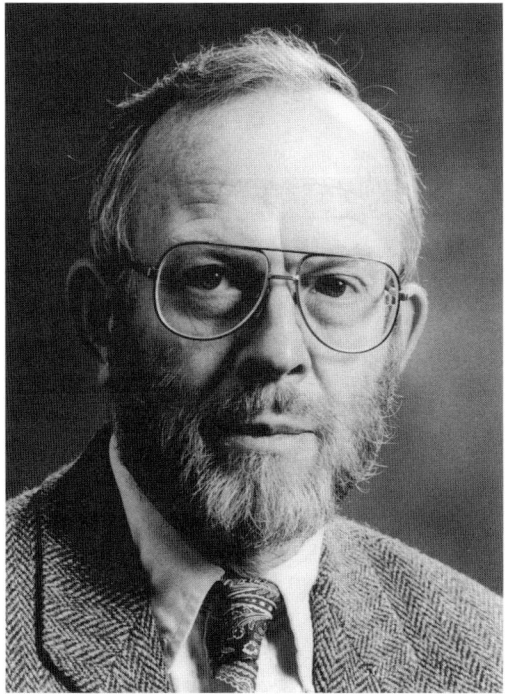

Fig. 8.4 Newton Ennis Morton.

certainly not to a problem as complex as the muscular dystrophies. Chung and Morton[35] selected 18 variables that they considered could be important (such as onset age, facial onset, scapulohumeral onset, pelvifemoral onset, calf pseudohypertrophy, etc.). They then used these as discriminant functions in the analysis of several hundred cases of muscular dystrophy from Wisconsin and the literature (they excluded Bell's data for the reasons we have mentioned earlier). Their results revealed four different groups: dominant facioscapulohumeral, X-linked Duchenne, and recessive and isolated limb girdle groups. In the limb girdle category, the isolated cases had significantly less parental consanguinity than familial cases, but the two groups were not clinically distinguishable. The data indicated that about 59% of limb girdle cases were caused by autosomal recessive genes. The four groups could not be subdivided further by discriminant methods. The authors concluded:

> Pedigree data and discriminant scores in conjunction provide the most accurate basis for classification of cases, with priority being given to the pedigree data (Ref. 35, page 357).

Their second paper[38] considered in more detail the genetics of muscular dystrophy using mainly the methods of segregation analysis. In many ways this was also a new departure in medical genetics. As the author says:

> During the course of this work there was an exciting interplay between collection of data which required more refined methods of genetic analysis than were then known, and development of techniques that required data that were not then available but are included in our Wisconsin material. The result has been a stringent test of the potentialities of modern methods of analysis in human genetics (Ref. 38, page 360).

Their findings confirmed that the facioscapulohumeral group was caused by an autosomal dominant gene which was completely penetrant in those who survived to the age of onset. The limb girdle group was composed of autosomal recessive cases in which heterozygotes were rarely, if ever, affected, and isolated cases. The latter, they considered, may be due to recessive genes in some cases but *not* dominant mutations since all 110 children of these cases were normal. Finally, the findings in the Duchenne group confirmed the X-linked mode of inheritance in this condition. Morton and Chung showed that, for a rare gene, the proportion of new mutants will be:

$m / (m + 1)$ for an autosomal dominant gene with sex limitation

and

$m u / (2u + v)$ for an X-linked recessive gene

where

m = coefficient of selection against affected males (i.e. unity in Duchenne)

u and v = mutation rates in eggs and sperm, respectively

Thus, if mutation in eggs and sperm is equal, then the expected proportion of new mutants approaches 0.5 for an autosomal dominant gene with sex limitation, and 0.33 for a lethal X-linked recessive gene. They arrived at a figure of 0.355 ± 0.050 and therefore concluded that the disorder is X-linked.

By a combination of detailed clinical and pedigree studies, as well as statistical analysis, several different types of the commoner dystrophies could now be distinguished.

References

1. Adams, R. D., Denny-Brown, D., Pearson, C. M. *Diseases of Muscle—A Study in Pathology*, 2nd edn. New York: Harper & Row, 1962: 348–69.
2. Emery, A. E. H. Genetic approach to the nosology of the muscular dystrophies. *Birth Defects: Original Article Series*, 1971; **7**: 15–17.
3. McKusick, V. A. On lumpers and splitters, or the nosology of genetic disease. *Perspectives in Biology and Medicine*, 1969; **12**: 298–312. (See also: *American Journal of Human Genetics*, 1978; **30**: 105–22.)
4. Stubbe, H. *History of Genetics*, 2nd edn. English translation, 1972. Cambridge, Mass. & London: MIT, 1965: 286–90.

5. McKusick, V. A., Walter S. Sutton and the physical basis of Mendelism. *Bulletin of the History of Medicine*, 1960; **34**: 487–97.
6. Shine, I., Wrobel, S. *Thomas Hunt Morgan—Pioneer of Genetics.* Lexington: University Press of Kentucky, 1976.
7. Milhorat, A. T., Wolff, H. G. Studies in diseases of muscle: XII. Heredity of progressive muscular dystrophy; relationship between age at onset of symptoms and clinical course. *Archives of Neurology and Psychiatry*, 1943; **49**: 641–54.
8. Minkowski, M., Sidler, A. Zur Kenntnis der Dystrophia musculorum progressiva und ihrer Vererbung. *Schweizerische Medizinische Wochenschrift*, 1928; **9**: 1005–9.
9. Macklin, M. T. The relation of the mode of inheritance to the severity of an inherited disease. *Human Biology*, 1932; **4**: 69–79.
10. Bell, J. On pseudohypertrophic and allied types of progressive muscular dystrophy. In: *Treasury of Human Inheritance*, Vol. 4 (Part 4). (Eugenics Laboratory Memoirs Series XXXII.) Cambridge: Cambridge University Press, 1943: 283–341.
11. Tyler, F. H., Wintrobe, M. M. Studies in disorders of muscle: I. The problem of progressive muscular dystrophy. *Annals of Internal Medicine*, 1950; **32**: 72–9.
12. Levison, H. Dystrophia musculorum progressiva. *Acta Psychiatrica et Neurologica Scandinavica*, 1951; Suppl. **76**.
13. Becker, P. E. *Dystrophia Musculorum Progressiva. Eine genetische und klinische Untersuchung der Muskeldystrophien.* Stuttgart: Georg Thieme Verlag, 1953.
14. Stevenson, A. C. Muscular dystrophy in Northern Ireland: I. An account of the condition in 51 families. *Annals of Eugenics (London)*, 1953; **18**: 50–91.
15. Lamy, M., de Grouchy, J. L'hérédité de la myopathie (forme basses). *Journal de Génétique Humaine*, 1954; **3**: 219–61.
16. Walton, J. N., Nattrass, F. J. On the classification, natural history and treatment of the myopathies. *Brain*, 1954; **77**: 169–231.
17. Sjövall, B. Dystrophia musculorum progressiva. *Acta Psychiatrica et Neurologica*, 1936; Suppl. **10**.
18. Tyler, F. H., Stephens, F. E. Studies in disorders of muscle: II. Clinical manifestations and inheritance of facioscapulohumeral dystrophy in a large family. *Annals of Internal Medicine*, 1950; **32**: 640–60.
19. Tyler, F. H. Inheritance of neuromuscular disease. *Neuromuscular Disorders: Research Publications of the Association for Research in Nervous and Mental Disease*, 1960; **38**: 357–67.
20. Walton, J. *The Spice of Life—From Northumberland to World Neurology.* London and New York: Royal Society of Medicine, 1993.
21. Nattrass, F. J. Recovery from 'muscular dystrophy'. *Brain*, 1954; **77**: 549–70.
22. Walton, J. N. Frederick John Nattrass. *Lives of the Fellows of the Royal College of Physicians of London (Munk's Roll)*, 1979; **7**: 421–4.
23. Mastaglia, F. L., Walton, J. N. (eds) *Skeletal Muscle Pathology*, 2nd edn. Edinburgh: Churchill Livingstone, 1992.
24. Walton, J. N. *et al.* (ed.) *Disorders of Voluntary Muscle*, 6th edn. Edinburgh: Churchill Livingstone, 1994.
25. Walton, J. N. Clinical aspects of human muscular dystrophy. In: G. H. Bourne and M. N. Golarz (eds). *Muscular Dystrophy in Man and Animals.* New York: Hafner Publishing Co., 1963: 263–321.

26. Walton, J. N. On the inheritance of muscular dystrophy, with a note on the blood groups by R. R. Race, and a note on colour vision and linkage studies by U. Philip. *Annals of Human Genetics (London)*, 1955; **20**: 1–38.
27. Walton, J. N. The inheritance of muscular dystrophy: further observations. *Annals of Human Genetics (London)*, 1956; **21**: 40–58.
28. Walton, J. N. The inheritance of muscular dystrophy. *Acta Genetica*, 1957; **7**: 318–20.
29. Mann, J. D., Cahan, A., Gelb, A. G. *et al.* A sex-linked blood group. *Lancet*, 1962; **i**: 8–10.
30. Haldane, J. B. S. The rate of spontaneous mutations of a human gene. *Journal of Genetics*, 1935; **31**: 317–26.
31. Tjio, J. H., Levan, A. The chromosome number of man. *Hereditas*, 1956; **42**: 1–6.
32. Ford, C. E., Jones, K. W., Polani, P. E., de Almeida, J. C., Briggs, J. H. A sex-chromosome anomaly in a case of gonadal dysgenesis (Turner's syndrome). *Lancet*, 1959; **i**: 711–13.
33. Thompson, M. W. Carrier detection in muscular dystrophy. *Lancet*, 1962; **ii**: 1120–21.
34. Morton, N. E. The development of linkage analysis. In: K. R. Dronamraju (ed.) *The History and Development of Human Genetics*. Singapore: World Scientific Publishing Co., 1992: 48–56.
35. Chung, C. S., Morton, N. E. Discrimination of genetic entities in muscular dystrophy. *American Journal of Human Genetics*, 1959; **11**: 339–59.
36. Box, J. F. *R. A. Fisher: The Life of a Scientist*. New York: John Wiley & Sons, 1978: 332–4.
37. Fisher, R. A. The use of multiple measurements in taxonomic problems. *Annals of Eugenics (London)*, 1936; **7**: 179–88.
38. Morton, N. E., Chung, C. S. Formal genetics of muscular dystrophy. *American Journal of Human Genetics*, 1959; **11**: 360–79.

Chapter 9

Recognition of other types of muscular dystrophy

By the 1950s the work of Walton, Morton, and others had led to the delineation of several of the more common and relatively distinct forms of dystrophy. But a number of other forms had been reported either previous to this or subsequently. All appeared to share the same features in their muscle histology and for this reason have been classified together as dystrophies. Clinically, however, they differ considerably and it is now clear that they do *not* share the same aetiology. In this chapter, attempts to resolve problems of heterogeneity are described as the situation appeared when the book was first published in 1995. In the final chapter, the results of further studies into the problem over the succeeding 15 years are summarized which previously would have been almost unbelievable.

Becker muscular dystrophy

We have seen previously that an X-linked form of muscular dystrophy, similar to Duchenne's disease but more benign, had occasionally been reported in the past (Chapters 6 and 8). However, Becker was the first to recognize that this was a *distinct* entity.

Peter Emil Becker (Figure 9.1) was born in 1908, in Hamburg, Germany where he went to school. It was actually during his school days that he developed interests in geology and art, interests he retained throughout his life. He later studied medicine at Marburg and Munich and, because of the freedom to change universities in Germany at the time, he also studied in Berlin and Vienna, and graduated from Hamburg.

He passed the State Medical Board examination in 1933 at a time when Hitler and National Socialism were gaining power in Germany but he never became a party member[1]. After internship he went on a 4-month trip to Indonesia as a ship's doctor and during his travels read a textbook in which a neurologist (Kurt Hiller) had written a chapter on muscular dystrophy. At this time, Becker was developing an interest in neurology and genetics, and the article attracted him because the classification of these diseases based purely on

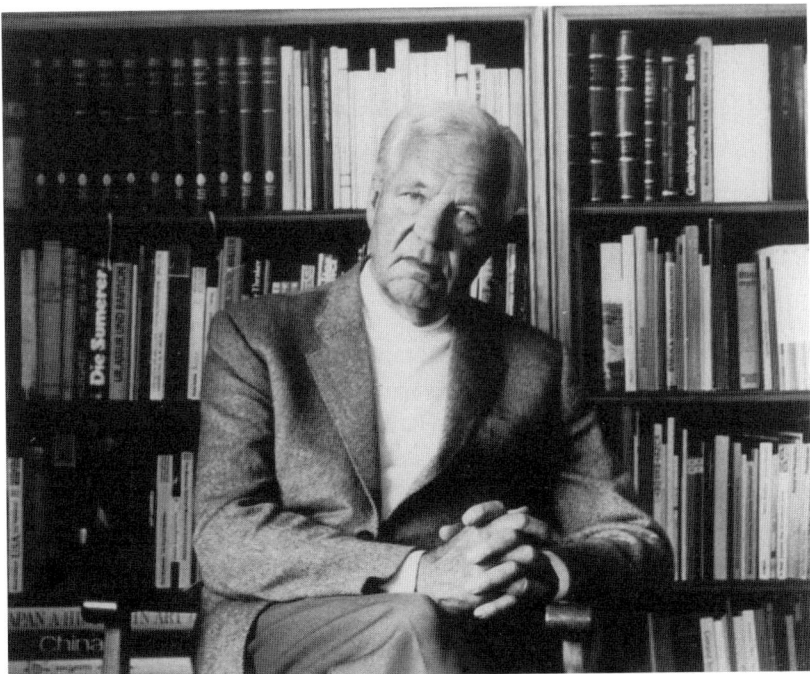

Fig. 9.1 Peter Emil Becker in his 76th year. (The eleven volumes of his *Handbook of Medical Genetics* can be seen at the left end of the top shelf.)

clinical criteria seemed to him extremely confusing. When eventually he began working in the Neurology Clinic at the University of Freiburg, he started to study the problem from a genetic point of view. In fact, Becker can be credited with having first proposed a classification of the dystrophies in which genetic parameters were emphasized[2,3]. This he published in 1940, dividing them into sex-linked recessive pelvic girdle, autosomal dominant shoulder girdle, and autosomal recessive pelvic girdle forms[4]. Later, in 1942 he wrote a monograph on the dystrophies but because of the war it was impossible to have it published and it did not appear until 1953[5].

After military service as a medical officer in the air force he returned to neurology and psychiatric practice, and in 1957 was appointed professor of human genetics at the University of Göttingen, where later, in 1961, he was elected dean of the faculty of medicine.

During his years in Göttingen he made a number of notable contributions to neurogenetics. He was the first to recognize, for example, the autosomal recessive form of myotonia congenita, which is commoner than the dominant Thomsen's disease and is now often referred to as Becker type myotonia congenita. He also edited a major text on human genetics. The first volume appeared in 1964 but eventually grew to 11 volumes (no longer *ein kurzes Handbuch*!), the last of which was published in 1975[6].

As Grimm[2,3] has pointed out, Becker belonged to a generation when it was still possible to achieve a great deal as an individual rather than as a member of a team. His individualism is clearly reflected by his scientific output of 122 publications, Becker being the sole author in 94, which nowadays would be impossible. Becker, a quietly spoken and cultured man, retired in 1975 and became emeritus professor, with more time then for his family, writing, and pursuit of his interests in geology and fine art. He devoted much of his time in retirement to researching the history of racial hygiene (*Rassenhygiene*), which he abhorred. He died in September 2000 after suffering a stroke in Göttingen at the age of 92.

How he came to study the form of dystrophy which now bears his name is recounted in his *Living Biography*[1]. One day, while still in practice, he received a letter from a Dr Franz Kiener, a psychologist in Regensburg, seeking advice on a muscular dystrophy which affected several of his relatives. The description he provided was similar to that of a family described earlier in 1937 by Kostakow and Derix[7]. This had attracted Becker's attention because, though only affecting males, the age of onset did not correspond with that expected in Duchenne muscular dystrophy. He had therefore assumed Kostakow and Derix may have received inaccurate historical information. Dr Kiener's family offered an opportunity to determine the precise age at onset and to study the clinical manifestations in greater detail. So Dr Kiener and Becker set out to visit the family in the Bavarian Upper Palatinate. The results confirmed the sex-linked mode of inheritance, that the onset was around adolescence with loss of ambulation only some years later, and a comparatively benign course with survival often into middle age. Otherwise, it was very similar to Duchenne muscular dystrophy, with calf pseudohypertrophy and predominantly pelvic girdle muscle weakness at the beginning, which only later affected the pectoral girdle musculature (Figure 9.2). They published their findings on the family in 1955[8] and a few years later Becker described two other large families with the same disorder[9]. Subsequently, the existence of this specific form of dystrophy was generally recognized and accepted as a distinct entity and became referred to as Becker muscular dystrophy. Recent molecular genetic studies now make it seem likely that previously described cases of so-called 'quadriceps myopathy' represent in fact the early stage of this type of dystrophy.

Emery–Dreifuss muscular dystrophy

In 1961 Dreifuss and Hogan described a large family in Virginia with muscular dystrophy[10]. In many respects it was similar to Duchenne's disease (with sex-linked

134 | RECOGNITION OF OTHER TYPES OF MUSCULAR DYSTROPHY

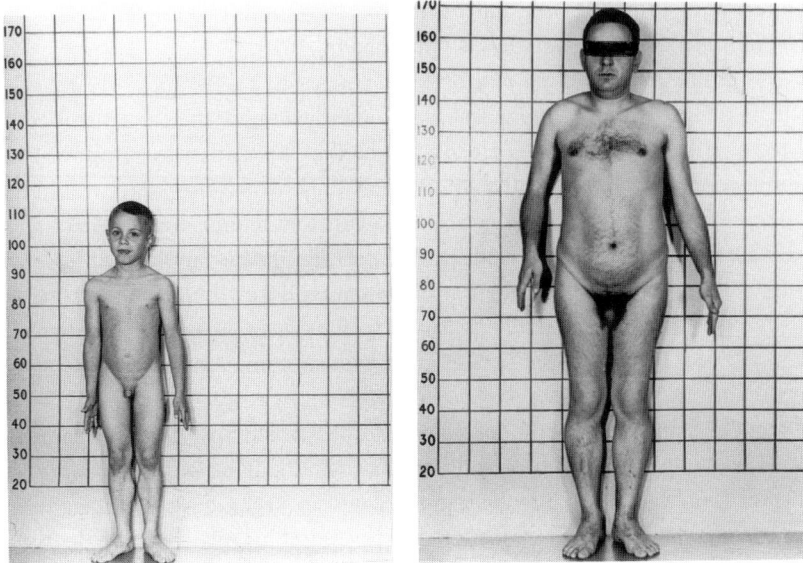

Fig. 9.2 A 6-year-old boy with preclinical Becker muscular dystrophy (note the enlarged calves) and his affected 26-year-old maternal uncle.

inheritance and onset in childhood) but differed in the absence of pseudohypertrophy, early contractures of the heel cords, and particularly in the 'inordinately slow and benign course of the condition'. In reviewing the literature of previously recorded cases of apparently benign sex-linked muscular dystrophy described by Kostakow and Derix, Walton and Nattrass and Becker, the authors proposed that inclusion of such families with Duchenne-type muscular dystrophy 'involves only a minor broadening of the concept of what constitutes the Duchenne type'. They therefore considered the disease in the Virginia family to be a benign form of Duchenne's disease. At the time, Fritz Dreifuss was an associate professor in neurology in the school of medicine, University of Virginia.

He was born in 1926, in Dresden, Germany, but in the early 1930s left for New Zealand where he obtained his schooling and subsequent medical training at the University of Otago, from which he graduated in 1950. Later he spent time at the National Hospital for Nervous Diseases in London and subsequently in 1959 accepted an appointment in the University of Virginia where he remained, eventually becoming the Thomas E. Worrell professor of epileptology and neurology (Figure 9.3). His main academic interests were always in adult and child neurology, and he was awarded many distinctions for his contributions to epilepsy. He was a past president of the American Epilepsy Society, the Epilepsy Foundation of America, and the International League Against Epilepsy. He listed his hobbies as writing, travelling, and 'combating

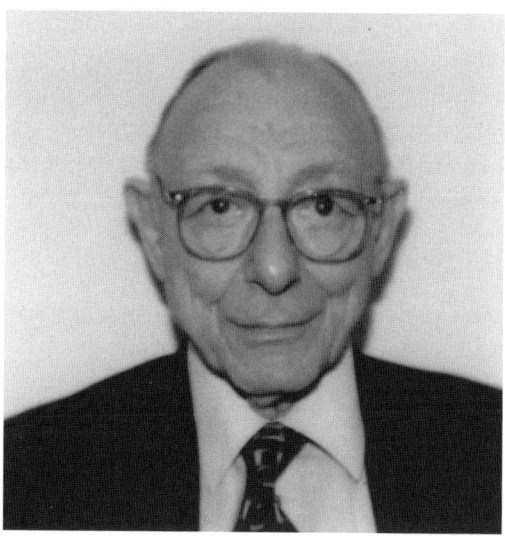

Fig. 9.3 Fritz E. Dreifuss.

needless bureaucracy' in health care. He died at home in Charlottesville, Virginia in October 1997, age 71.

At the time when Dreifuss reported this interesting Virginia family, one of the authors (AEHE) was studying neuromuscular disease for a PhD degree at Johns Hopkins University. So, when in 1962 my supervisor, Dr Victor McKusick, suggested I study the Dreifuss family for possible linkage to the newly discovered Xg blood group locus, I seized on the opportunity.

As Grimm has said about Becker, in those early days it was still possible to do a great deal on one's own. So, with the car loaded with an ECG machine and a spectrophotometer for enzyme analysis, I set off for Virginia to examine the members of the family in detail. In a single long weekend trip with almost the entire family gathered in the local schoolhouse (where the 55-year-old proband was a teacher), it was possible for me to examine everyone, carry out ECG studies, and measure their serum levels of creatine kinase. A few months later I returned to check some of the clinical findings, but all the essential and important work was done at the first visit. This second visit, however, allowed me to record some more of the old English folk songs of the Virginia/Kentucky mountain people!

On going over the data it seemed that this was quite a different disease from that described by Duchenne. Furthermore, although many were still somewhat reluctant to accept the existence of Becker muscular dystrophy, reading of the literature led me to think that the Virginia family was yet another type of X-linked dystrophy. Details of the family were published a few years later, after

I had returned to England, when we suggested with some trepidation that this represented another form of X-linked muscular dystrophy in which the clinical features were distinctive and consistent[11]. Incidentally, linkage studies with colour vision and the Xg blood group were uninformative.

I revisited the family 25 years later and was able to record the changes in the progress of the disease in affected members over the intervening period[12].

This relatively benign form of dystrophy, with onset in early childhood and thereafter usually only slowly progressive, is characterized by the triad of:

1. *Early* contractures, often *before* there is any significant weakness, of the elbows, Achilles tendons, and postcervical muscles (with limitation of neck flexion, but later forward flexion of the entire spine becomes limited)
2. Slowly progressive muscle wasting and weakness with a humeroperoneal distribution (i.e. proximal in the upper limbs and distal in the lower limbs) early in the course of the disease. Later weakness also affects the proximal limb girdle musculature
3. A cardiomyopathy, usually presenting as cardiac conduction defects ranging from sinus bradycardia, prolongation of the PR interval, to complete heart block.

Cardiac involvement usually becomes evident as muscle weakness progresses, but may exceptionally occur before there is any significant weakness. Provided that the diagnosis is made sufficiently early, the insertion of a cardiac pacemaker can be life-saving (Figure 9.4). The disorder has since been described in many other families throughout the world. It can also be inherited as an autosomal dominant trait[13].

The eponymous association was suggested by Rowland in 1979, though it seems the disorder may have been first described by Cestan and Lejonne of Paris in two affected brothers in 1902[14] and the rarer autosomal dominant form in a family of French Canadian descent in 1941[15], though in both instances the clinical presentation is not quite the same.

The locus for the X-linked form is located at Xq28. The gene has been identified and encodes a new protein which has been called 'emerin', the precise function of which has yet to be established[16].

Other rare forms of X-linked muscular dystrophy

The *scapuloperoneal* syndrome with predominant muscle wasting and weakness of the shoulder girdle and peroneal muscles, but without early contractures and cardiac conduction defects, remains nosologically uncertain[17]. The often quoted large affected family studied by Oransky in 1927[18], when restudied 50 years later, led the investigators to suggest that the disease in this family

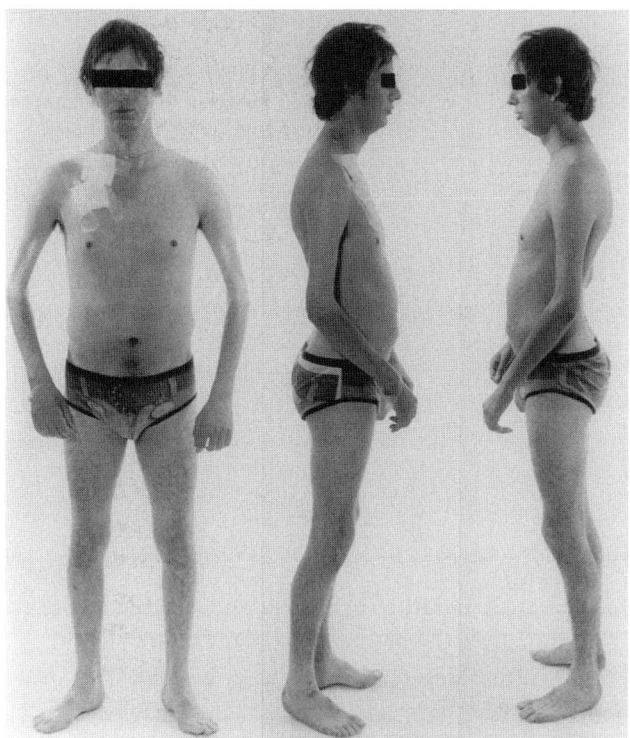

Fig. 9.4 A 17-year-old male with Emery–Dreifuss muscular dystrophy. Note the flexion contractures of the elbows, and wasting of the lower legs. A cardiac pacemaker has been inserted.

might be related to facioscapulohumeral muscular dystrophy[19]. Families with the scapuloperoneal syndrome had certainly been described but whether or not the disease was myopathic in many of these families is difficult to assess because the appropriate investigations (electromyography and muscle biopsy) had often not been carried out. However, a detailed and careful study by Thomas and colleagues has shown that an autosomal dominant *dystrophic* form of the syndrome does exist[20].

In the past this condition may have been confused with Emery–Dreifuss muscular dystrophy. However, in the scapuloperoneal syndrome, onset is usually much later (in adult life), *early* contractures do *not* occur, and cardiac *conduction* defects are not a consistent feature. Furthermore, whereas Emery–Dreifuss dystrophy is usually X-linked and less commonly autosomal, usually myopathic and not neurogenic, scapuloperoneal syndrome is autosomal and not X-linked, and is usually neurogenic and only occasionally myopathic. Some distinguishing features are summarized in Table 9.1.

Table 9.1 Some distinguishing features between Emery–Dreifuss muscular dystrophy and the scapuloperoneal syndrome

	Emery–Dreifuss muscular dystrophy	Scapuloperoneal syndrome
Genetics		
X-linked	++	–
Autosomal dominant	+	++ (or sporadic)
Clinical		
Onset	Early childhood	Adulthood
Contractures	Early	Late
Cardiac conduction defects	+	–
Basis		
Myopathic	++	+
Neurogenic	–	++

++, More frequent; +, less frequent; –, absent.

Several other rare X-linked muscle diseases have been described (Barth's syndrome, myotubular myopathy, and myopathy associated with autophagy), but in each of these disorders the myopathology is unique and not compatible with dystrophy.

However, several rare families, each with an X-linked dystrophy but clinically different from the Duchenne, Becker, and Emery–Dreifuss types, have been described[21–24]. These are listed in Table 9.2 along with some distinguishing features. Since each of these conditions has so far been reported only in single families, their nosological status remains unclear.

Limb girdle muscular dystrophies

We have seen already that several early studies had pointed to the existence of a limb girdle form of dystrophy. But this was clearly heterogeneous. In some cases it was primarily a disease of childhood but not in others. A division into childhood and adult forms therefore seems justified although the nosology of limb girdle muscular dystrophy even now is still not entirely clear and will be discussed in detail in Chapter 13.

Limb girdle muscular dystrophy of childhood

In some early studies there were reports of occasional families with a Duchenne-like dystrophy but which affected brothers and sisters or just sisters or occurred sporadically in little girls (Chapters 6 and 8). In some of these families the parents were cousins (for example, cases 14 and 15 in Gowers[25] and family D41 in

Table 9.2 Some families with X-linked muscular dystrophies reportedly manifesting distinctive clinical features

Onset (usual)	Predominant weakness	Early contractures	Mental handicap	Cardio-myopathy	Pseudo-hypertrophy	Reference
Early adolescence	Proximal	–	–	+	+++	Mabry et al.[21]
10–?32	Proximal	+/–	–	+	+/–	Wadia et al.[22]
Early childhood	Scapuloperoneal	–	++	+	–	Bergia et al.[23]
Late childhood	'Scapulo-back'	–	–	–	–	Ji et al.[24]

++, More frequent; +, less frequent; –, absent.

Stevenson[26]), which suggested autosomal recessive inheritance. This is particularly clear in the two extensive inbred families later recorded by Kloepfer and Talley[27], but the earliest and most detailed review of the condition was by Dubowitz in 1960[28]. This study was important for several reasons. Having reviewed in detail reports of similar cases in the earlier literature, Dubowitz carefully compared the clinical findings in these and his own two cases (whose parents were cousins) with those in X-linked Duchenne muscular dystrophy. He then considered how the disease in little girls could have occurred and concluded that the only logical explanation was autosomal recessive inheritance. This publication marked Victor Dubowitz's entry into the field of neuromuscular diseases, where he has ever since made many important contributions (Figure 9.5).

He was born in 1931 and educated in Beaufort West, South Africa, otherwise noted as the place that Chris Barnard, the pioneering cardiac surgeon, grew up. Dubowitz attended medical school in Cape Town, where he graduated in 1954. After junior hospital appointments at Groote Schuur Hospital he came to London in 1956 for further medical training and by one of those freaks of chance accepted a short locum appointment at Queen Mary's Hospital for Children at Carshalton where there were many children with muscular dystrophy and related disorders. At this time he had not planned to become a paediatrician, but the disease intrigued and increasingly interested him and the locum appointment extended to 2 years!

At the same time, through the encouragement and support of Professor Tony Pearse, Dubowitz gained invaluable training and experience in histopathology and histochemistry. Subsequently, he assembled the data he had collected on children with muscular dystrophy for an MD degree from which

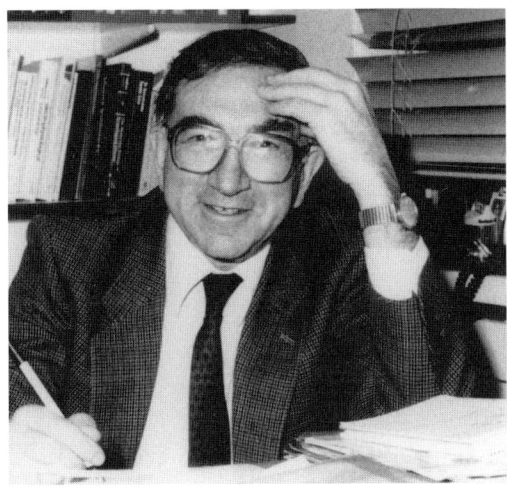

Fig. 9.5 Victor Dubowitz.

originated his article on the disease in little girls[28]. In 1972 he became professor of paediatrics at the Royal Postgraduate Medical School and director of the Jerry Lewis Muscle Research Centre at the Hammersmith Hospital; later, in 1995 he became founder and president of the World Muscle Society. Since his retirement in 1996, he has been emeritus professor of paediatrics and still pursues his interests in muscle disease, editorship of the journal *Neuromuscular Disorders*, and presidency of the World Muscle Society, as well as being an acclaimed sculptor! With his wife, Lilly, he developed the scoring system for assessing neurological development in the infant which is now universally accepted and which is often referred to as the Dubowitz score or simply 'Dubowitzing' the patient. He has published over 300 scientific papers, largely on neuromuscular diseases, and eight books.

The autosomal recessive limb girdle muscular dystrophy of childhood is rare in Europe and North America, but seems more common in Brazil[29] and particularly prevalent in certain Arabic communities[30]. It has been variously referred to as 'autosomal recessive Duchenne-like muscular dystrophy' or 'severe childhood autosomal recessive muscular dystrophy'.

Clinically, this disorder is indistinguishable from Duchenne muscular dystrophy and the serum level of creatine kinase can be grossly elevated in both. However, whereas most boys with the X-linked condition have significantly taller R waves in the right praecordial lead of the electrocardiogram, this is not found in the autosomal recessive condition[31,32]. The basic biochemical defect in the two conditions, however, is now known to be quite different: a deficiency of muscle dystrophin in the X-linked disease, and a deficiency of a 50-kDa dystrophin-associated glycoprotein called *adhalin*, after the Arabic for muscle, in at least some cases of the autosomal recessive disease[33]. The defective protein was subsequently shown to be a sarcoglycan.

Autosomal recessive childhood muscular dystrophy is itself heterogeneous, for families have been described in the past where the onset was in childhood but the subsequent course was relatively benign (for example, family D37 in Stevenson[26] and family M10 in Blyth and Pugh[34]). A disorder with onset in late childhood and thereafter relatively slowly progressive was subsequently described in Switzerland[35], among the Amish population of North America[36], and on the Island of Réunion[37]. As we shall see in Chapter 13, the situation has become much more complex in regard to these various forms of what are now referred to as limb girdle dystrophies.

Limb girdle muscular dystrophy of adulthood

Sporadic adult cases of limb girdle weakness beginning in the pelvic girdle and lower limb musculature are most likely to be due to spinal muscular atrophy, Becker muscular dystrophy, or manifestations in a female carrier of Duchenne muscular dystrophy. The so-called limb girdle syndrome of adults may also result from a variety of other genetic or non-genetic causes apart from muscular dystrophy. When all such possibilities are excluded, *true* limb girdle muscular dystrophy with adult onset appears to be relatively rare[38] (Figure 9.6).

However, there is no doubt that the disorder does exist and has been recognized for many years, the early literature being reviewed by Nevin[39]. Often sporadic, it can be inherited as an autosomal recessive or autosomal dominant trait. In the latter case, in some families it could apparently be limited to females[40] and in others to males[41]. In most families, however, both sexes are equally affected[42].

The manifesting carrier of Duchenne muscular dystrophy

Female carriers of Duchenne muscular dystrophy may occasionally manifest features of the disease itself. These range from pseudohypertrophy of the calf muscles, first recorded by Meryon in 1864, to marked limb girdle muscle weakness, first recorded by Gowers in 1879 (Chapter 6). But neither author drew particular attention to these features. However, enlargement of the calves in a female carrier was emphasized and illustrated by Kryschowa and Abowjan in their study of a large Moscow family in 1934[43]. Similar cases, with or without limb girdle weakness, were reported in several subsequent studies (reviewed in Emery and Walton[44]). Such manifestations were attributed to preferential inactivation of the X-chromosome carrying the normal gene in these carriers[45],

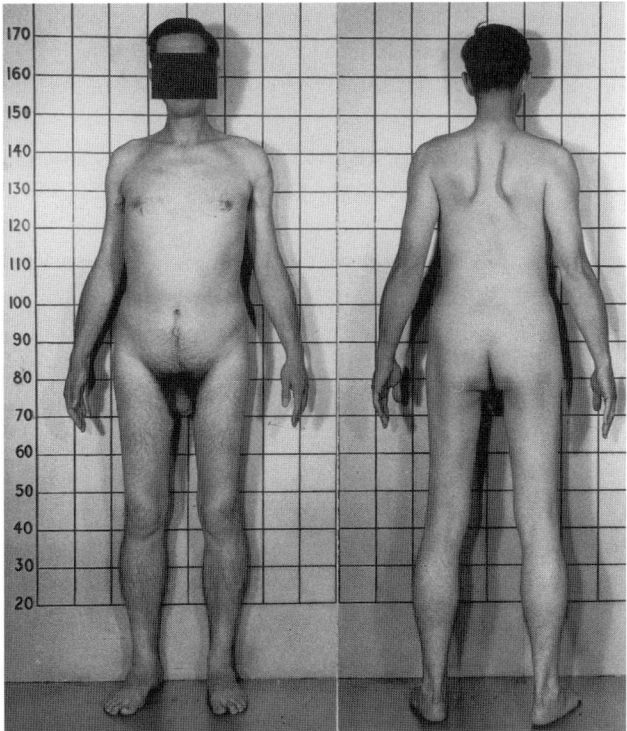

Fig. 9.6 Limb girdle muscular dystrophy with onset in late adolescence. A sister was similarly affected. Note the winging of the scapulae and possible wasting of the thigh muscles.

which is now supported by recent evidence from molecular studies. Rarely, a cardiomyopathy may be the only clinical manifestation in a female carrier.

In manifesting carriers, but not in healthy carriers, muscle dystrophin is reduced on Western blot and shows variation both within and between muscle fibres on immunohistochemistry (Chapter 12).

Distal muscular dystrophies

In this form of dystrophy, muscle weakness predominantly affects the *distal* limb muscles—those of the forearms and hands (Figure 9.7) and the lower legs. But this too is very heterogeneous. The earliest description of the condition is often attributed to Gowers[46].

The earliest and most extensive study of the condition was that of Welander in Sweden[47,48], involving 249 examined cases in 72 families. Onset was almost always after the age of 40, and usually began in the hands, affecting fine movements of the fingers. Later, the lower legs became affected. The disorder was inherited as an autosomal dominant trait and she recognized two forms of

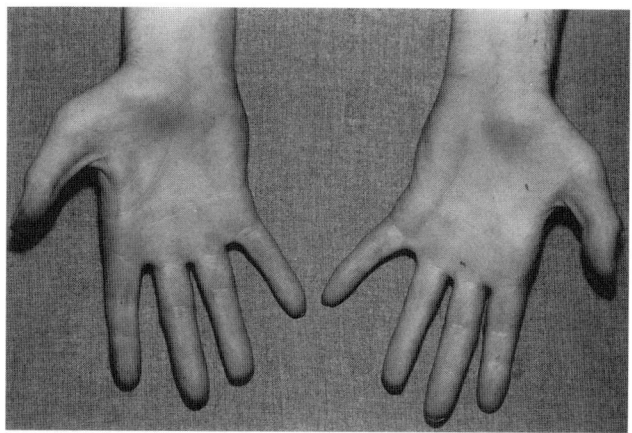

Fig. 9.7 Distal muscular dystrophy. Note the wasting of the small muscles of the hands.

the disease. Firstly, *typical* cases in which only the distal muscles were affected and the disease was slowly progressive. These cases were considered to be heterozygotes. Secondly, *grossly atypical* cases, in which the proximal muscles also became affected and the disease pursued a more rapid course. These cases were considered to be homozygotes. Since Welander's publications there have been reports of affected families in which the clinical features were somewhat different and therefore represent separate disease entities[49–54] (Table 9.3). A simplified current classification of these diseases is summarized in Chapter 13.

Table 9.3 Some different types of distal muscular dystrophy

	Inheritance	Onset (usual)	Reference
Late adult onset			
	AD	UL	Welander[47,48]
	AD[a]	LL	Markesbery et al.[49]
Early adult onset			
	AR[b]	LL (Posterior)	Miyoshi et al.[50]
	AR	LL (Anterior)	Nonaka et al.[51]
Juvenile onset			
	AD	UL & LL (simultaneously)	Biemond[52]
Infantile onset			
	AD	LL	Magee and De Jong[53]

[a]Finnish tibial muscular dystrophy[54]; [b]serum creatine kinase levels very high. AD, autosomal dominant; AR, autosomal recessive; UL, upper limb; LL, lower limb.

Ocular and oculopharyngeal muscular dystrophies

Ocular muscular dystrophy, presenting as ptosis with ophthalmoplegia, is a recognized disease entity, but establishing the diagnosis may not always be clear on the basis of external ocular muscle histology alone. Furthermore, an ever-increasing number of other conditions associated with ophthalmoplegia are now being recognized, such as certain mitochondrial disorders (progressive external ophthalmoplegia and the Kearns–Sayre syndrome) and congenital myopathies (myotubular myopathy)[55].

The onset of ocular muscular dystrophy is usually in early adult life but may occasionally begin in infancy or even middle age. Ptosis is an early complaint and as a result the forehead is constantly wrinkled and the head tilted backwards to see beneath the drooping eyelids. This is sometimes referred to as the Hutchinsonian facies (Figure 9.8) after one of the earliest descriptions of ophthalmoplegia[56]. Eventually all eye movements become restricted but if both eyes are not equally affected then occasionally there may be some diplopia.

From a historical point of view the earliest clinical description of ptosis and ophthalmoplegia was given by Albrecht von Gräfe (or Graefe) (1828–1870) in 1868[57], a German ophthalmic surgeon whose name is now eponymously

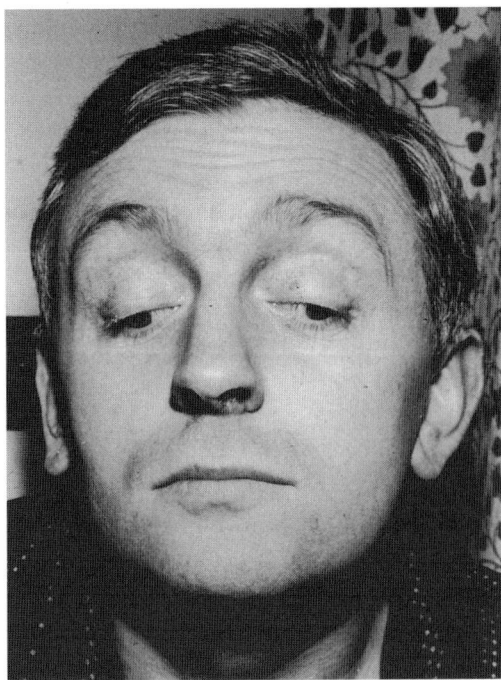

Fig. 9.8 Ocular muscular dystrophy.

associated with the eye sign in exophthalmia. In 1890, Ernst Fuchs (1851–1930) of Vienna provided a more detailed clinical description, including the muscle histology[58]. He first thought the histology might reflect a neurogenic basis, but subsequently decided that it was myopathic. Later, it became clear that weakness may also extend to the muscles of the neck and upper limbs, and the uniqueness of this type of dystrophy was emphasized[59].

It can be inherited as an autosomal dominant trait. The term oculopharyngeal muscular dystrophy is reserved for the disorder in which ocular involvement is associated with progressive dysphagia. This form of muscular dystrophy can also be inherited as an autosomal dominant trait and a large proportion of such cases have been of French Canadian extraction. This was first reported by Taylor in 1915[60]. Many cases in the United States can be traced back to French Canadians, the founder having arrived in Canada from France in 1634. The disorder, however, is not restricted to North America and Canada, but also occurs in France as well as various other European countries[61]. A similar condition, but with early onset, has been reported in Israel, inherited as an autosomal recessive trait[62].

Congenital muscular dystrophies

The early history of this type of dystrophy, which is present from birth, has been reviewed[63], and the first detailed report is that of Howard in the early nineteen-hundreds[64].

Four distinct forms of congenital muscular dystrophy were recognized, although it seems likely that there is heterogeneity even within some of these forms, and recent research has revealed additional forms. In all cases, the muscle pathology is that of dystrophy and all are inherited as autosomal recessive traits.

Firstly, there is the form characterized by exclusive involvement of skeletal muscle with hypotonia and weakness from birth, but with no apparent brain or eye abnormalities. Arthrogryposis may occur[63]. This is the commonest form in most countries outside Japan (Figure 9.9). In some cases the disease is progressive and motor development is severely affected, whereas in others the disease is less severe. The more severe cases are associated with a deficiency of *merosin*, a major component of the muscle extracellular matrix[65], now referred to as *laminin α2* (Chapter 13).

Another form has been described mainly in Finland and is associated with ocular (myopia, glaucoma, retinal atrophy) and central nervous system abnormalities (mental retardation, epilepsy, hydrocephalus). Hence it is sometimes referred to as muscle eye brain (MEB) disease[66]. There is some debate as to its

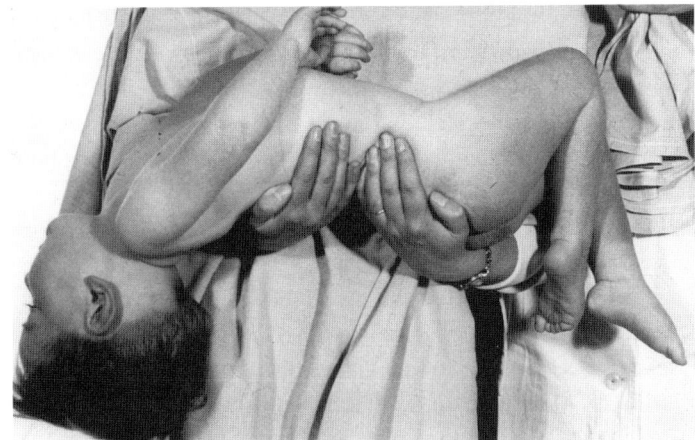

Fig. 9.9 Congenital muscular dystrophy in a 3-year-old boy. He has generalized hypotonia and retarded motor development and still cannot sit without support.

relationship with the Walker–Warburg syndrome and whether this is the same or a different condition.

A third, rare, form is associated with hyperextensibility of distal joints, contractures of proximal joints, high arched palate, hyperhidrosis, and posterior protrusion of the calcaneus, and is sometimes referred to as Ullrich disease[67,68].

Finally, in 1960 Fukuyama, then in the department of paediatrics in Tokyo, described a distinctive form of congenital muscular dystrophy which now bears his name[69–71].

Yukio Fukuyama (Figure 9.10) was born in Miyazaki, Japan in 1928. After high school he studied medicine at Tokyo University, graduating in 1952.

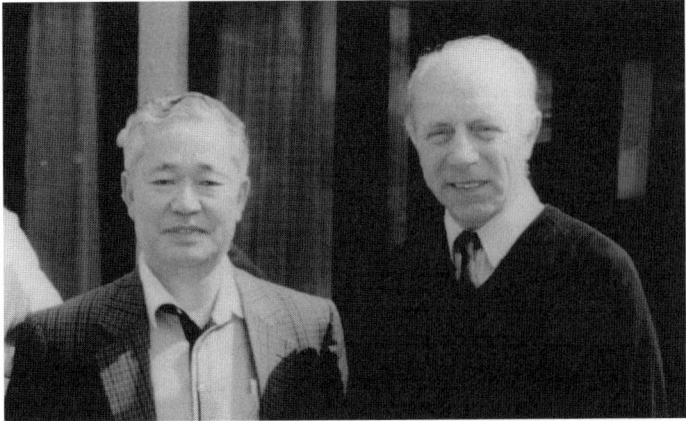

Fig. 9.10 Professor Yukio Fukuyama and the author (AEHE) at a 1993 meeting of the European Neuromuscular Centre in Baarn, The Netherlands.

After junior hospital appointments, he entered the graduate school of medicine where he carried out research under the guidance of the late Professor Tadao Takatsu, the renowned paediatrician. The latter immediately recognized Fukuyama's talents and promise, and encouraged him to specialize in child neurology. At the time this speciality hardly existed and almost all children with neurological problems were seen by general paediatricians. He became increasingly interested in infants and children with hypotonia and weakness, which included a great variety of conditions such as acute poliomyelitis, cerebral palsy, mental retardation, and, of course, Werdnig–Hoffmann's disease and muscular dystrophies. The investigation of such cases was now becoming more reliable, with the introduction of new diagnostic techniques, most notably electromyography (EMG) and serum enzyme studies. According to Simpson, in his history of electromyography:

> The many nerve and spinal injuries and the epidemics of poliomyelitis during and after the Second World War forced the development of electromyography in the assessment of paralyzed muscles in man (Ref. 72, page 84).

From the 1940s onwards the pioneering work of the Scandinavian Fritz Buchthal established the value of the technique in the diagnosis of myopathies and their differentiation from neurogenic disorders. Also at about this time Ebashi in Tokyo introduced a reliable method for measuring serum creatine kinase activity and demonstrated its value in diagnosing muscular dystrophy (Chapter 10).

Fukuyama applied both these techniques, along with muscle biopsy, to his paediatric patients with hypotonia and weakness, and in this way established a paediatric neurological diagnostic unit. In retrospect he now feels that it was the establishment of this armamentarium of diagnostic tools which led to his recognition of the distinctive form of congenital muscular dystrophy that now bears his name.

Fukuyama has played a major role in developing the speciality of child neurology in Japan. He has made a number of important and influential studies, most notably of infantile spasms, and has published widely on many other neurological problems of childhood[73]. He is now emeritus professor at the Tokyo Women's Medical College and continues with his lecturing and writing. What little spare time he has he devotes to philately and watching his favourite sport—baseball.

After Duchenne muscular dystrophy, Fukuyama type congenital muscular dystrophy is the next most frequent form of muscular dystrophy in Japan, but has rarely been reported elsewhere in the world. Although affected children learn to crawl, few are ever able to walk unaided. Calf pseudohypertrophy is common, as are joint contractures. All are mentally retarded, often severely so, and some have epilepsy, but there are no major ocular abnormalities. Many die in childhood but some have occasionally survived into their twenties.

Conclusions

The only unifying feature in all these various form of muscular dystrophy is a similar muscle pathology. But muscle as a tissue is limited in its response to injury, whether due to an environmental insult, such as viral infection, or a genetic defect as in the dystrophies. The similarity of the muscle pathology in the various dystrophies is therefore in no way an indication of a shared aetiology. In fact, evidence is accumulating that they are all caused by very different genetic defects (Chapter 13). Only time will tell, however, if all these different defects perhaps share a common feature in pathogenesis by, for example, affecting the integrity of the muscle cell membrane but in different ways. At present this is difficult to envisage because diseases included under this rubric vary so considerably in their onset, severity, and distribution of muscle involvement. At one extreme we have the rapidly progressive form of congenital muscular dystrophy which is present at birth with generalized muscle involvement and can lead to death in infancy or early childhood. At the other extreme there is ocular muscular dystrophy where onset is in adult life, and the disease is often limited to the extraocular muscles and may be no more than a minor inconvenience.

Among the various forms of dystrophy the only one related to Duchenne muscular dystrophy is Becker muscular dystrophy: the genetic defect in both conditions resides at Xp21, and affects the muscle protein dystrophin. However, this brief review of the relevant history of many other forms of dystrophy and their recognition in the history of the disease in general, will at least help place Duchenne muscular dystrophy in perspective, and perhaps explain why, for so long, there was so much confusion about nosology.

References

1. Becker, P. E. Living history biography: Peter Emil Becker. *American Journal of Medical Genetics*, 1985; **20**: 699–709.
2. Grimm, T. Peter Emil Becker zum 85. Geburtstag. *Medizinische Genetik*, 1993; **4**: 358–63.
3. Grimm, T. Peter Emil Becker on his 85th birthday. *Neuromuscular Disorders*, 1995; **5**: 243–7.
4. Becker, P. E. Die Einteilung der Muskeldystrophien (Ein Beitrag zur Systematik der 'Heredodegenerationen'). *Nervenarzt*, 1940; **13**: 209–14.
5. Becker, P. E. *Dystrophia Musculorum Progressiva, Eine genetische und klinische Untersuchung der Muskledystrophien*. Stuttgart: Georg Thieme Verlag, 1953.

6. Becker, P. E. (ed.) *Humangenetik. Ein kurzes Handbuch*. Vol. 1–11. Stuttgart: Georg Thieme Verlag, 1964–75.
7. Kostakow, S., Derix, F. Familienforschung in einer muskeldystrophischen Sippe und die Erbprognose ihrer Mitgleider. *Deutsches Archiv für klinische Medizin*, 1937; **180**: 586–606.
8. Becker, P. E., Kiener, F. Eine neue X-chromosomale Muskeldystrophie. *Archiv für Psychiatrie und Zeitschrift Neurologie*, 1955; **193**: 427–48. (See also: *Acta Genetica*, 1957; **7**: 303–10.)
9. Becker, P. E. Two new families of benign sex-linked recessive muscular dystrophy. *Revue Canadienne de Biologie*, 1962; **21**: 551–66.
10. Dreifuss, F. E., Hogan, G. R. Survival in X-chromosomal muscular dystrophy. *Neurology*, 1961; **11**: 734–7.
11. Emery, A. E. H., Dreifuss, F. E. Unusual type of benign X-linked muscular dystrophy. *Journal of Neurology, Neurosurgery and Psychiatry*, 1966; **29**: 338–42.
12. Emery, A. E. H. X-linked muscular dystrophy with early contractures and cardiomyopathy (Emery–Dreifuss type). *Clinical Genetics*, 1987; **32**: 360–7.
13. Emery, A. E. H. Emery–Dreifuss syndrome. *Journal of Medical Genetics*, 1989; **26**: 637–41.
14. Cestan, R., Lejonne, P. Une myopathie avec rétractions familiales. *Nouvelle Iconographie de la Salpêtrière*, 1902; **15**: 38–52. (See also: 1904; **17**: 343–53.)
15. Hauptmann, A., Thannhauser, S. J. Muscular shortening and dystrophy— a heredofamilial disease. *Archives of Neurology and Psychiatry*, 1941; **46**: 654–64.
16. Bione S., Maestrini E., Rivella S. *et al*. Identification of a novel X-linked gene responsible for Emery–Dreifuss muscular dystrophy. *Nature Genetics*, 1994; **8**: 323–7.
17. Munsat, T. L., Serratrice, G. Facioscapulohumeral and scapuloperoneal syndromes. In: L. P. Rowland and S. DiMauro (eds) *Handbook of Clinical Neurology, Vol. 18(62): Myopathies*. Amsterdam: Elsevier Science, 1992: 161–77.
18. Oransky, W. Über einen hereditären Typus progressiver Muskeldystrophie. *Deutsche Zeitschrift für Nervenheilkunde (Leipzig)*, 1927; **99**: 147–55.
19. Kazakov, V. M., Bogorodinsky, D. K., Skorometz, A. A. The myogenic scapulo-peroneal syndrome. Muscular dystrophy in the K. kindred: clinical study and genetics. *Clinical Genetics*, 1976; **10**: 41–50.
20. Thomas, P. K., Schott, G. D., Morgan-Hughes, J. A. Adult onset scapuloperoneal myopathy. *Journal of Neurology, Neurosurgery and Psychiatry*, 1975; **38**: 1008–15.
21. Mabry, C. C., Roeckel, I. E., Munich, R. L., Robertson, D. X-linked pseudohypertrophic muscular dystrophy with a late onset and slow progression. *New England Journal of Medicine*, 1965; **273**: 1062–70.
22. Wadia, R. S., Wadgaonkar, S. U., Amin, R. B., Sardesai, H. V. An unusual family of benign 'X' linked muscular dystrophy with cardiac involvement. *Journal of Medical Genetics*, 1976; **13**: 352–6.
23. Bergia, B., Sybers, H. D., Butler, I. J. Familial lethal cardiomyopathy with mental retardation and scapuloperoneal muscular dystrophy. *Journal of Neurology, Neurosurgery and Psychiatry*, 1986; **49**: 1423–6.
24. Ji, X-W., Tan, J., Chen, X-Y., Yi, S-X., Liang, H. New type of X-linked progressive muscular dystrophy involving shoulder girdle and back. *American Journal of Medical Genetics*, 1990; **37**: 209–12.

25. Gowers, W. R. *Pseudo-hypertrophic Muscular Paralysis: A Clinical Lecture.* London: J. & A. Churchill, 1879.
26. Stevenson, A. C. Muscular dystrophy in Northern Ireland: I. An account of the condition in 51 families. *Annals of Eugenics (London)*, 1953; **18**: 50–91.
27. Kloepfer, H. W., Talley, C. Autosomal recessive inheritance of Duchenne-type muscular dystrophy. *Acta Genetica*, 1957; **7**: 314–18.
28. Dubowitz, V. Progressive muscular dystrophy of the Duchenne type in females and its mode of inheritance. *Brain*, 1960; **83**: 432–9.
29. Zatz, M., Passos-Bueno, M. R., Rapaport, D. Estimate of the proportion of Duchenne muscular dystrophy with autosomal recessive inheritance. *American Journal of Medical Genetics*, 1989; **32**: 407–10.
30. Ben Hamida, M., Fardeau, M., Attia, N. Severe childhood muscular dystrophy affecting both sexes and frequent in Tunisia. *Muscle and Nerve*, 1983; **6**: 469–80.
31. Skyring, A., McKusick, V. A. Clinical, genetic, and electrocardiographic studies in childhood muscular dystrophy. *American Journal of Medical Sciences*, 1961; **242**: 534–47.
32. Emery, A. E. H. Abnormalities of the electrocardiogram in hereditary myopathies. *Journal of Medical Genetics*, 1972; **9**: 8–12.
33. Matsumura, K., Tomé, F. M. S., Collin, H. *et al.* Deficiency of the 50K dystrophin-associated glycoprotein in severe childhood autosomal recessive muscular dystrophy. *Nature*, 1992; **359**: 320–2.
34. Blyth, H., Pugh, R. J. Muscular dystrophy in childhood, the genetic aspect. *Annals of Human Genetics*, 1959; **23**: 127–63.
35. Moser, H., Wiesmann, U., Richterich, R., Rossi, E. Progressive Muskeldystrophie, VIII. Häufigkeit, Klinik und Genetik der Typen I und II. *Schweizerische Medizinische Wochenschrift*, 1966; **96**: 169–74.
36. Jackson, C. E., Strehler, D. A. Limb-girdle muscular dystrophy: clinical manifestations and detection of preclinical disease. *Pediatrics*, 1968; **41**: 495–502. (See also: *Pediatrics*, 1961; **28**: 77–84.)
37. Beckmann, J. S., Richard, I., Hillaire, D. *et al.* A gene for limb-girdle muscular dystrophy maps to chromosome 15 by linkage. *Comptes Rendus de l'Académie des Sciences, Serie III (Paris)*, 1991; **312**: 141–8.
38. Yates, J. R. W., Emery, A. E. H. A population study of adult onset limb girdle muscular dystrophy. *Journal of Medical Genetics*, 1985; **22**: 250–7.
39. Nevin, S. Two cases of muscular degeneration occurring in late adult life, with a review of the recorded cases of late progressive muscular dystrophy (late progressive myopathy). *Quarterly Journal of Medicine*, 1936; **29**: 51–68.
40. Henson, T. E., Muller, J., De Myer, W. E. Hereditary myopathy limited to females. *Archives of Neurology*, 1967; **17**: 238–47.
41. De Coster, W., De Reuck, J., Thiery, E. A late onset autosomal dominant form of limb-girdle muscular dystrophy. A clinical, genetic and morphological study. *European Neurology*, 1974; **12**: 159–72.
42. Gilchrist, J. M., Pericak-Vance, M., Silverman, L., Roses, A. D. Clinical and genetic investigation in autosomal dominant limb-girdle muscular dystrophy. *Neurology*, 1988; **38**: 5–9.

43. Kryschowa, N., Abowjan, W. Zur Frage der Heredität der Pseudohypertrophie Duchenne. *Zeitschrift für die gesamte Neurologie*, 1934; **150**: 421–6.
44. Emery, A. E. H., Walton, J. N. The genetics of muscular dystrophy. *Progress in Medical Genetics*, 1967; **5**: 116–45.
45. Emery, A. E. H. Clinical manifestations in two carriers of Duchenne muscular dystrophy. *Lancet*, 1963; **i**: 1126–1128. (See also: Pegoraro, E. et al. *American Journal of Human Genetics*, 1994; **54**: 989–1003.)
46. Gowers, W. R. A lecture on myopathy and a distal form. *British Medical Journal*, 1902; **ii**: 89–92.
47. Welander, L. Myopathia distalis tarda hereditaria. *Acta Medica Scandinavica*, 1951; **141**(Suppl. 265): 1–124.
48. Welander, L. Homozygous appearance of distal myopathy, *Acta Genetica (Basel)*, 1957; **7**: 321–5.
49. Markesbery, W. R., Griggs, R. C., Leach, R. P., Lapham, L. W. Late onset hereditary distal myopathy. *Neurology*, 1974; **24**: 127–34. (See also: *Neurology*, 1977; **27**: 727–35.)
50. Miyoshi, K., Kawai, H., Iwasa, M., Kusaka, K., Nishino, H. Autosomal recessive distal muscular dystrophy as a new type of progressive muscular dystrophy. *Brain*, 1986; **109**: 31–54.
51. Nonaka, I., Sunohara, N., Ishiura, S., Satayoshi, E. Familial distal myopathy with rimmed vacuole and lamellar (myeloid) body formation. *Journal of the Neurological Sciences*, 1981; **51**: 141–55. (See also: *Annals of Neurology*, 1985; **17**: 51–9.)
52. Biemond, A. Myopathia distalis juvenilis hereditaria. *Acta Psychiatrica Neurologica Scandinavica*, 1955; **30**: 25–38.
53. Magee, K. R., De Jong, R. N. Hereditary distal myopathy with onset in infancy. *Archives of Neurology*, 1965; **13**: 387–90.
54. Udd, B. Limb-girdle type muscular dystrophy in a large family with distal myopathy: homozygous manifestation of a dominant gene. *Journal of Medical Genetics*, 1992; **29**: 383–9.
55. Rowland, L. P. Progressive external ophthalmoplegia and ocular myopathies. In: L. P. Rowland and S. Di Mauro (eds) *Handbook of Clinical Neurology. Vol. 18 (62): Myopathies*. Amsterdam: Elsevier Science, 1992: 287–329.
56. Hutchinson, J. On ophthalmoplegia externa or symmetrical immobility (partial) of the eyes, with ptosis. *Medico-Chirurgical Transactions*, 1879; **62**: 307–29.
57. von Gräfe, A. Verhandlungen ärztlicher Gesellschaften. *Berliner klinische Wochenschrift*, 1868; **5**: 125–7.
58. Fuchs, E. Ueber isolirte doppelseitige Ptosis. *von Graefe's Archiv für Ophthalmologie*, 1890; **36**: 234–59.
59. Kiloh, L. G., Nevin, S. Progressive dystrophy of the external ocular muscles (ocular myopathy). *Brain*, 1951; **74**: 115–43.
60. Taylor, E. W. Progressive vagus-glossopharyngeal paralysis with ptosis. A contribution to the group of family diseases. *Journal of Nervous and Mental Disease*, 1915; **42**: 129–39.
61. Brunet, G., Tomé, F. M. S., Samson, F., Robert, J. M., Fardeau, M. Dystrophie musculaire oculo-pharyngée recensement des familles Françaises et étude généalogique. *Revue Neurologique*, 1990; **146**: 425–9.

62. Fried, K., Arlozorov, A., Spira, R. Autosomal recessive oculopharyngeal muscular dystrophy. *Journal of Medical Genetics*, 1975; **12**: 416–418.
63. Banker, B. Q., Victor, M., Adams, R. D. Arthrogryposis multiplex due to congenital muscular dystrophy. *Brain*, 1957; **80**: 319–34.
64. Howard, R. A case of congenital defect of the muscular system (Dystrophia muscularis congenita) and its association with congenital talipes equino-varus. *Proceedings of the Royal Society of Medicine (London)*, 1907–8; **1**: 157–66.
65. Tomé, F. M. S., Evangelista, T., Leclerc, A. *et al.* Congenital muscular dystrophy with merosin deficiency. *Comptes Rendus de l'Académie des Sciences (Paris)*, 1994; **317**: 351–7.
66. Santavuori, F., Leisti, J., Kruus, S. Muscle, eye and brain disease: a new syndrome. *Neuropädiatrie*, 1977; **8** (Suppl.): 553. (See also: Raitta, J. *et al. Acta Ophthalmologica*, 1978; **56**: 465–72.)
67. Ullrich, O. Kongenitale, atonisch-sklerotische Muskel-dystrophie. *Monatsschrift für Kinderheilkunde*, 1930; **47**: 502–10. (See also: *Zentralblatt für die gesamte Neurologie und Psychiatrie*, 1930; **126**: 171–201.)
68. Furukawa, T., Toyokura, Y. Congenital, hypotonic-sclerotic muscular dystrophy. *Journal of Medical Genetics*, 1977; **14**: 426–9.
69. Fukuyama, Y., Kawazura, M., Haruna, H. A peculiar form of congenital progressive muscular dystrophy. Report of 15 cases. *Paediatria Universitatis Tokyo*, 1960; **4**: 5–8.
70. Fukuyama, Y., Osawa, M., Suzuki, H. Congenital progressive muscular dystrophy of the Fukuyama type—clinical, genetic, and pathological considerations. *Brain and Development*, 1981; **3**: 1–29.
71. Fukuyama, Y., Ohsawa, M. A genetic study of the Fukuyama type congenital muscular dystrophy. *Brain and Development*, 1984; **6**: 373–90.
72. Simpson, J. A. The development of electromyography and neurography for diagnosis. *Journal of the History of the Neurosciences*, 1993; **2**: 81–105.
73. Kamoshita, S. Yukio Fukuyama. In: S. Ashwal (ed.) *The Founders of Child Neurology*. San Francisco: Norman Publishing, 1990: 726–31.

Chapter 10

Biochemical diagnosis and carrier detection

By the late 1950s, the X-linked mode of inheritance of Duchenne muscular dystrophy had been firmly established and it was now clear that healthy females could carry the mutant gene and thereby have affected sons. But unless a mother had an affected maternal relative as well as an affected son there was no certainty as to her carrier status. If a mother had two affected sons she was likely to be a carrier but there was also the remote possibility that she and her husband could be heterozygous for the autosomal recessive dystrophy which resembled Duchenne's disease. Also, if she had only one affected son and no one else in the family was affected she might possibly be a carrier, but on the other hand she might not, her affected son being the result of a new mutation. Finally, the carrier status of sisters of affected boys was never certain until they themselves had an affected son. A search therefore began to find a test which would detect female carriers of the disease.

The obvious approach at this time was to find a significant biochemical or other abnormality in affected boys (preferably demonstrable in an accessible tissue such as blood) and then determine if this same abnormality occurred, but doubtless to a lesser extent, in female carriers. It was generally recognized that the closer such an abnormality might be to the basic defect in the disease, the more successful it would be in carrier detection. But there was an important biological consideration which was not always appreciated at the time.

In the early 1960s, Mary Lyon of Harwell[1,2] proposed that in any cell (apart from oocytes) of a normal female, only one of her X chromosomes was active, the other being inactive. This process of random inactivation occurred early in development and affected either X chromosome, but once a particular X chromosome in a particular cell was inactivated, the same X chromosome became inactive in all its descendant cells. This became known as the Lyon hypothesis, for which a great deal of supportive evidence has since accumulated. It has important implications when considering carrier detection tests in X-linked disorders. In occasional carriers by chance the active X chromosome in most cells might be the one bearing the normal gene. Such carriers would then be very difficult to detect unless by some biochemical method that employed cloned cells to identify two populations of cells, and this was not attempted until many years later. Any other type of test would never be able to detect all carriers. Over the next few years claims for detection rates approaching 100% were sometimes made but clearly for these reasons this could never be true. Furthermore, it would be impossible by such tests to determine the false positive rate.

Serum enzymes

Jean-Claude Dreyfus (Figure 10.1) was born in Rouen in 1916 where he attended school, and later became a medical student in Paris. He graduated in 1941 but in 1942 was dismissed from his hospital appointment because he was Jewish and sent to Buchenwald. After the war his interest in muscle disease was initially fired by the influential professor of paediatrics in Paris, Robert Debré. Debré had started studying the biochemistry of muscle disease in the 1930s and foresaw the importance of the subject at a time when it was attracting very little attention. In 1945 he created a laboratory at the Hôpital des Enfants-Malades to be specifically devoted to the subject and invited Dreyfus and Georges Schapira to develop the field. Schapira was born in 1912 and obtained his MD degree in Paris in the same year as Dreyfuss; later, he also obtained a PhD in biochemistry and was one of the first in the new generation of clinical chemists. Dreyfus retired to live in Paris, where he died in 1995.

It was the collaboration between Dreyfus and Schapira, along with the latter's wife, Fanny Schapira, which proved so important in the early biochemical

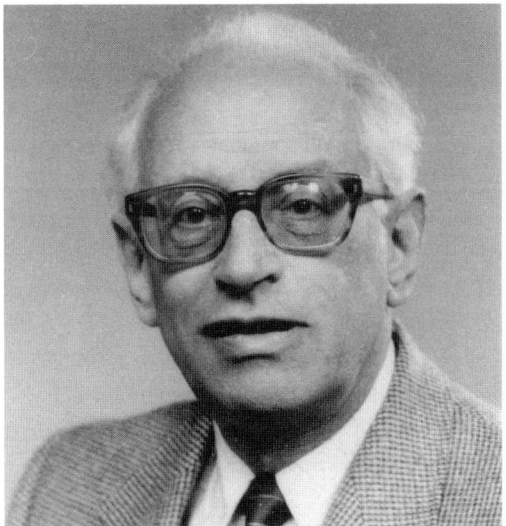

Fig. 10.1 Jean-Claude Dreyfus.

studies of dystrophy, and particularly in the development of serum enzyme tests for detecting preclinical cases and carriers of Duchenne dystrophy. Their fruitful research into the biochemistry of muscle disease lasted many years, and for their work Dreyfus and Schapira were jointly awarded the Grand Prix de la Fondation pour la Recherche Médicale Française.

Dreyfus and Schapira began by studying muscle glycolysis in dystrophy since at the time this seemed an obvious way to look for the cause of the disease. However, in 1949 Sibley and Lehninger[3] published a convenient method for determining serum aldolase activity and subsequently found elevated levels in patients with various cancers and other disorders, the latter including two patients with muscular dystrophy[4]. The recognition by Dreyfus and Schapira of the importance of this chance finding pays great credit to their perspicacity since Sibley and Lehninger's paper was almost exclusively concerned with cancer. Dreyfus and the Schapiras subsequently confirmed the finding in a series of patients with muscular dystrophy[5]. This was to prove a singularly important observation. Up to this time the only *consistent* reported biochemical abnormalities in dystrophy were generalized aminoaciduria and an increased urinary excretion of creatine and decreased excretion of creatinine, changes which were accepted as merely being the result of muscle breakdown.

Following their original publication in 1953[5], over the next few years Dreyfus and his colleagues investigated the serum levels of several enzymes in dystrophy[6] and found that the level was 2.4 times normal for phosphohexoisomerase, 3.3 for glutamic oxalacetic transaminase, 3.8 for lactate dehydrogenase, 5.2 for glutamic pyruvic transaminase, and approaching 10 times normal for aldolase. The reason for these differences was not clear at the time, but this increase in serum enzyme activity represented the first biochemical abnormality detectable in blood in dystrophy. Furthermore, they found that the levels in Duchenne muscular dystrophy were much higher than in other forms of dystrophy. Finally, and most significantly, such elevations in serum enzyme activities did not occur to anywhere near the same extent in neurogenic disorders such as spinal muscular atrophy.

These early studies of Dreyfus and his colleagues stressed the importance of serum enzyme levels in the diagnosis of dystrophy as well as the potential for *preclinical diagnosis.* But they were also aware that their findings could have a bearing on the pathophysiology and cause of the disease[7]. This we shall return to later.

The problem with using the serum levels of these enzymes for diagnosis, however, was their lack of specificity and even with aldolase there was overlap with normal values. A more specific and sensitive test was required. This was provided by creatine kinase.

This enzyme, which is particularly abundant in muscle tissue, catalyses the transfer of a phosphate group from adenosine triphosphate to creatine, a reaction exploited in muscle contraction. In 1958 Dr Setsuro Ebashi and colleagues, including Dr Hideo Sugita, decided to examine serum levels of creatine kinase activity in dystrophy. Their results were published the following year[8] and indicated that this was clearly the most sensitive test for dystrophy. These findings were soon confirmed by Dreyfus[9] and his colleagues, and the use of this enzyme in diagnosis was another landmark in the history of Duchenne muscular dystrophy.

Subsequently, other groups throughout the world substantiated these findings. Even at birth, and before the disease becomes clinically evident, serum levels of creatine kinase were found to be considerably elevated—up to 100 times higher. In the early stages of Becker muscular dystrophy, similarly high levels were found. Very few other conditions are associated with such high levels, and it therefore became an essential diagnostic test for these disorders.

In the same year that they reported significantly elevated serum levels of creatine kinase in muscular dystrophy patients, the Japanese investigators also reported that a proportion of healthy *female carriers* of Duchenne muscular dystrophy also had raised levels[10], and the following year this too was confirmed by the Paris group[11]. Both Ebashi and Sugita have made many other contributions to neuromuscular research ever since. Professor Setsuro Ebashi (1922–2006) graduated in medicine from Tokyo University in 1944 and, on retirement, became professor emeritus, University of Tokyo. Over the years he received many honours and awards for his research, including foreign membership of the Royal Society of London and the American Physiological Society (Figure 10.2).

Professor Hideo Sugita (born 1930) graduated in medicine in 1954, also from Tokyo University. From 1961 to 1963 he was a research fellow in neurology with Frank Tyler at the University of Utah, at which time he taught the author (AEHE) the vagaries of creatine kinase assay. He retired in 1998 and is now president emeritus of the National Centre of Neurology and Psychiatry in Tokyo, but remains actively involved in the ethical and financial aspects of intractable diseases. He is a foreign member of the Royal Society of Medicine of London and the Gaetano Conte Academy of Italy (Figure 10.3).

Carrier detection

The reports of the Japanese and French groups of significantly raised levels of serum creatine kinase in female carriers of Duchenne muscular dystrophy was excitedly welcomed by all working in the field. After all, this now provided a means of determining the carrier status of female relatives *before* they had an

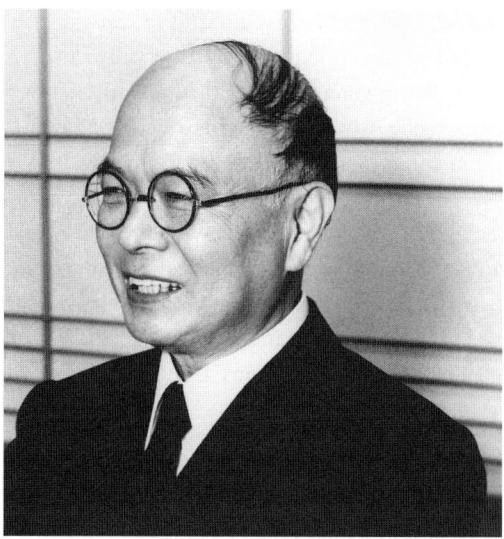

Fig. 10.2 Professor Setsuro Ebashi.

affected son. Its importance cannot be over-emphasized and it had a profound effect on genetic counselling. Over the next few years various groups determined the detection rate in known carriers. Overall, this turned out to be around 70%[12]. But this meant that 30% of definite carriers did not have a significantly raised level. This posed a serious problem for, if a suspected carrier had a level within the normal range, then there was no certainty as to her carrier status. As a result, various attempts were made to improve the detection rate, though it had to be appreciated that this could never approach 100% (for reasons mentioned earlier). Since the serum level of creatine kinase is raised by physical exertion,

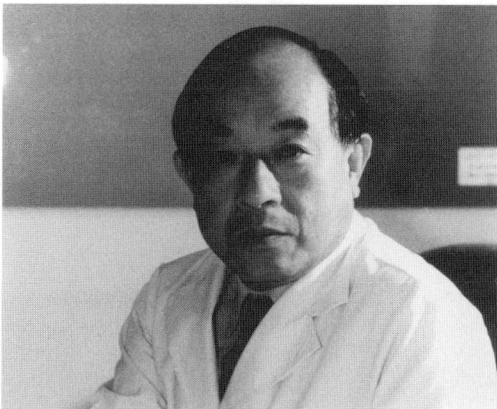

Fig. 10.3 Professor Hideo Sugita.

attempts were made to determine if standardized exercise might improve the detection rate[12]. Others combined the results of the creatine kinase test with other serum enzyme levels, such as pyruvate kinase, or serum proteins such as myoglobin or haemopexin. Abnormalities in muscle histology and histochemistry were reported in some carriers, and the results of such investigations were combined with serum enzyme levels to improve the detection rate. Yet others suggested that electromyography might provide a valuable adjunct to other tests in carrier detection. Such work occupied many investigators right up to the time the defective gene was identified in the mid 1980s[13]. However, none of these approaches proved to be a significant improvement on the serum level of creatine kinase alone, provided the test was carried out by an experienced investigator.

Bayesian statistics

Another problem was that serum levels of creatine kinase in both normal women and carriers were not normally distributed but positively skewed. Methods for normalizing the data were therefore important. Furthermore, it became obvious that it would be more informative to base risk (or probability) estimates on pedigree data as well as serum creatine kinase data. But there seemed no simple way of combining information on the particular level of creatine kinase which was within the normal range with, say, the fact that a woman's affected son might be the result of a new mutation since no one else in the family was affected. Credit for having solved this problem should go to Edmond A. (Tony) Murphy. He was born in 1925 in Swansea, Wales, did his medical training at Queen's University Belfast, and by the late 1950s had joined Victor McKusick in the Moore Clinic at Johns Hopkins (Figure 10.4). His ScD

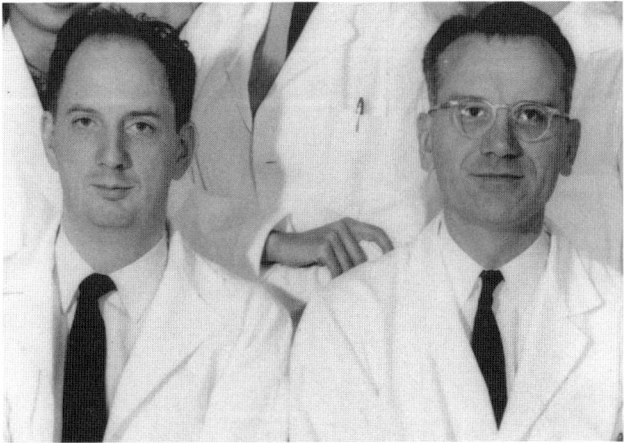

Fig. 10.4 E. A. (Tony) Murphy (left) and Victor A. McKusick, photographed in the Moore Clinic around 1964.

thesis in 1964, entitled *An Exploration of Some Effects of Incomplete Penetrance on the Ascertainment of Recessive Characteristics*, reflected Murphy's fascination with statistical problems in medical genetics. The muscular dystrophies in fact provided him with a group of disorders that illustrated very well some of these problems.

His work, he stated, continued to be his major hobby, and understanding the pathogenesis of genetic disease remained a passion with him throughout his life, along with his love for the piano (which he claimed to play with 'ashamed mediocrity… mostly from Haydn to Fauré') (Figure 10.5), foreign languages, and medical philosophy. He became a full professor with a joint appointment in biostatistics and medicine in 1974. Upon his retirement with emeritus status in 1994, he went to live with his niece and nephew near Barcelona, Spain, where he died in January 2009. He never married.

When he began his work at Hopkins, it became evident that Murphy was one of those rare people who could accommodate more than one discipline: he was a physician as well as an accomplished mathematical statistician. He argued that the answer to many important problems in medical genetics could

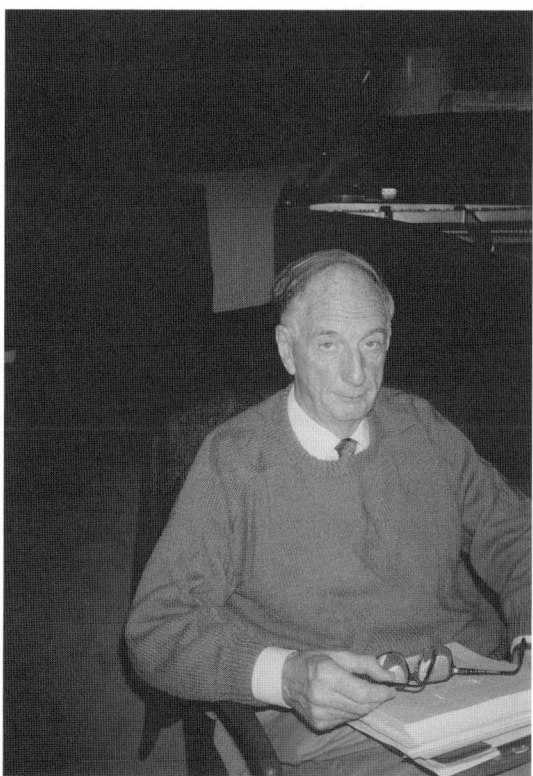

Fig. 10.5 Edmond A. (Tony) Murphy.

be found in the method of calculating probabilities first introduced by Thomas Bayes (1702–1761), an English clergyman and mathematician.

When considering the probability of an individual having a particular genotype (preclinical case or a heterozygous carrier), it had been customary to base such calculations only on 'anterior' information; that is, the *prior* probability based on knowledge of the individual's antecedents and sibs. But Murphy emphasized that this ignored information based on the individual's phenotype (clinical findings and test results) and that of any of the individual's offspring. Such information could be included in so-called *conditional* probabilities. In the case of Duchenne dystrophy, the conditional probabilities would be of a woman being a carrier or not depending on her serum creatine kinase level and, for example, the number of normal sons she may have had. The product of the prior and conditional probabilities was termed the *joint* probability. The final *posterior* probability of an individual having a particular genotype was the *joint* probability of getting the observed information given the genotype in question (e.g. a carrier), divided by the sum of this probability and the joint probability of getting the observed information if the individual was normal (e.g. not a carrier). The expression of posterior probabilities in terms of prior and conditional probabilities is attributed to Bayes, whose theorem was published posthumously by his wife in 1763[14].

The use of Bayesian statistics in risk calculations and similar problems in medical genetics was first introduced by Murphy at the 3rd International Congress of Human Genetics in Chicago in 1966[15]. Details were subsequently published in 1969[16] and much expanded in his *Principles of Genetic Counselling*[17]. We demonstrated its particular value in a lethal X-linked disorder such as Duchenne muscular dystrophy[18]. The use of Bayesian methods in genetic risk calculation has been widely used in counselling ever since. But in the case of Duchenne muscular dystrophy the problem still remained that, although risk estimates could be refined in this way, it was never going to be possible to completely reassure a woman at risk that she was definitely *not* a carrier. This would only become possible with the advent of DNA technology.

However, the fact that muscle enzymes were detectable at increased levels in the serum of patients with dystrophy was not only of practical value in diagnosis and counselling, but suggested that the muscle membrane was perhaps defective in some way. At this time, Zierler showed that when isolated mouse or rat muscle was incubated in Ringer solution, aldolase leaked into the medium, and this was particularly marked with muscle from a dystrophic mouse[19,20]. That the muscle membrane in dystrophy was in some way 'leaky' was an important observation. It had been suggested by Meryon many years previously (Chapter 3) that the sarcolemma was broken down and destroyed in the disease, and there was now biochemical evidence which seemed to support this idea. A rational approach to investigating the cause and pathogenesis of the disease was beginning.

References

1. Lyon, M. F. Gene action in the X-chromosome of the mouse. *(Mus musculus* L.). *Nature*, 1961; **190**: 372–3.
2. Lyon, M. F. Sex chromatin and gene action in the mammalian X-chromosome. *American Journal of Human Genetics*, 1962; **14**: 135–48.
3. Sibley, J. A., Lehninger, A. L. Determination of aldolase in animal tissues. *Journal of Biological Chemistry*, 1949a; **177**: 859–72.
4. Sibley, J. A., Lehninger, A. L. Aldolase in the serum and tissues of tumour-bearing animals. *Journal of the National Cancer Institute*, 1949b; **9**: 303–9.
5. Schapira, G., Dreyfus, J. C., Schapira, F. L'élévation du taux de l'aldolase sérique, test biochimique des myopathies. *Semaine des Hôpitaux, Paris*, 1953; **29**: 1917–20.
6. Dreyfus, J-C., Schapira, G., Schapira, F., Démos, J. Activités enzymatiques du muscle humaine. *Clinica Chimica Acta*, 1956; **1**: 434–49. (See also: Dreyfus, J-C., Schapira, G., Schapira, F. Serum enzymes in the physiopathology of muscle. *Annals of the New York Academy of Sciences*, 1958; **75**: 235–49.)
7. Dreyfus, J-C., Schapira, G. *Biochemistry of Hereditary Myopathies*. Springfield, Illinois: Charles C. Thomas, 1962.
8. Ebashi, S., Toyokura, Y., Momoi, H., Sugita, H. High creatine phosphokinase activity of sera of progressive muscular dystrophy. *Journal of Biochemistry*, 1959; **46**: 103–4.
9. Dreyfus, J-C., Schapira, G., Démos, J. Étude de la créatine-kinase sérique chez les myopathes et leurs familles. *Revue Française Étude Clinique et Biologique*, 1960; **5**: 384–6.
10. Okinaka, S., Sugita, H., Momoi, H., Toyokura, Y., Kumagai, H., Ebashi, S., Fujie, Y. Serum creatine phosphokinase and aldolase activity in neuromuscular disorders. *Transactions of the American Neurological Association*, 1959; **84**: 62–64 (84th Annual Meeting, Atlantic City).
11. Schapira, F., Dreyfus, J-C., Schapira, G., Démos, J. Étude de l'aldolase et de la créatine kinase du sérum chez les mères de myopathes. *Revue Française Études Clinique et Biologique*, 1960; **5**: 990–4.
12. Emery, A. E. H. The use of serum creatine kinase for detecting carriers of Duchenne muscular dystrophy. In: A. T. Milhorat (ed.) *Exploratory Concepts in Muscular Dystrophy and Related Disorders*. Amsterdam: Excerpta Medica, 1967: 90–7.
13. Emery, A. E. H. *Duchenne Muscular Dystrophy*, 2nd edn. Oxford: Oxford University Press, 1993: 217–28.
14. Bayes, T. An essay toward solving a problem in the doctrine of chances. *Philosophical Transactions*, 1763; **53**: 376–418.
15. Murphy, E. A., Mutalik, G. S., Eldridge, R. The application of Bayesian methods in genetic counselling. *Proceedings of the 3rd International Congress of Human Genetics, Chicago*, 1966; 70.
16. Murphy, E. A., Mutalik, G. S. The application of Bayesian methods in genetic counselling. *Human Heredity*, 1969; **19**: 126–51.

17. Murphy, E. A., Chase, G. A. *Principles of Genetic Counselling.* Chicago: Year Book Medical Publishers, 1975.
18. Emery, A. E. H., Morton, R. Genetic counselling in lethal X-linked disorders. *Acta Genetica (Basel)*, 1968; **18**: 534–42.
19. Zierler, K. L. Muscle membrane as a dynamic structure and its permeability to aldolase. *Annals of the New York Academy of Sciences*, 1958a; **75**: 227–34.
20. Zierler, K. L. Aldolase leak from muscle of mice with hereditary muscular dystrophy. *Bulletin of the Johns Hopkins Hospital*, 1958b; **102**: 17–20.

Chapter 11

Pathogenesis of Duchenne dystrophy

Over the years the history of Duchenne muscular dystrophy has been replete with suggestions as to its cause. Early on, some believed a defect in muscle nutrition might be responsible as was implied in the term *dystrophy* (from the Greek, 'faulty nutrition'). Another suggestion was the possibility of a circulating toxic factor which in some way damaged the muscle. But little, if any, supporting evidence was ever forthcoming for any of these ideas. By the early 1960s it was clear that the answer would only come from carefully planned and executed research.

Until the advent of DNA technology in the 1980s, the tools for investigating the possible cause of muscular dystrophy were limited to electromyography, muscle histology, and histochemistry and biochemistry. Each of these techniques was used by their proponents in attempts to understand the basic underlying defect in the disease.

As we shall see in Chapter 13, current ideas of pathogenesis are now firmly centred on biochemical and related pathways. But at the beginning, the field was dominated by neurologists and, since neurological practice is often concerned with *locating the site* of a pathological lesion within the nervous system, so the emphasis in seeking the cause of dystrophy often centred on the possible *location* of the defect—be it in the nerve supply to the muscle, or its blood supply, or in the muscle itself.

Many geneticists, however, held a different philosophy: because the basic defect was genetic and the same genes were present in every cell of the body, so the defect might be expressed by any tissue, given the right conditions for its expression. However, for almost 20 years most research was directed toward a search for a possible location of the basic defect and primary abnormality.

Neurogenic basis of dystrophy

Stemming from the early work of Buchthal and Kugelberg in the 1940s[1,2], the diagnostic importance of electromyography gradually became established. The technique usually involved recording motor units or action potentials using a fine concentric needle electrode inserted into the muscle. From the 1950s, methods of amplifying and recording these potentials improved[3] and within 10 years this was established as an important diagnostic technique. In particular, it could be used to differentiate muscular dystrophy from neurogenic causes of muscle wasting and weakness. In dystrophy the characteristic features on electromyography were action potentials of reduced duration and amplitude, and an increased frequency of polyphasics.

One refinement was to use the technique to estimate the number of functioning motor units in a muscle. This could be achieved by determining the average amplitude of a *single* motor unit potential produced by stimulating the nerve supply to the muscle, and then comparing this with the amplitude of the potential produced by a *maximal* stimulus of the nerve, the muscle responses being recorded in this instance using surface electrodes. An estimate of the number of motor units in the muscle was obtained by dividing the maximal amplitude by the average amplitude of single potentials. Using this technique, McComas and colleagues from Newcastle published a paper in the journal *Nature* in 1970 in which they claimed that in the *extensor digitorum brevis* muscle of the foot there was a significant reduction in the number of motor units in Duchenne dystrophy[4]. The authors suggested that this indicated a loss of functioning motor neurones in dystrophy, and that 'the primary abnormality in muscular dystrophy may lie in the motor nerve supply'. So developed the concept of the so-called *sick motor neurone* with the implication that the disease might be due to a deficiency of some neurotrophic factor. Such a mechanism, its advocates argued, might also explain the association of the disease with intellectual impairment.

This report stimulated much research activity but the concept soon faced serious problems, most notably that the methodology used by McComas and the interpretation of his results were questionable. In fact, many of the papers presented at the *Third International Congress on Muscle Diseases* held in Newcastle in September 1974 addressed such matters[5]. Over the next few years a consensus emerged that a neurogenic basis for the disorder was most unlikely.

Vascular hypothesis

Since Duchenne's time, the idea had occasionally been entertained that the disease might have a vascular basis. In the early 1960s, Démos and colleagues in France claimed to have demonstrated abnormalities in the blood supply to the muscles in affected boys as well as in some carriers, though no one succeeded in reproducing these findings. Later, King Engel in the United States was impressed by the apparent *clustering* of necrotic muscle fibres in the disease and suggested this might be due to local ischaemia, and reproduced similar findings in experimental animals by a variety of techniques, including aortic ligation and the injection of vasoactive agents[6]. However, the validity and relevance of these findings to the cause of dystrophy were also seriously questioned at the Congress in Newcastle[7], and most investigators later abandoned the idea of a vascular basis for the disorder.

The neurogenic and vascular hypotheses are of historical interest but neither added anything to our knowledge of pathogenesis. This would benefit more from the biochemical study of affected muscle tissue.

Muscle biochemistry

As the possible neurogenic or vascular basis of the disease was being investigated, others turned their attention to the possible biochemical defect in the disorder. After all, this seemed to offer the most logical and direct approach to the problem.

At this point mention should be made of the help provided by the study of various animal analogues. The first of these was a mouse mutant described by Michelson in 1955 (she was then a student working at the Jackson Memorial Research Laboratory, Bar Harbor, Maine), which became known as the Bar Harbor *dy* 129 strain[8]. But results from this mutant have sometimes been misleading since we now know that it is equivalent to a congenital rather than Duchenne form of muscular dystrophy in humans. In 1984 an X-linked mouse mutant *(mdx)* was discovered by Bulfield. This more closely resembled Duchenne muscular dystrophy[9], but the disorder identified in the dog was recognized as being perhaps a better model[10]. Biochemical and other studies in these last two animal models have benefited a great deal our understanding of the disease in humans. Currently, however, there are at least 12 other naturally occurring or genetically engineered mouse models of the muscular dystrophies[11].

The basis for studying the biochemistry of affected muscle, and in particular the search for an *enzymatic defect,* stemmed from the work of Archibald Garrod (1857–1936) and the biochemical basis of inherited diseases[12,13]. Garrod's influential work, embodied in the Croonian Lectures at the beginning of the century and subsequently expanded in his book[14], developed the idea of *inborn errors of metabolism*. Ultimately this led to Beadle and Tatum's concept of *one gene—one enzyme* in the 1940s[15,16] (although the work initiated by Pauling in 1949[17] on haemoglobin defects broadened the concept to *one gene—one polypeptide*). The work of Garrod, Beadle, and Tatum established that metabolic processes proceed in steps, each step being controlled by an enzyme which itself is the product of a particular gene. A defect in the latter would therefore produce a *metabolic block* with the accumulation of metabolites before the block and a reduction in metabolites after the block. The investigation of the basic cause of a genetic disease thought to have a metabolic basis, therefore, involved searching for the accumulation of a metabolite which would then provide a clue as to the specific enzymatic defect in the disorder. For example, in 1934 Asbjörn Fölling (1888–1972) observed increased amounts of phenyl pyruvic acid in the urine of children with a condition later to be called phenylketonuria. This provided a clue as to the possible enzymatic defect in the disorder which was subsequently identified by G. A. Jervis in 1953[18].

In the late 1950s, among the influential texts of the period was Harris' *Human Biochemical Genetics*[19], where he states:

> The unusual concentrations of metabolites in the body fluids and excretions, and the various clinical signs and symptoms with which they might be associated, could all ultimately be traced back to the inability to perform [a] single step in the metabolic sequence (Ref. 19, page 5).

Even then Harris recognized that not every metabolic condition could be simply the result of an enzyme deficiency, and that some could be due to other mechanisms such as defects in renal tubular reabsorption, end organ unresponsiveness, and so on. Nevertheless, it was generally accepted that:

> the manifold biochemical and clinical characteristics of many inherited metabolic disorders can be ultimately traced back to the effects of a single specific enzyme deficiency remains the most plausible and satisfactory general way of thinking about them (Ref. 19, page 286).

In Duchenne dystrophy this philosophy motivated many investigators until the gene product was identified in 1987 by an entirely different approach.

Unfortunately, many of the early studies of the biochemistry of dystrophic muscle were confounded by lack of adequate and appropriate controls. Furthermore, although by the 1960s it was clear that muscular dystrophy could no longer be considered a single disease entity, some investigators nevertheless persisted in presenting findings in cases of *progressive muscular dystrophy*. Another, and serious, problem which was not always appreciated in early studies was that as the disease progressed and functioning muscle tissue degenerated and was replaced by connective tissue (collagen), certain constituents might *appear* to be reduced when expressed in terms of total muscle weight, when in fact levels in *functioning* muscle might actually be normal. When this problem was recognized, investigators began to concentrate their attention on minimally affected muscle with little fibrosis and, more importantly, to express results in terms of a specific reference base such as *non-collagen* protein. Only in this way were more relevant and meaningful results obtained.

Early biochemical studies of affected muscle were reported by a number of groups, including Dreyfus in France, Pennington in England, Sugita in Japan, and particularly Carl Pearson in the United States, who, with his colleagues, carefully and systematically studied a variety of enzymes. Although no specific enzymatic or protein defect was ever identified by this approach, a picture of the biochemical changes in affected muscle did gradually emerge.

Whereas the levels of activity of some enzymes remained more or less normal, others were reduced (such as aldolase, lactate dehydrogenase, and creatine kinase) as a result of efflux from diseased muscle fibres into the circulation (Chapter 10). On the other hand, the activity of some enzymes in muscle actually *increased* in the disease (NADP-linked dehydrogenases and various proteases). This latter could be attributed to the invasion of affected muscle tissue by macrophages and fibroblasts which contain these enzymes. Finally, dystrophic muscle was found in some ways to resemble *fetal muscle*, most notably in certain isoenzyme patterns such as those of lactate dehydrogenase. The most likely explanation for this was *de-differentiation* of affected muscle owing to the reactivation of genes normally active only in fetal development, presumably as a result of attempts by dystrophic muscle to regenerate.

Around this period various groups were also studying the behaviour and biochemical profiles of muscle tissue and fibroblasts in culture. The effects of innervating cultured muscle cells were also studied in co-cultures of, for example, Duchenne muscle and rodent spinal cord. These highly technical and ingenious studies have been reviewed by Valerie Askanas and King Engel[20], who have been among the major contributors to this field. But though a great deal was learnt about the growth and development of muscle tissue in culture, no specific biochemical defect was revealed by these studies. A most intriguing observation, however, was an increase in intracellular calcium in cultured Duchenne muscle[21]. This had been demonstrated earlier by histochemical studies of biopsied muscle.

Contribution of muscle pathology

The earliest detailed study of the microscopic appearance of skeletal muscle was made by William Bowman (1816–1892) in 1840–1841[22]. Bowman proposed that muscle tissue was composed of *fasciculi* (fibres), each of which in turn contained numerous *fibrillae* (fibrils). In transverse section the former were not round and tubular as previously thought, but polygonal in shape due to 'mutual pressure'.

He also described the appearance of transverse striations and, most importantly, the 'membranaceous sheath of the most exquisite delicacy, investing every fasciculus from end to end, and isolating its fibrillae from all the surrounding structures', for which he coined the term *sarcolemma*. Edward Meryon may well have known of Bowman's work, though he does not quote it, for he repeatedly refers to the breakdown of the sarcolemma in granular degeneration of muscle or muscular dystrophy. He states quite clearly:

> the striped elementary primitive fibres were found to be completely destroyed, the sarcous element being diffused, and in many places converted into oil globules and granular matter, *whilst the sarcolemma or tunic of the elementary fibre was broken down and destroyed* [italics ours](Ref. 23, page 76).

The history of the microscopic findings in normal skeletal muscle has been reviewed[24], as has the history of the histopathology of dystrophy[25]. The latter, apart from some minor detail, has been little improved upon since the early descriptions published at the beginning of the last century.

From the 1950s, *Diseases of Muscle: A Study in Pathology*, written by Adams, Denny-Brown, and Pearson, and first published in 1953, became one of the standard works of reference on the subject. The pathological changes in muscle tissue are detailed but, in the second edition, published in 1962, the authors had to admit:

> the difficulty of determining primary changes in this disease. Once degeneration of a muscle fiber begins, all parts of it appear to be involved (Ref. 25, page 362).

And Walton also concluded around this time:

> routine studies of dystrophic muscle with the conventional light microscope have probably revealed by now most of the secrets which we can ever hope to discover with this technique...(Ref. 26, page 399).

However, subsequent studies by light microscopy and particularly electron microscopy, although not revealing the basic cause of the disease, did throw significant light on pathogenesis.

In the *preclinical* stage of Duchenne muscular dystrophy, before there are any clinical manifestations of the disease, there are already significant abnormalities in muscle pathology. These were first reported by Pearson in 1962[27]. These changes included increased variation in fibre size and an increase in the number of rounded fibres which stained more densely with eosin and were therefore referred to as *eosinophilic* or *hyaline* fibres. At this stage, however, there was no obvious necrosis. At first some considered such fibres to be artefacts produced during tissue preparation and sectioning. But gradually it became accepted that such changes did indeed represent an early manifestation of the disease process. A few years later, the careful and detailed light and electron microscopic studies of Cullen and Fulthorpe[28] indicated that these were hypercontracted fibres, and they suggested that these might be due to *increased intracellular calcium*. It was subsequently proposed that, owing to a postulated defect in the sarcolemma, the resultant influx of calcium led to mitochondrial calcium overload and cell death[29], as well as to further muscle damage as a result of calcium-activated protease activity[30]. An increase in muscle intracellular calcium in Duchenne dystrophy was subsequently confirmed by the elegant studies of Bodensteiner and Engel[31]. That this was a significant and early manifestation of the disease would later be supported when similar histochemical changes were also found in muscle from affected male fetuses in the second trimester of pregnancy[32].

Engel, with his co-workers at the Mayo Clinic, has over the years contributed significantly to our understanding of the pathogenesis of Duchenne dystrophy. Apart from demonstrating unequivocal evidence of increased muscle intracellular calcium[31], he also showed by careful immunocytochemical methods that many of the cells which invaded necrotic fibres in dystrophy were in fact T cells[33]. Also, that maybe 'abnormal muscle fiber components in Duchenne muscular dystrophy instigate a secondary autoimmune response'[34]. This may prove to have important therapeutic implications.

Andrew Engel was born in Budapest, Hungary in 1930, but after his early schooling emigrated to Canada and subsequently entered McGill University where he graduated in Medicine in 1955. After junior hospital appointments he was appointed in 1960 resident in internal medicine, and later in neurology, at the Mayo Clinic, an internationally renowned centre for neurology. After a 3-year period as fellow in neuropathology at Columbia University he returned to the Mayo Clinic in 1965 where he has remained ever since. He is currently 3M-McKnight professor of neuroscience in the College of Medicine, consultant in neurology and director of the muscle laboratory at the Mayo Clinic. He has received many awards and distinctions, perhaps the most prestigious being the Duchenne–Erb Prize in Germany, the Jerry Lewis Research Award of the MDA, and the Wartenberg Award of the American Academy of Neurology (Figure 11.1).

He first became interested in the pathogenesis of muscular dystrophy in the early 1970s around the time that McComas proposed the neurogenic hypothesis and King Engel proposed the vascular hypothesis for Duchenne dystrophy. At the time he felt his own light microscopic and electron microscopic observations supported neither of these ideas. Instead he became more interested in the possibility of a defect in the sarcolemma. Looking back on this work it now seems unbelievable that any should have doubted the relevance of his findings, so clearly based on very careful observations. But at the time there

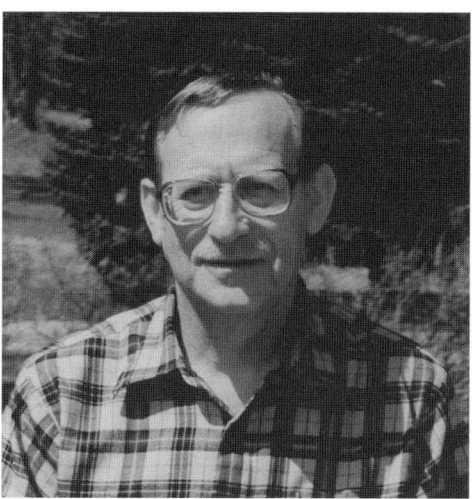

Fig. 11.1 Andrew G. Engel.

were those who felt Engel's findings were no more than artefact. However, as Engel now comments 'After the discovery of dystrophin and its subsarcolemmal localization, the idea that the sarcolemmal defects were artefacts was not mentioned again!' His contribution on the proposed defect in the sarcolemma merits special consideration.

The term *sarcolemma* had been used to describe the membrane surrounding the muscle fibre as seen on light microscopy, but electron microscopy revealed a more complex structure. Each muscle fibre was bounded by a plasma membrane (*plasmalemma*) and an outer basement membrane (*basal lamina*). The latter, along with the endomysium, constituted the sarcolemma (though often this term is also used when referring to the plasma and basement membranes together).

An early electron microscopic study of muscular dystrophy by Milhorat[35] showed that the plasma membrane was denuded in *necrotic* fibres. But this was perhaps not unexpected. The importance of the work of Engel and colleagues was that defects in the plasma membrane were found in *non-necrotic* fibres[36]. This was far more difficult to demonstrate and of much greater significance to pathogenesis. They observed areas of myofibril rarefaction under the fibre surface (which because of their shape were referred to as *delta lesions*). On electron microscopy, the plasma membrane over these areas of rarefaction was disrupted, indistinct or totally absent. However, the basement membrane overlying those regions from which the plasma membrane had disappeared was invariably preserved.

These observations suggested to the investigators that such membrane lesions could well be an ineffective barrier to the ingress of extracellular fluid.

They then proceeded to demonstrate the focal penetration of peroxidase into the fibre interior in the regions of the delta lesions. The authors concluded, with prescience:

> if the cause of the structural defects resided in the membrane itself (as it very well might), it could be caused by an abnormal lipid component or by a defective structural protein in the membrane. Further studies directed at the molecular architecture of the muscle fibre plasma membrane will clarify these questions (Ref. 36, page 1120).

They concluded that the basic abnormality in Duchenne dystrophy probably resided in the plasma membrane of the muscle fibre!

Thus, from the mid 1970s attention turned away from muscle tissue itself as being the possible site of the basic defect in the disease to the muscle membrane.

Muscle histology in the numerous forms of dystrophy now recognized presents a wide spectrum of abnormalities, although the muscle membrane itself remains an important component in many[37].

A defect in membranes

The idea that the muscle membrane was 'leaky' had been held for some time (Chapter 10), and now electron microscopy confirmed this[36]. However, the biochemical investigation of the membrane was not at all easy because of the difficulty of isolating it uncontaminated from other muscle constituents. This had confounded the results of many early studies regarding, for example, the lipid composition of the membrane. Two enzymes associated with the membrane are (Na^+ and K^+)ATPase and adenyl cyclase, and the earliest biochemical abnormality reported in 'pure' sarcolemmal samples in Duchenne dystrophy was in 1973 of an apparent reduction in ATPase activity[38]. The following year it was also reported that there was less than normal stimulation of adenyl cyclase activity by sodium fluoride or adrenaline[39]. But at the time it would be fair to say that not all were wholly convinced by such findings or of their relevance to the cause of Duchenne dystrophy.

In June 1976 the Muscular Dystrophy Association of America sponsored an international conference in Durango, Colorado, on the pathogenesis of muscular dystrophies. The meeting was organized by members of the Scientific Advisory Committee of MDA guided by L. P. ('Bud') Rowland, whose knowledge and wisdom were, and still continue to be, much in demand at such gatherings. He subsequently edited the proceedings[40]. At this meeting the *neurogenic hypothesis* was further discussed and largely rejected. But what was most important was the emphasis on a possible membrane defect in dystrophy and to many the high point was a presentation by Allen Roses of

Duke University Medical Center[41]. This presentation was greeted exuberantly at the time by the entertainer Jerry Lewis, who was attending the meeting and who for 20 years had devoted most of his life to raising money for research into muscular dystrophy. 'This is the sort of research we want!' he declaimed. The reason was clear to most of the audience, including Rowland himself, who said 'For more than a decade, the mood of investigators was pessimistic because the dystrophies seemed totally resistant to analysis'. Roses' paper suggested an entirely new approach. He argued, as had other genetically oriented investigators before:

> Muscular dystrophy researchers have been sidetracked in attempts to prove myopathic, neurogenic or vascular etiological theories while a major principle of genetic disease has been virtually ignored. The muscular dystrophies are inherited diseases in which inborn errors lead to a variety of clinical manifestations in several tissues. Independent expression in a variety of somatic tissues is possible and to be expected. Muscle is the major target organ for whatever biochemical defects exist in the muscular dystrophies. Whether or not a particular tissue presents clinical symptoms or signs may depend on the relative importance of the specific biochemical defect for the function of that tissue. Whether muscle is affected independently of nerve or blood supply, or whether nerve is involved leading to a secondary muscle disorder leads us no closer to the biochemical defect (Ref. 41, page 648).

We ourselves had searched for a defect in glycolysis and fatty acid oxidation in *leukocytes* in Duchenne dystrophy but found no abnormality. Roses, on the other hand, had investigated the biochemistry of *erythrocyte membranes* and found an abnormality of the membrane-associated protein, spectrin, specifically an apparent increase in spectrin band II phosphorylation[42–44]. This finding had instant appeal because it provided a biochemical basis for any proposed membrane defect and also demonstrated that the basic genetic defect could be expressed in tissues other than muscle.

Allen D. Roses was born in 1943 in Paterson, New Jersey, and took a Bachelor of Science degree (summa cum laude) in chemistry at the University of Pittsburgh before graduating in medicine from the University of Pennsylvania in 1967. After junior hospital appointments he eventually became chief resident in neurology at Duke University Medical Center in 1970. For 5 years until 1972 he served as a captain in the US Air Force Reserve. After being chief resident he remained at Duke University, becoming the Jefferson-Pilot professor of neurobiology and genetics, but left in 1997 to join GlaxoSmithKline for 10 years. He has now returned to Duke University to resume his professorship and head Duke's new Deane Drug Discovery Institute.

His interest in neuromuscular disorders began in the early 1970s as a result of a stimulating and productive collaboration with Stanley Appel. From the very beginning they were interested in the biochemistry of membranes and their main focus of attention at first was myotonic dystrophy. It was their interest in protein kinase activity in erythrocyte membranes which led Roses to study Duchenne muscular dystrophy. This disorder had been one of their *control* neurological diseases but in which, to their complete surprise, they found an abnormality in spectrin band II phosphorylation, and only in this disorder.

Later he returned to the study of myotonic dystrophy as well as research into late onset genetic disorders, most notably Alzheimer's disease. He has received many awards for his research, perhaps somewhat belatedly. He has been elected a foreign member of the Association of British Neurologists, and is a recipient of the Metropolitan Life Foundation Award for Excellence in Medical Research as well as the Potamkin Award of the American Academy of Neurology. He was an enthusiastic aerobics instructor for many years and is also a collector of early American copper coins and somewhat of an expert on red wines. He had triple bypass surgery following a serious myocardial infarction in 1990, but fully recovered to continue his personal and professional life with as much enthusiasm as ever (Figure 11.2).

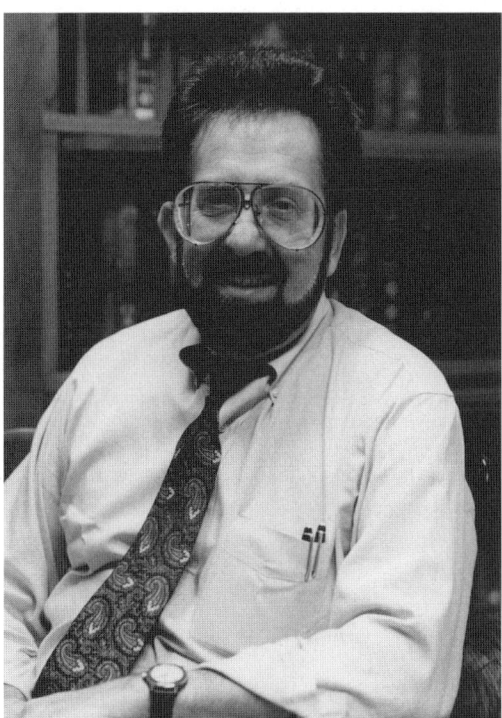

Fig. 11.2 Allen D. Roses.

The work of Roses and colleagues was an important and much needed stimulus to research at the time, and a number of membrane-associated abnormalities were subsequently reported in Duchenne muscular dystrophy. These included: (1) in erythrocytes, echinocyte formation, a reduction in intramembranous particles, increased Ca-ATPase activity, reduced deformability, and increased osmotic fragility; (2) in lymphocytes, reduced 'capping'; (3) in fibroblasts, reduced intercellular adhesiveness; and (4) in muscle, reduced intramembranous particles.

These various findings were later extensively and critically reviewed by Rowland[45] and in many cases the findings proved controversial. Either a reported abnormality was not reproducible in different laboratories (the technology was difficult and often new to those working in dystrophy) or it proved not to be limited to boys with Duchenne muscular dystrophy. But the approach of researchers had changed. The membrane was now the focus of attention. However, the basic defect would not be identified by these biochemical or physiochemical techniques but by an entirely new approach: that of so-called *reverse genetics*. Before this was possible, however, it was first necessary to locate and then isolate the defective gene in Duchenne muscular dystrophy.

References

1. Buchthal, F., Clemmesen, S. On the differentiation of muscle atrophy by electromyography. *Acta Psychiatrica et Neurologica Scandinavica*, 1941; **16**: 143–81.
2. Kugelberg, E. Electromyograms in muscular disorders. *Journal of Neurology, Neurosurgery and Psychiatry*, 1947; **10**(NS): 122–33.
3. Simpson, J. A. The development of electromyography and neurography for diagnosis. *Journal of the History of the Neurosciences*, 1993; **2**: 81–105.
4. McComas, A. J., Sica, R. E. P., Currie, S. Muscular dystrophy: evidence for a neural factor. *Nature*, 1970; **226**: 1263–4.
5. Bradley, W. G., Gardner-Medwin, D., Walton, J. N. (eds) *Recent Advances in Myology: Proceedings of the Third International Congress on Muscle Diseases*. Amsterdam: Excerpta Medica, 1975.
6. Engel, W. K. The vascular hypothesis. In: W. G. Bradley, D. Gardner-Medwin and J. N. Walton (eds) *Recent Advances in Myology: Proceedings of the Third International Congress on Muscle Diseases*. Amsterdam: Excerpta Medica, 1975: 166–73.
7. Bradley, W. G., Gardner-Medwin, D., Walton, J. N. (eds) *Recent Advances in Myology: Proceedings of the Third International Congress on Muscle Diseases*. Amsterdam: Excerpta Medica, 1975: 173–7.
8. Michelson, A. M., Russell, E. S., Harman, P. J. Dystrophia muscularis: a hereditary primary myopathy in the house mouse. *Proceedings of the National Academy of Sciences USA*, 1955; **41**: 1079–84.
9. Bulfield, G., Siller, W. G., Wight, P. A. L., Moore, K. J. X chromosome-linked muscular dystrophy (mdx) in the mouse. *Proceedings of the National Academy of Sciences USA*, 1984; **81**: 1189–92.

10. Valentine, B. A., Winand, N. J., Pradhan, D. et al. Canine X-linked muscular dystrophy as an animal model of Duchenne muscular dystrophy: a review. *American Journal of Medical Genetics*, 1992; **42**: 352–6.

11. Bushby, K., Lochmuller, H., Lynn, S., Straub, V. Interventions for muscular dystrophy: molecular medicines entering the clinic. *Lancet*, 2009; **374**: 1849–56.

12. Scriver, C. R., Childs, B. *Garrod's Inborn Factors in Disease*. Oxford: Oxford University Press, 1989.

13. Bearn, A. G. *Archibald Garrod and the Individuality of Man*. Oxford: Clarendon Press, 1993.

14. Garrod, A. E. The Croonian Lectures on Inborn Errors of Metabolism. *Lancet*, 1908; **ii**: 1–7, 73–9, 142–8, 214–20. (See also: Garrod, A. E. *Inborn Errors of Metabolism*, 2nd edn. Oxford: Oxford University Press, 1923.)

15. Beadle, G. W., Tatum, E. L. Genetic control of biochemical reactions in *Neurospora*. *Proceedings of the National Academy of Sciences USA*, 1941; **27**: 499–506.

16. Beadle, G. W. Biochemical genetics. *Chemical Reviews*, 1945; **37**: 15–96.

17. Pauling, L., Itano, H. A., Singer, S. J., Wells, I. C. Sickle cell anemia, a molecular disease. *Science*, 1949; **110**: 543–8.

18. Jervis, G. A. Phenylpyruvic oligophrenia: deficiency of phenylalanine oxidizing system. *Proceedings of the Society of Experimental Biology and Medicine*, 1953; **82**: 514–15.

19. Harris, H. *Human Biochemical Genetics*. Cambridge: Cambridge University Press, 1959.

20. Askanas, V., Engel, W. K. Cultured normal and genetically abnormal human muscle. In: L. P. Rowland and S. DiMauro (eds) *Handbook of Clinical Neurology, Vol. 18(62): Myopathies*. Amsterdam: Elsevier, 1992: 85–116.

21. Mongini, T., Ghigo, D., Doriguzzi, C. Free cytoplasmic Ca^{++} at rest and after cholinergic stimulus is increased in cultured muscle cells from Duchenne muscular dystrophy patients. *Neurology*, 1988; **38**: 476–80.

22. Bowman, W. On the minute structure and movements of voluntary muscle. *Philosophical Transactions of the Royal Society*, 1840; **130**: 457–501; 1841; **131**: 69–72.

23. Meryon, E. On granular and fatty degeneration of the voluntary muscles. *Medico-Chirurgical Transactions*, 1852; **35**: 73–84. (See also: Meryon, E. *Practical and Pathological Researches on the Various Forms of Paralysis*. London: John Churchill and Sons, 1864: 211.)

24. Fulthorpe, J. J. Microscopy in the study of skeletal muscle pathology. *Microscopy & Analysis*, 1993; No. 35 (May): 9–11.

25. Adams, R. D., Denny-Brown, D., Pearson, C. M. *Diseases of Muscle: A Study in Pathology*, 2nd edn. New York: Harper and Row, 1962.

26. Walton, J. N. Muscular dystrophy and its relation to the other myopathies. *Research Publications, Association for Research in Nervous and Mental Disease*, 1960; **38**: 378–421.

27. Pearson, C. M. Histopathological features of muscle in the preclinical stages of muscular dystrophy. *Brain*, 1962; **85**: 109–20.

28. Cullen, M. J., Fulthorpe, J. J. Stages in fibre breakdown in Duchenne muscular dystrophy—an electron-microscopic study. *Journal of the Neurological Sciences*, 1975; **24**: 179–200.

29. Wrogemann, K., Pena, S. D. J. Mitochondrial calcium overload: a general mechanism for cell-necrosis in muscle diseases. *Lancet*, 1976; **i**: 672–4.
30. Duncan, C. J. Role of intracellular calcium in promoting muscle damage: a strategy for controlling the dystrophic condition. *Experientia*, 1978; **34**: 1531–5.
31. Bodensteiner, J. B., Engel, A. G. Intracellular calcium accumulation in Duchenne dystrophy and other myopathies: a study of 567,000 muscle fibres in 114 biopsies. *Neurology*, 1978; **28**: 439–46.
32. Emery, A. E. H., Burt, D. Intracellular calcium and pathogenesis and antenatal diagnosis of Duchenne muscular dystrophy. *British Medical Journal*, 1980; **280**: 355–7.
33. Engel, A. G., Arahata, K. Mononuclear cells in myopathies. *Human Pathology*, 1986; **17**: 704–21.
34. Engel, A. G., Arahata, K., Biesecker, G. Mechanisms of muscle fiber destruction. In: G. Serratrice *et al.* (eds) *Neuromuscular Diseases*. New York: Raven Press, 1984: 137–41.
35. Milhorat, A. T., Shafiq, S. A., Goldstone, L. Changes in muscle structure in dystrophic patients, carriers and normal siblings seen by electron microscopy; correlation with levels of serum creatinephosphokinase (CPK). *Annals of the New York Academy of Sciences*, 1966; **138**: 246–92.
36. Mokri, B., Engel, A. G. Duchenne dystrophy: electron microscopic findings pointing to a basic or early abnormality in the plasma membrane of the muscle fiber. *Neurology*, 1975; **25**: 1111–20. (See also: Lotz, B. P., Engel, A. G. Are hypercontracted muscle fibers artifacts and do they cause rupture of the plasma membrane? *Neurology*, 1987; **37**: 1466–75.)
37. Dubowitz, V., Sewry, C. A. *Muscle Biopsy—A Practical Approach*, 3rd edn. London, New York: Saunders/Elsevier, 2007.
38. Dhalla, N. S., McNamara, D.B., Balasubramanian, V., Greenlaw, R., Tucker, F. R. Alterations of adenosine triphosphatase activities in dystrophic muscle sarcolemma. *Research Communications in Chemical Pathology and Pharmacology*, 1973; **6**: 643–50.
39. Mawatari, S., Takagi, A., Rowland, L. P. Adenyl cyclase in normal and pathologic human muscle. *Archives of Neurology*, 1974; **30**: 96–102.
40. Rowland, L. P. (ed.) *Pathogenesis of Human Muscular Dystrophies*. Amsterdam: Excerpta Medica, 1977.
41. Roses, A. D. Erythrocytes in dystrophies. In: L. P. Rowland (ed.) *Pathogenesis of Human Muscular Dystrophies*. Amsterdam: Excerpta Medica, 1977: 648–55.
42. Roses, A. D., Herbstreith, M. H., Appel, S. H. Membrane protein kinase alteration in Duchenne muscular dystrophy. *Nature*, 1975; **254**: 350–1.
43. Roses, A. D., Appel, S. H. Erythrocyte spectrin peak II phosphorylation in Duchenne muscular dystrophy. *Journal of the Neurological Sciences*, 1976; **29**: 185–93.
44. Roses, A. D., Herbstreith, M., Metcalf, B., Appel, S. H. Increased phosphorylated components of erythrocyte membrane spectrin band II with reference to Duchenne dystrophy. *Journal of the Neurological Sciences*, 1976; **30**: 167–78.
45. Rowland, L. P. Biochemistry of muscle membranes in Duchenne muscular dystrophy. *Muscle and Nerve*, 1980; **3**: 3–20.

Chapter 12

The search for the gene

So far the thinking behind much research in muscular dystrophy could be summed up as—find a specific biochemical defect, perhaps an enzyme defect, and then in some way trace this back to the responsible mutant gene. By the late 1950s this had been achieved with remarkable success in the case of sickle-cell anaemia involving standard biochemical techniques such as electrophoresis, chromatography, and amino acid sequencing. The work of Pauling, Itano, Ingram, and others showed how the protean clinical manifestations of this disease could be traced back to a point mutation in the sixth codon of the β-globin gene, much later to be located on chromosome 11. But there were very few other examples like this. However, in the 1970s an entirely new technology opened up the possibility of finding the basic biochemical defect in a disorder by first identifying the mutant gene itself. This therefore became known as reverse genetics or, more appropriately, positional cloning, and involved the techniques of recombinant DNA technology or genetic engineering. It generated a quantum leap in the study and understanding of genetic disorders.

Recombinant DNA technology

The first steps toward recombinant DNA technology were taken in 1944 when Avery, MacLeod, and McCarty[1], working at the Rockefeller Institute in New York, first showed that genetic information was stored in nucleic acid. It turned out that there were two different nucleic acids: deoxyribonucleic acid (DNA) and ribonucleic acid (RNA), and in 1953 Watson and Crick proposed the now well known double helical structure of DNA[2]. Genetic information was stored in the DNA molecule in the form of triplet codes, or codons, derived from the four constituent bases of DNA (adenine, thymine, guanine, and cytosine). The first successful attempt to break the genetic code was made by Nirenberg and Matthaei in 1961 while working at the National Institutes of Health[3]. By 1966 the complete genetic code for all 20 amino acids, as well as for start and stop codons, had been established. In 1970, Khorana and colleagues succeeded in the *in vitro* synthesis of a gene from its constituent bases[4].

It also became established that genetic information was transferred from DNA to RNA (so-called messenger RNA or mRNA) by a process referred to as *transcription*. The mRNA then migrated to the cytoplasm where the genetic information was *translated* into protein synthesis.

These various early developments provided the foundation for recombinant DNA technology, the real story of which began in 1970 with the discovery by Hamilton Smith at Johns Hopkins University of a group of enzymes, referred to as *restriction enzymes*, which occurred naturally in certain microorganisms[5,6]. Their importance lay in the fact that they cleaved DNA at sequence-specific sites and it was the specificity exhibited by each enzyme that proved particularly important in the subsequent development of recombinant DNA technology.

Also around this time, Howard Temin[7], and independently David Baltimore[8], discovered another enzyme which subsequently proved to be of immense value in the new technology. This enzyme, referred to as *reverse transcriptase*, catalysed the synthesis of DNA from RNA. Thus this enzyme provided a valuable method for making in the laboratory a complementary copy of a gene (referred to as cDNA) from mRNA extracted from a relevant tissue. For example, reticulocytes contain only globin mRNA, and therefore, if treated with reverse transcriptase, it is possible in this way to create a globin cDNA gene copy.

Another important development occurred in 1972 when methods were first described for joining (or recombining) DNA fragments, produced by restriction enzymes, from two different organisms to produce a hybrid molecule. Hence the term *recombinant DNA*. There then followed the introduction of *plasmid* vectors which could carry fragments of human DNA. The first constructed plasmid vector was reported by Stanley Cohen in 1973 and became known as pSC101[9]. Later, various other vectors were introduced which could be used to carry human DNA which, when taken up by a bacterium and the latter then grown in culture, would produce *clones,* each containing multiple copies of the same incorporated DNA fragment.

Another important technique introduced around this time by E. M. ('Ed') Southern, then in Edinburgh[10], involved separating DNA fragments on agarose gel by electrophoresis, then transferring these fragments to a cellulose nitrate filter by, in effect, 'blotting', the filter being laid over the gel. The DNA fragments in this way became firmly bound to the filter. This technique is now referred to as a *Southern blot*. An appropriately labelled DNA fragment used as a probe will hybridize with, and thereby detect and locate, any complementary sequences among DNA fragments on a Southern blot. With various modifications this technique would later prove of immense value in diagnosing various dystrophies.

Another important development of relevance to the history of muscular dystrophy was the construction of so-called *gene libraries*. This is the cloning in appropriate vectors of fragments of DNA, from the entire human genome, which are then stored. The pioneers of this development were Tom Maniatis and his colleagues in the United States, who reported the first successful construction of a human gene library in 1978[11].

As these technological developments were occurring, new ideas about the structure and arrangement of genes were taking place. Until the mid 1970s it had generally been assumed that genes consisted of continuous coding sequences and were discrete but contiguous entities. But in 1977 it was shown in higher organisms[12] that most genes were interrupted by so-called *introns*, the remaining parts of the gene (separated by these introns) being referred to as *exons*. Subsequently it was shown that during transcription functional mRNA was derived only from exons, which were spliced together, the precursor RNA from introns being excised. The reason for this still remains unknown.

In 1977 two new methods for *sequencing* DNA were reported which were both quicker and more accurate than previous methods. One was developed by Sanger at Cambridge[13] and the other by Maxam and Gilbert at Harvard[14]. When these methods were applied to fragments of DNA it was discovered that genes were not contiguous with each other, but were separated by large stretches of DNA which appeared to have no function. For this reason these stretches of DNA were referred to by some as *junk DNA*. This intergenic DNA in fact constituted over 90% of the total DNA. Of considerable interest was the finding that there were sequence variations in this intergenic DNA which, however, had no phenotypic effects on the individual. It was speculated by David Botstein and colleagues that these variations might be detectable using restriction enzymes, since they might conceivably result in the loss of an existing recognition site or in the acquisition of a new site. Such variations would be detectable by different fragment lengths and therefore different mobilities on an electrophoretic gel. Since these variations were assumed to be frequent in the population, they were referred to as *restriction fragment length polymorphisms*, or *RFLPs*. Such RFLPs would define arbitrary genetic sites though were not necessarily associated with any specific disease gene. Botstein speculated that such RFLPs should be inherited as simple Mendelian co-dominant markers and be distributed throughout the genome and therefore by chance the locus for any disease gene should be found near to at least one such RFLP. That is, the disease gene would be *linked* to an RFLP. Since there were straightforward molecular techniques for locating the approximate positions of RFLPs on chromosomes, so the location of a disease gene to which an RFLP was found to be linked would also be located. These ideas were summarized in a now classical paper by Botstein and colleagues published in 1980[15].

It began prophetically:

> We describe a new basis for the construction of a genetic linkage map of the human genome.

A few months later, after carefully searching Maniatis' gene library, Wyman and White reported that they had found a clearly defined RFLP which was frequent in the population and was inherited as a simple Mendelian trait[16]. Since then several hundreds of RFLPs have been located throughout the genome, occurring about once every 100–200 base pairs. The use of such DNA polymorphisms continues, as we shall see later in Chapter 13.

Localizing the Duchenne gene

Until the advent of recombinant DNA technology and the recognition of RFLPs, there were few common genetic markers and even the chromosomal location of these was quite unknown except for those which were inherited as X-linked traits: colour blindness, glucose-6-phosphate dehydrogenase (G6PD) deficiency, and the Xg blood group.

The first reported genetic linkage in humans was in 1937 between two X-linked traits, in this case colour blindness and haemophilia[17] (the methodology of linkage analysis was later much refined by the *lod* score method pioneered by Morton; Chapter 8). In 1955 Ursula Philip[18] reported a family in which crossing over occurred between colour blindness and Duchenne dystrophy, suggesting the two loci were far apart (see Chapter 8). Ten years later, in 1965 the then newly discovered Xg blood group locus was also found not to be closely linked to Duchenne dystrophy[19]. This remained the extent of our knowledge for almost 20 years. However, around 1980 Kay Davies and others realized that the answer to locating the Duchenne gene could be provided by the new molecular techniques and in particular the use of linked RFLPs. At the time Davies was working as a research fellow in the biochemistry department of St Mary's Hospital Medical School, London, under the guidance of Professor Robert ('Bob') Williamson. The latter was an exuberant and enthusiastic advocate of the new biotechnology and provided much inspiration. Davies was well aware of developments in molecular biology, and made this very clear in a review she wrote at this time in which she emphasized the importance of the approach proposed by Botstein[20].

Kay Davies was born in Stourbridge, England in 1951 and had been an undergraduate at Somerville College, Oxford where she graduated with a degree in chemistry in 1973, later followed by a DPhil in 1976 on the structure and function of chromatin in the slime mould *Physarum*. It was around this time that her interest in genetics was kindled. After a period of further research in Oxford she accompanied her husband, also a scientist, to Paris where, as a Royal Society European postdoctoral fellow, she continued her work on protein structure, though she admits she was often distracted by the pleasures of playing tennis, skiing, and mountain walking. However, in 1980, on her return to Britain, she was appointed by Williamson to work on cystic fibrosis in his newly established Molecular Biology Unit. During the next 2 years she became infected by Williamson's enthusiasm for the molecular approach to human disease. She also became increasingly interested in muscular dystrophy, another of Williamson's interests, who at the time was recruiting affected families for his DNA studies. When, in 1984, she was appointed by Sir David Weatherall as a senior research fellow in his department of medicine in Oxford she turned her attention entirely to muscle disease with what proved to be phenomenal success.

Over the years she has made numerous and important contributions not only in muscular dystrophy but also in spinal muscular atrophy and the fragile X syndrome, for which she has received many international awards. She is founding co-editor of the journal *Human Molecular Genetics* and was vice president of HUGO (Human Genome Organisation), as well as being a member of many other scientific and advisory committees. She has become a much respected and liked member of the scientific community. For a time she was director of the MRC Clinical Sciences Centre in London but in 1994 she admits she had 'looked into the corridors of power and even enjoyed doing a high level [administrative] job. However once it began to take me away from science, I knew I would have to leave.' She returned to her much-loved Oxford, later to become Dr Lee's professor of anatomy and now director of the MRC Functional Genomics Unit, and has also become a Fellow of the Royal Society and Dame of the British Empire (Figure 12.1).

Knowing that the gene was on the X chromosome, Davies and her colleagues proceeded to construct a library of cloned fragments derived from the X chromosome[21]. In essence they did this by first isolating a concentrate of X chromosome using the technique of fluorescence-activated cell sorting of a human cell line containing several X chromosomes (48, XXXX). The sorted chromosomes were then digested with a restriction enzyme (in this case *Eco RI*) and then cloned in a vector. To identify those clones which contained human X chromosome sequences, DNA from selected clones was labelled and hybridized on a Southern blot with digested DNA from a mouse–human hybrid cell line (HORL 9X) which contained mouse chromosomes but *only* the human X chromosome. Pure mouse DNA was used as a control. If a clone contained

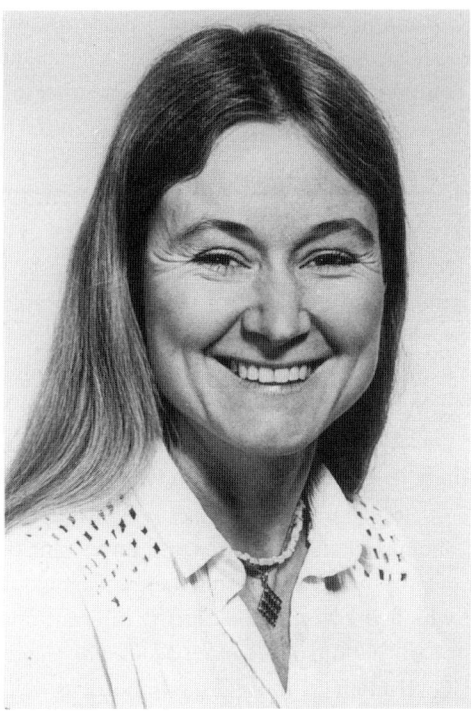

Fig. 12.1 Kay E. Davies.

human X sequences it would hybridize with the hybrid DNA but not with pure mouse DNA. By also using DNA from a cell bank of normal males, if the selected clone (used as a probe) detected by chance an X-linked RFLP this would be reflected in the variation in fragment sizes and therefore their mobilities on a gel (Figure 12.2). The isolation from the X chromosome of such a probe allowed it now to be used to detect possible linkage with Duchenne muscular dystrophy. This seems remarkably straightforward, but at the time it was an ingenious approach to the problem and proved an important breakthrough.

There was now a need for families with Duchenne dystrophy in which the disease affected more than one individual, and preferably in at least two generations, to test selected probes for possible linkage. Over the years Peter Harper in Cardiff had been collecting and studying such families, and it was therefore natural that Davies and Williamson should turn to him for collaboration.

Peter Harper was born in 1939 in Barnstaple, Devon, and studied medicine at Oxford where he graduated in 1964. Although always at heart a clinician, like his father before him he became increasingly interested in medical genetics.

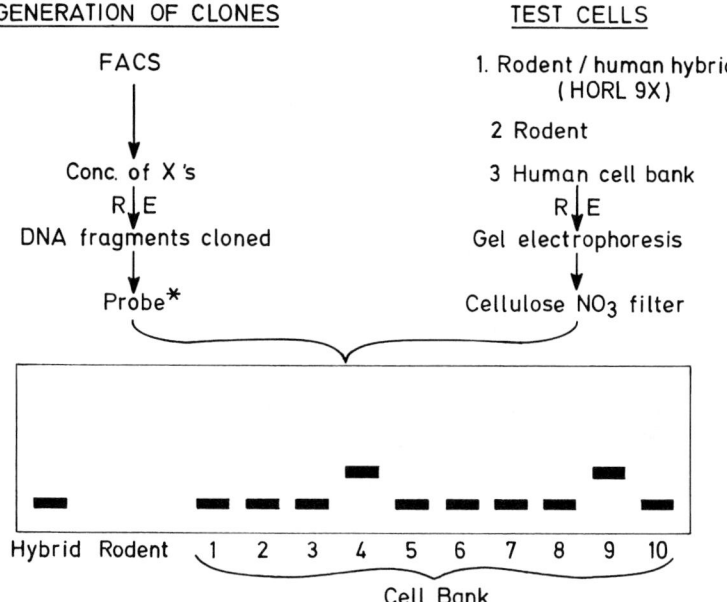

Fig. 12.2 Generation and identification of X chromosome probes and the detection of an X-linked restriction fragment length polymorphism. FACS, Fluorescent Activated Cell Sorter; RE, restriction enzyme; *labelled probe.

Along with his father and Howell Evans he published in 1970 details of a familial syndrome of oesophageal cancer associated with tylosis[22]. While spending 2 years as a postdoctoral fellow with Dr Victor McKusick at Johns Hopkins Hospital, Harper made an important study of the congenital form of myotonic dystrophy which he showed was almost always inherited through an affected mother[23]. He was by now becoming interested in neuromuscular diseases and, most importantly, in genetic linkage[24], a subject which was increasingly attracting the attention of many medical geneticists at this time. He later became professor of human genetics, Cardiff University, until he retired in 2004, becoming university research professor (emeritus), and was subsequently knighted for his contributions to the subject (Figure 12.3).

Around 1981, when approached by Bob Williamson and Kay Davies to collaborate, Harper was now a professor and had working with him in his department in Cardiff Joanne Murray, a young PhD student. In collaboration with Bob Williamson's group, and using patient material provided by Harper, Murray began to search for linkage between the disease gene and the probes they had previously isolated. In November 1982 (the paper had actually been first submitted for publication in July) they reported that one of the probes (RC8) detected a polymorphism (now called DXS9) which proved to be linked

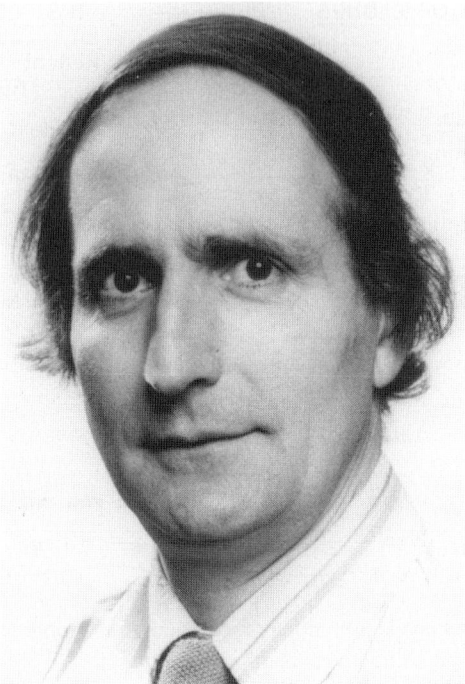

Fig. 12.3 Peter S. Harper.

to the disease gene. This was the first gene for a disease where the biochemical defect was unknown to be found linked to an RFLP[25], and there was little doubt about Murray's PhD being accepted! Just a few months later another probe (L1.28), isolated by Peter Pearson's group in Leiden, The Netherlands, was found to detect another polymorphism (now called DXS7). This was also found to be linked to the disease gene but on the opposite side to that detected by RC8[26]. Thus these two markers were *flanking* the disease gene.

But the question now to be answered was the actual location of these flanking markers on the X chromosome. This was attempted by hybridizing the probes on a Southern blot with enzyme-digested DNA from a panel of rodent–human hybrid cell lines, each containing different structurally abnormal human X chromosomes (previously characterized cytogenetically). The results indicated that the Duchenne gene appeared to be located 'in the middle of the short arm of the X chromosome'[25]; that is, around a position referred to as Xp21.

While these molecular studies were proceeding, two other lines of evidence also indicated that this was the likely locus for the gene. Firstly, a young boy had been described who not only had Duchenne muscular dystrophy but also chronic granulomatous disease, a form of retinitis pigmentosa and the McLeod syndrome (reduced antigenicity of the red cell Kell blood group). This appalling constellation of all these X-linked conditions in the same individual suggested that perhaps a large deletion had removed the responsible genes because they were contiguous. High resolution chromosome banding studies did reveal a suspicious reduction in the region of band Xp21, but this was not convincingly reported until some time later[27]. More convincing evidence of the location of the Duchenne gene came from reports of certain girls with severe Duchenne muscular dystrophy. From the time of the original report by Walton in the 1950s (Chapter 8), it had become customary to check that any girl with the disease did not also have Turner's syndrome with an abnormal sex chromosome constitution. However, this proved not to be so in the cases reported in the late 1970s. Unfortunately, the earliest of these reports in 1977 was published in abstract form only[28,29], but in 1979 others were reported in full[30,31]. Each of these cases proved to have an X/autosome translocation, and, though the autosome involved was different in each case, the breakpoint on the X chromosome was always in the region of Xp21. The most likely explanation was therefore that the translocation had in some way disrupted the normal gene at Xp21 which thereby resulted in the disease. (In such X/autosome translocation carriers, X inactivation is not random, the normal X chromosome tending to be preferentially inactivated.)

Thus, by 1982 evidence from three different sources all indicated that the disease locus was at Xp21 (Figure 12.4). Later, gene loci for other X-linked diseases would be located by these same techniques of RFLP linkage, cytological identification of deletions in rare affected boys, and X/autosome translocations in affected girls.

Duchenne and Becker muscular dystrophies shown to be allelic

Since Duchenne and Becker muscular dystrophies were both X-linked and also very similar in their clinical presentations, if differing in their severity, Becker himself had considered it likely that they would prove to be *allelic*; that is, due to different mutations but at the same locus. However, there had been suggestions subsequently that, although Duchenne dystrophy was definitely not closely linked to either colour blindness or to G6PD deficiency, Becker dystrophy might be. If true, this would suggest that they were not allelic disorders. But the evidence for linkage between Becker muscular dystrophy and these two markers was not very convincing, the statistical confidence limits being wide.

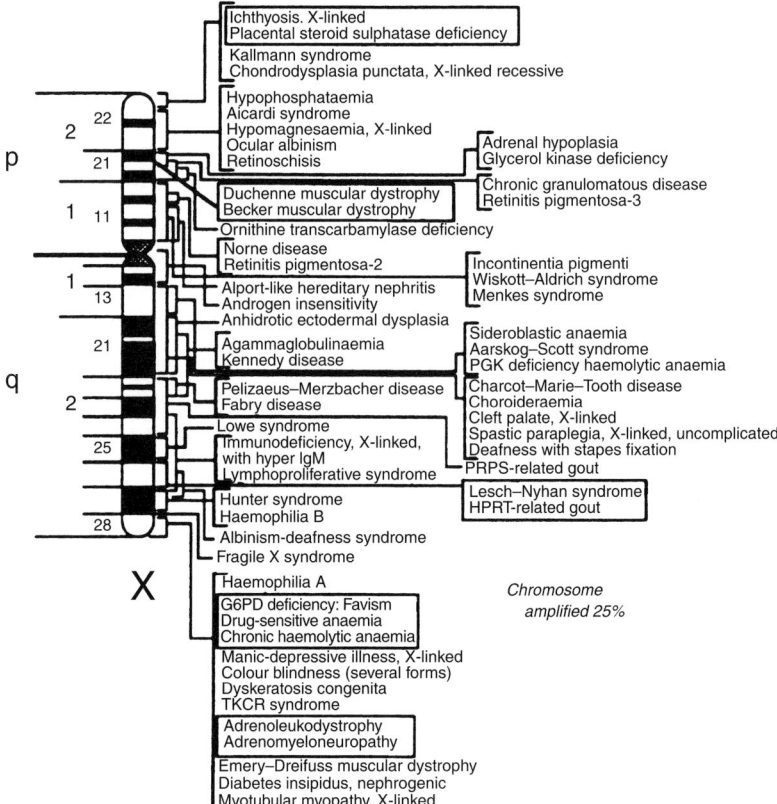

Fig. 12.4 Gene map of the X chromosome and its banding pattern. (Reproduced with kind permission of the late Dr. Victor McKusick.)

At the time that the DNA markers linked to Duchenne dystrophy were discovered, Helen Kingston, a young medical graduate in Harper's department, was studying Becker dystrophy for her MD degree thesis. To determine if the two disorders were allelic she carried out linkage studies on her families using these same markers. She first found that the polymorphism detected by probe L 1.28 was linked to Becker dystrophy at a distance comparable to that of Duchenne dystrophy. This placed the locus of the former disorder on the short arm of the X chromosome and not on the long arm where colour blindness and G6PD deficiency were located. It also suggested that Duchenne and Becker dystrophies were either closely linked to each other or possibly allelic[32].

In a subsequent study published the following year[33], she and her colleagues, using both the polymorphisms DXS9 and DXS7, found that the locus for Becker dystrophy showed roughly similar genetic distances from these two markers as did Duchenne dystrophy. It was now fairly clear that the two disorders were in fact allelic and this would be supported as more DNA markers in the region were identified in future. That they were allelic was later confirmed by molecular studies which showed that the gene defects in these two disorders were definitely the result of mutations at the same locus.

DNA markers for carrier detection and prenatal diagnosis

Immediately that linked DNA markers were discovered it became obvious that this information, combined with serum creatine kinase data, could be used to refine the likelihood of a woman being a carrier of Duchenne muscular dystrophy. However, as a result of crossing-over (or recombination) during meiosis, the farther a marker from the disease gene, the greater the likelihood of a diagnostic error. The frequency of recombination is related to the distance between the genes concerned—1% recombination being equivalent to a map distance of one map unit or one centiMorgan (cM), so named after Thomas Hunt Morgan who, in the 1930s, had pioneered work on gene mapping in the fruit fly *Drosophila* (Chapter 8). Molecular studies indicated that 1 cM was roughly equal to 1000 kilobases (kb) or 10^6 base pairs of DNA. In the case of DXS9 and DXS7, both these markers were roughly 15 cM from the Duchenne locus and the error rate with either was therefore of the order of 15%. However, provided *both* polymorphisms were segregating in a family, and since they flanked the disease gene, the error rate could be reduced to the product of their respective map distances from the disease gene—that is, to around 2%.

The first published report of combining serum creatine kinase information with data from these two linked DNA markers (made possible by the use of Bayesian statistics, Chapter 10) was published in the same year that the second marker had been reported by Davies and her colleagues[34]. It concerned a family with one affected boy whose sister was concerned about her carrier status. Within a few weeks there appeared a more detailed account involving three informative families[35]. However, this latter report emphasized that 'The margins of error involved for these probes, which are still a moderate distance from the Duchenne muscular dystrophy locus, make this approach inappropriate at present for antenatal diagnosis.'

Antenatal diagnosis (now referred to as *prenatal diagnosis*) for genetic disease had begun in the late 1960s. This had been made possible through the technique of amniocentesis, developed some 10 years previously for the management of pregnancies with rhesus incompatibility, the procedure then usually being carried out after 30 weeks' gestation. But in the 1960s it was suggested that the procedure be extended to the diagnosis of genetic disease by studying amniotic fluid cells obtained by amniocentesis carried out during the second trimester of pregnancy. These cells, of fetal origin, could be separated off from the amniotic fluid and cultured. In this way cytogenetic[36,37] and certain biochemical disorders[38] could be diagnosed prenatally. The subject developed considerably over the next 20 years and became an important aspect of medical genetics[39]. But in the case of Duchenne muscular dystrophy there was no associated biochemical abnormality and in the early days of prenatal diagnosis only fetal sexing was possible: if the mother was a carrier she could be offered termination of pregnancy if a fetus was male. This was very unsatisfactory because there was a high probability, at least 50%, that such a fetus might be normal.

However, closely linked DNA markers, which could be studied in cultured amniotic fluid cells, offered a high probability of being able to diagnose an *affected* male fetus *in utero*. By 1985, 11 RFLPs linked to Duchenne dystrophy and located on either side of the locus had become available and several were closer than the original markers. The margin of error was therefore much reduced and the first use of the technology in prenatal diagnosis was reported in 1985 by the Leiden group[40].

However, there were problems in the use of linked RFLPs for carrier detection and prenatal diagnosis. Apart from errors due to recombination, it depended on a particular polymorphism being present in the family and being informative. A solution would only be possible with *gene-specific probes* and this would depend on identifying and isolating the responsible gene itself.

Isolation of the Duchenne gene

Within a year or two of the first linked DNA markers being found, many other probes were identified, several proving much closer to the disease locus. The possibility therefore of isolating the gene itself by '*chromosome walking*' was attractive but likely to be very difficult. In fact, two very different approaches were to lead to the gene being isolated by teams led by Kunkel in the United States and Worton in Canada.

Louis ('Lou') Kunkel came of an illustrious family of scientists. His grandfather, Louis O. Kunkel, had been a distinguished botanist and his father, Henry Kunkel, an eminent immunologist, both at Rockefeller University. Lou Kunkel is very proud of being the only direct descent third generation member of the US National Academy of Sciences.

He was born in New York in 1949 but later the family moved away from the city and he spent many holidays on his grandfather's farm where he acquired a love of nature and an interest in genetics. He raised and bred German bearded irises with his father and at a very young age so learned many of the principles of genetics. He still breeds irises, some of which his father originated 30 years ago. He cherishes the idea of one day having a farm himself.

He attended Gettysburg College in Pennsylvania and through summer vacation research with Alec Bearn at Cornell Medical School, he met Victor McKusick. This was around the time of the Vietnam War and there was the ever-present concern of having to do military service. In the hope of delaying his call-up he had applied to various graduate schools in botany in his final year in college. These graduate programmes would begin in September of 1971, but Kunkel's A1 draft status would no doubt have resulted in his induction into the army upon his graduation in June. He was therefore very delighted to be invited to join Victor McKusick's graduate programme in human genetics at Johns Hopkins, with official enrolment beginning in the summer, thus deferring his being drafted immediately after graduating from college. At Johns Hopkins he worked for a time with Kirby Smith and the likeable but sometimes irascible S. H. ('Ned') Boyer, who was a great teacher and stimulator, and with whom one of us (AEHE,) had worked for a time some 10 years previously. Here Kunkel became interested in isolating DNA sequences from the human Y chromosome. This was a very successful and productive period which generated two important publications on the subject[41,42].

But he now admits, that although 'during my graduate studies I became familiar with human genetics as only a student who attended Moore Clinic and Genetics conferences with Victor McKusick could…', he was beginning to feel that human genetics was 'too descriptive and that molecular approaches were needed'. From this history it is none the less evident that the former, by clearly defining a disease entity, was first necessary before the latter could possibly provide any meaningful information about molecular pathology. However, having obtained his PhD at Hopkins in 1978, he left, eventually joining Samuel Latt at Harvard Medical School to work on the human X chromosome then being isolated using a newly acquired cell sorter. His postdoctoral research fellowship required financing and so it was decided to approach the Muscular Dystrophy Association, because of Kunkel's interest in the X chromosome, Duchenne muscular dystrophy, of course, being an X-linked trait. When the fellowship was awarded he says his fate with muscular dystrophy was sealed, and when the fellowship expired he wrote a research proposal to the MDA to clone the Duchenne gene, and later he was given a research contract for this work. But he admits quite honestly that his involvement with dystrophy at the beginning was somewhat luck and 'based on paying my salary'. In any case, his research proved enormously successful and he has been honoured by many awards, including the Duchenne–Erb Prize in Germany, the

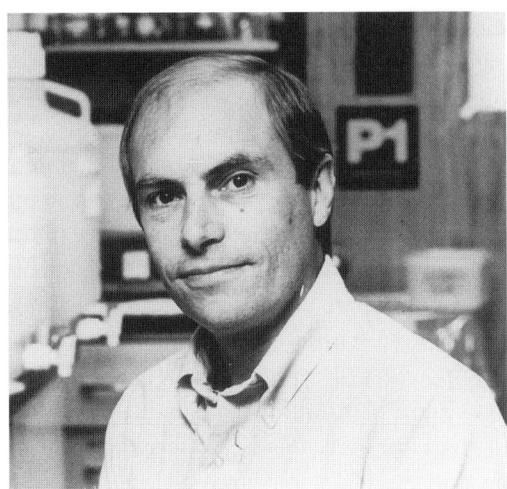

Fig. 12.5 Louis M. Kunkel.

Royal Society Wellcome Foundation Prize in England, Gairdner Foundation International Award, and, in 1990, he was elected a member of the National Academy of Sciences. He has remained at Harvard ever since and is now tenured professor of pediatrics and genetics and director of the program in genomics at the Children's Hospital Boston (Figure 12.5).

The strategy Kunkel adopted in cloning the Duchenne gene was in essence simple: isolate chromosomal DNA from the reported case with a cytologically recognizable deletion at Xp21, and then hybridize this with normal chromosomal DNA. Any unhybridized DNA would represent the deleted region in the affected boy's DNA and therefore presumably include the normal counterpart of the disease gene. How this was achieved, however, was ingenious but complicated, and required detailed knowledge and expertise in recombinant DNA technology. The DNA of the affected boy was sheared by sonication, so producing fragments with *irregular* ends.

Normal DNA (from a 49, XXXXY cell line) was cleaved with the restriction enzyme *Mbo 1*. This enzyme produced irregular *sticky ends*, so called because they combine with similar ends produced by the same enzyme on other DNA fragments. The two sets of fragments, with the patient's DNA much in excess, were mixed together and then heated to disassociate all the DNA strands. They were then allowed to reassociate in the presence of phenol (so-called phenol-enhanced reassociation technique or PERT), which increased the rate of DNA–DNA reassociation reactions several thousand-fold. Under the particular conditions, most of the reassociated molecules would have sheared ends and a few would be hybrid molecules with one sheared end and one *Mbo 1* sticky end. But those sequences from the control and *not* present in the patient's DNA because they were deleted, could not hybridize with the patient's DNA but only with themselves and therefore would have *two Mbo 1* sticky ends. Only the last could be inserted into an appropriately cleaved plasmid vector and be cloned. In this way a library of probes (so-called PERT probes) was produced. Presumably some of these would contain at least part of the Duchenne gene. Using these as probes, one (PERT 87) was found which detected submicroscopic *deletions* in a proportion of affected boys. Since none of these had any of the original patient's diseases except Duchenne muscular dystrophy, so the PERT 87 probe must have corresponded to at least part of the Duchenne gene[43]. Tragically, BB (Bruce Bryer), the affected boy whose DNA had helped so much in the search for the gene, died following a car accident at Christmas 1983, 2 years before Kunkel's publication.

At this time Worton's group in Toronto had also been tackling the problem but from a very different angle. Ron Worton had had a remarkably varied career and certainly at the beginning few would ever have imagined he would be among the first to isolate a disease gene. He was born in 1942 in Winnipeg, Canada, where he attended school. Later, as an undergraduate at the University of Manitoba, he took an honours degree in mathematics and physics, but then decided he did not want to be a physicist after all. Instead he became interested in cancer research, working on lithium fluoride crystals and in fact he was one of the first to use this material to calibrate a betatron for radiotherapy. Thus he began to move increasingly toward medical research and later, in Toronto in 1969, took his PhD in medical biophysics. He continued postdoctoral research at Yale where he came into contact with Frank Ruddle, who, with Victor McKusick, was pioneering and advocating the importance of gene mapping. One of Ruddle's particular interests was the use of somatic cell hybrids and in 1971 he introduced Worton to the then new technology of chromosome banding. It was around this time that Worton's interest was captured by genetics and when he returned to Canada he took up a junior position in the newly established department of genetics at the Hospital for Sick Children, Toronto. Dr M. W. (Peggy) Thompson was on the staff and was already well known for her work in muscular dystrophy.

Furthermore, in 1977 by one of those fortunate chance events which seem to recur in this history, Christine Verellen, a paediatrician from Belgium, came to Toronto with her husband, who had already accepted a fellowship in neonatology at the hospital. It was Verellen who in that year had just described the case of a girl with Duchenne dystrophy and an X/autosome translocation[28]. Worton was immediately intrigued by her description of the case. He encouraged Verellen to try to demonstrate non-random X-inactivation to explain the disease in the little girl and to try to map the breakpoints of the translocation.

This was his introduction to muscular dystrophy which he admits had not interested him previously. Having completed most of her research, Verellen, however, returned to Belgium in 1979 and it was in this year that Lindenbaum's full report of a similar case appeared[30], which further stimulated Worton's interest. Verellen and Worton were pretty confident that in her case the breakpoint in chromosome 21 was through a block of ribosomal genes and even then he felt that this might provide a means of somehow identifying the Duchenne gene. Later, in 1982, Worton heard that Roy Schmickel had succeeded in cloning ribosomal genes, but at the time Worton admits he knew little molecular biology and so he convinced his department chairman, Lou Siminovitch, to allow him to relinquish his position as director of the cytogenetic laboratory so that he could take a year's sabbatical to learn the technology. On returning to the Hospital for Sick Children in 1983, he recruited Peter Ray who had a good background in the new technology and so began an exciting and fruitful period of collaboration in isolating the Duchenne gene. Like Kunkel, Worton has been honoured with the Gairdner Foundation International Award. He has also been elected a Fellow of the Royal Society of Canada and received an honorary degree from the Université Catholique de Louvain. He was geneticist-in-chief at the Hospital for Sick Children, and professor in the department of molecular and medical genetics until 2007; he is now scientific director emeritus of the Ottawa Hospital Research Institute and professor emeritus in the department of medicine (Figure 12.6).

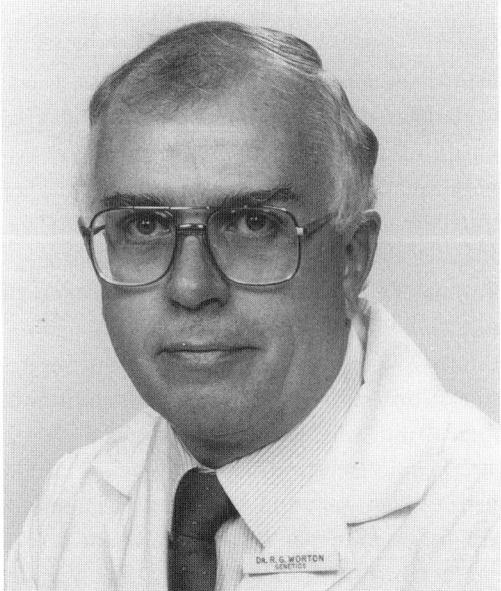

Fig. 12.6 Ronald G. Worton.

In isolating the Duchenne gene the first step Worton took was to show that in Verellen's case the translocation did indeed split the block of genes encoding ribosomal RNA on the short arm of chromosome 21[44]. He then proceeded to use ribosomal RNA gene probes to identify the junctional fragment in clones derived from the region of the translocation site. The region spanning the translocation breakpoint, and which presumably contained at least a part of the Duchenne locus, was then cloned. A sequence derived from this was found to detect an RFLP which proved to be very closely linked to the disease. This probe (referred to as XJ) also failed to hybridize with DNA from some patients with Duchenne dystrophy, indicating that in these boys there was a deletion of the region corresponding to the probe[45]. Most importantly, in many cases the XJ probe detected a deletion in cases in which PERT 87 probes also detected a deletion. Kunkel's paper was submitted in April and published in July of 1985; Worton's paper, however, was submitted in October and did not appear until December of 1985. But clearly both these very different and quite independent approaches had been successful, and in the history of Duchenne muscular dystrophy should therefore share the credit for having first isolated the responsible gene. Both the PERT 87[46], and later, the XJ probes were used to detect tightly linked RFLPs in the region, and these would be used for more precise carrier detection and prenatal diagnosis in future.

More information about the deletions in affected boys and particularly about the nature of the Duchenne gene itself now began to emerge. In a characteristically generous gesture Kunkel had made his probes available to investigators throughout the world. He collated this information, which was then published in a paper which must be unique in the history of medical science, there being no less than 76 co-authors[47]! In fact, a significant factor in the success of molecular research in Duchenne dystrophy has been the spirit of collaboration among all those working in the field. The conclusions of this collaborative study were that similar deletions were found to occur in both Duchenne and Becker dystrophies, that they were frequent and often larger than 140 kb, and that recombination between PERT 87 (now DXS164) and Duchenne dystrophy was around 5%. This indicated that the gene locus was very much larger than any previously studied locus. Furthermore, within a year or two it became clear that up to 70% of cases of Duchenne and Becker dystrophies had gene deletions or, rarely, duplications. The remaining 30% have been shown to be caused by a variety of point mutations which can now be detected by various molecular techniques.

The next step was to characterize the gene and its protein product. Using PERT[48] and XJ[49] probes, relevant mRNA transcripts in muscle were identified. The corresponding cDNAs were then cloned and sequenced[50,51].

Eventually, after much effort in sequencing cDNAs and studying their structure and organization, it turned out that the gene was, as suspected, very large. It proved to be some 2400 kb in length (about 0.1% of the total human genome), and in 1994 was still the largest gene so far identified in humans, taking up to 24 hours to be transcribed. Its large size, by presenting a greater target for mutagenic agents, would account for the relatively high mutation rate, of around 1 in 10,000 male births. In 2010 it is now known that the gene consists of 86 exons. The actual coding sequences of the gene represent less than 1% of its nucleotide composition, which is transcribed into a 14 kb mRNA.

Dystrophin—the gene product

The protein product of the Duchenne locus was further studied by techniques using specific polyclonal antibodies developed by Hoffman[52]. Eric Hoffman was born in 1958 in Woodbury, New Jersey. During his school years he spent a year in Denmark as a foreign exchange student, which was no doubt a prelude to his later love of international travel. He attended Gettysburg College and majored with honours in both biology and music. He then went to Baltimore for graduate research at Johns Hopkins University where he obtained his PhD in 1986. His research had centred on gene promoters in *Drosophila* and their role in gene regulation. However, like many others around this time, he was beginning to feel that applying the new molecular techniques to human disease held more attraction. So, he approached Kunkel (a fellow alumnus of Gettysburg College) who, recognizing Hoffman's talents, appointed him to a postdoctoral fellowship in his laboratory to work on muscular dystrophy. Within a year of obtaining his doctorate, Hoffman succeeded, in collaboration with the group, in identifying the protein product of the Duchenne gene. He has remained working in the field ever since, contributing much to our understanding of the details of the pathogenesis of Duchenne muscular dystrophy, and the relationship of the disease to that in various animal models. In 1990 he became assistant professor in the University of Pittsburgh School of Medicine, and in 1999 he moved to Washington, D.C. to establish the center for genetic medicine at Children's National Medical Center and is now chairman, department of integrative systems biology, George Washington University School of Medicine. Despite his achievements and impressive list of publications, he insists on finding time for his hobbies of choir singing and stained glass-making (Figure 12.7).

When he joined Kunkel's group he became responsible for transcriptional studies of the Duchenne gene. Using polyclonal antibodies directed against fusion proteins produced in bacteria from cDNAs, Hoffman and his colleagues

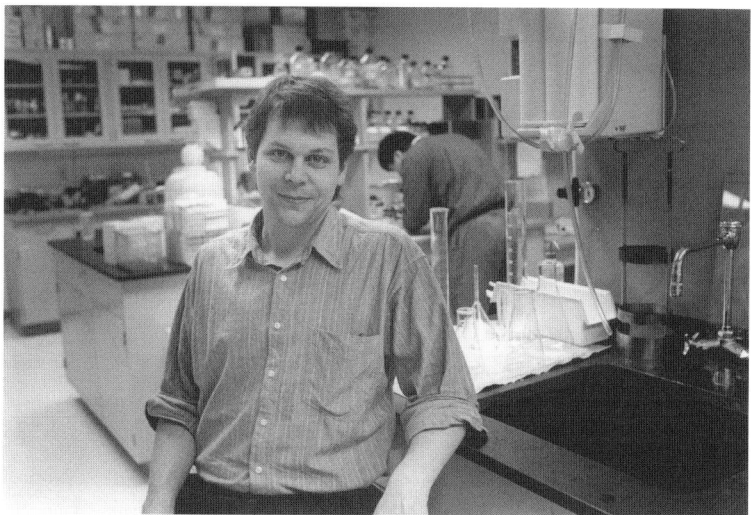

Fig. 12.7 Eric P. Hoffman.

identified the protein product of the Duchenne locus, which they termed *dystrophin*[52]. At the time some felt this was perhaps an inappropriate term since the protein proved to be absent in Duchenne muscular dystrophy, and only present in normal muscle. From the nucleotide sequence of the gene, the predicted amino acid constitution of its product suggested a rod-shaped cytoskeletal protein with some similarities to spectrin, and *not* an enzyme after all. It turned out to have a molecular weight of 427 kDa and consisted of 3685 amino acids. In summary, it was shown at the time to be composed of four domains:

- N-terminal domain composed of 240 amino acids and with homology to α-actinin
- Central rod domain of around 3000 amino acids consisting of 25 triple helical repeats similar to spectrin
- Cysteine-rich domain composed of 280 amino acids
- C-terminal domain composed of 420 amino acids.

It constituted only 0.002% of muscle protein[52] and was therefore most unlikely to have ever been identified by more conventional biochemical techniques. Duchenne muscular dystrophy was the *first* disorder in which the protein defect was identified by molecular techniques in a disease in which there was *no prior knowledge as to its basic cause*. It was therefore a triumph for *reverse genetics*.

The use of polyclonal antibodies to dystrophin developed by Hoffman when attached to suitable markers now allowed some quantitation of the protein on electrophoresis (Western immunoblot). The results of such studies revealed that dystrophin was virtually absent in Duchenne dystrophy, abnormal (in size or amount) in Becker dystrophy, but normal in all other muscular dystrophies, including limb girdle, Emery–Dreifuss, and oculopharyngeal muscular dystrophies, as well as in a variety of neurogenic disorders[53]. It now became clear that many adult patients previously thought to have limb girdle muscular dystrophy or spinal muscular atrophy had in fact Becker muscular dystrophy. For this reason terms such as *Xp21 myopathies* or *dystrophinopathies* were sometimes used.

The tissue distribution and localization of dystrophin and its function were now important problems to be solved. That its structure had suggested similarities to cytoskeletal proteins such as spectrin and α-actinin directed interest once again to the sarcolemma. Using histochemical methods with appropriately labelled polyclonal antibodies to dystrophin, groups in Japan[54], Canada[55], and in the United States[56] reported independently that in biopsy specimens dystrophin was localized at the sarcolemma in normal muscle but was virtually absent in Duchenne muscular dystrophy. These findings were soon corroborated by many other investigators.

Subsequently dystrophin was shown to be a costameric protein forming a lattice which encircled the muscle fibre. It could therefore be imagined that the deficiency of dystrophin in Duchenne dystrophy would somehow destabilize the integrity of the sarcolemma and so account for its breakdown. However, this proved to be an oversimplification.

Dystrophin-associated glycoproteins

In one of those seminal papers which have highlighted the history of Duchenne muscular dystrophy, Campbell showed that dystrophin was not directly inserted into the sarcolemma but via a glycoprotein complex. This was to prove important in understanding the pathogenesis not only of Duchenne and Becker dystrophies, but also several other forms of dystrophy.

Kevin Campbell was born in Brooklyn, New York in 1952 and eventually went to Manhattan College in the Bronx, where he was particularly impressed by the lectures on the physiology and biochemistry of muscle. Later, he went on to graduate school at the University of Rochester where he gained his PhD in 1978 on the biochemical characterization of muscle sarcoplasmic membranes. He continued this work as a postdoctoral fellow with David MacLennan at the University of Toronto, but in 1981 he returned to the United States to take up an appointment at the University of Iowa where he has remained ever since. He became distinguished professor of physiology and biophysics in 1989 and is now professor of internal medicine and neurology and director, Wellstone Muscular Dystrophy Co-operative Research Center.

Although his interest in muscle began as an undergraduate, it was toward the end of his graduate studies that he developed a specific interest in neuromuscular diseases when his own father was diagnosed as having myasthenia gravis. At the time there seemed no way of switching to medical research, but his eventual aim was one day to contribute to research in muscle disease. He was therefore immediately excited and attracted by the work of Kunkel and others in the mid 1980s which suggested a possible defect in a muscle cytoskeletal protein in Duchenne dystrophy. After all, Campbell's entire career up to this point had been the study of the biochemical properties of muscle membranes (Figure 12.8).

Just 2 years after the gene product had been identified and termed dystrophin, Campbell and Kahl[57] published their paper in *Nature*. They found that, though not a glycoprotein itself, dystrophin was intimately associated with glycoprotein, forming a *dystrophin-associated-glycoprotein* (DAG) complex. They suggested

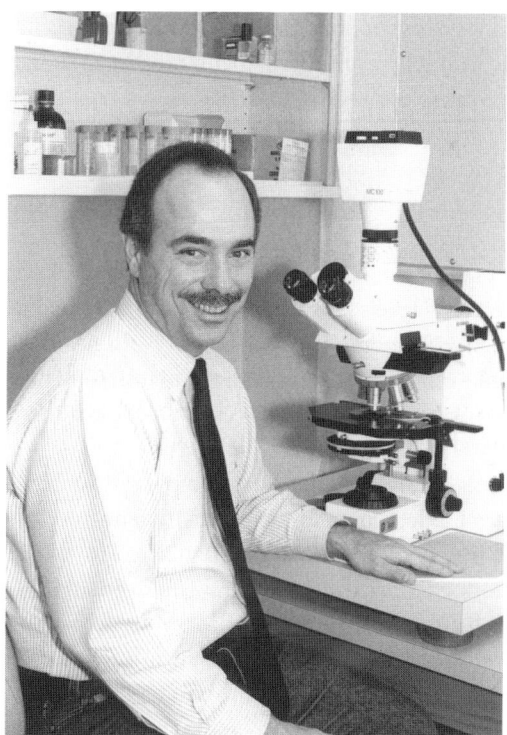

Fig. 12.8 Kevin P. Campbell.

that dystrophin was not directly attached to the sarcolemma but via glycoproteins in the membrane. Campbell's later studies confirmed and extended these findings. The C-terminal domain of dystrophin was attached to a complex of glycoproteins[58], which in their turn were related to the extracellular matrix. This will be discussed further in Chapter 13.

All the glycoproteins associated with dystrophins were found to be significantly reduced in Duchenne muscular dystrophy but to a lesser degree in Becker muscular dystrophy. Furthermore, in various collaborative studies, Campbell and colleagues have shown that *individual components* of this complex are absent in certain disorders: 50 kDa DAG (adhalin) in one form of autosomal recessive muscular dystrophy[59] and merosin (the M laminin isoform in muscle) in a form of congenital muscular dystrophy[60]. This was unlikely to be the end of the story. In fact, later it was shown that several other muscular dystrophies were also found to be associated with various components of this complex system (Chapter 13).

Genotype–phenotype correlations

The virtual absence of dystrophin on Western blot analysis in Duchenne dystrophy was confirmed by immunohistochemical studies on muscle biopsy specimens[54–56], which also revealed the occasional positive fibre (revertant) (Figure 12.9). It was calculated that the probability of Duchenne muscular dystrophy exceeded 99% if there was an absence of dystrophin, whereas the probability of Becker muscular dystrophy exceeded 95% if dystrophin was present but of abnormal size (larger or smaller) and/or reduced abundance[61].

Quantitation of dystrophin showed that levels less than 5% suggested severe Duchenne dystrophy, levels between 5 and 12% intermediate severity, and levels greater than 12% mild Becker dystrophy[62]. In healthy female carriers, muscle dystrophin was usually normal but in manifesting carriers dystrophin abnormalities were often detectable on Western blot but particularly on immunohistochemistry (Figure 12.9).

At the gene level there appeared to be no simple relationship in affected boys between the *size* of a deletion and the clinical phenotype. What did become clear, however, was that the *site* and particularly the *type* of mutation was important. Deletions affecting the central rod domain of dystrophin were more likely to lead to a milder (Becker) phenotype, whereas those which affected the C-terminal domain were more likely to lead to a severer (Duchenne) phenotype. More importantly, those mutations that disrupted the normal DNA nucleotide triplet sequences or reading frame (frame-shift) were more likely to result in Duchenne dystrophy, whereas those that did not disrupt but

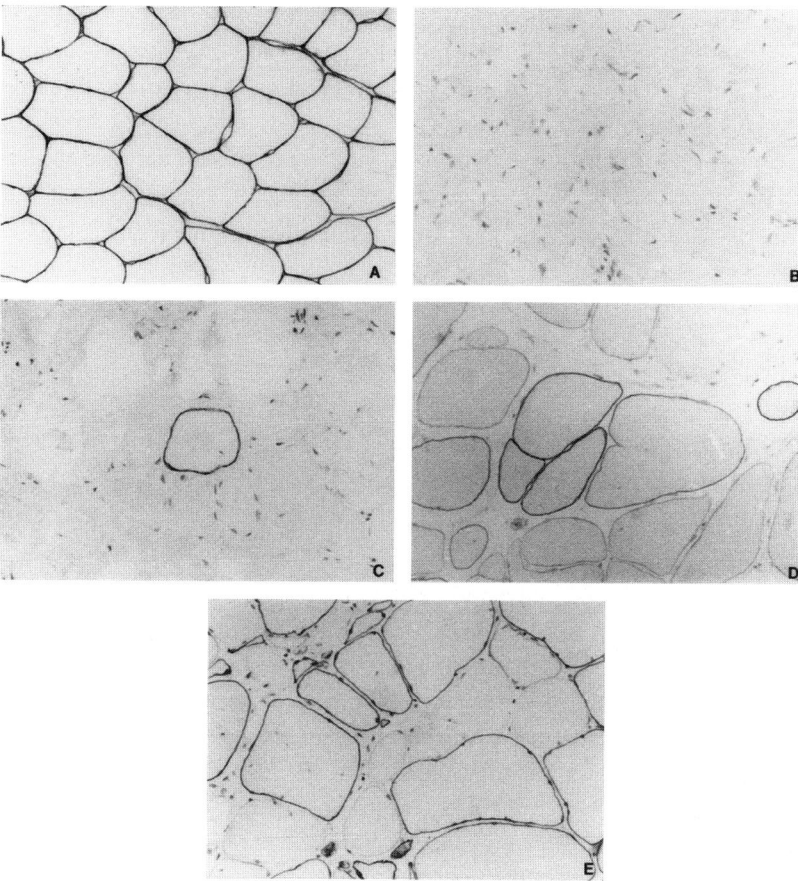

Fig. 12.9 Skeletal muscle sections with immunolabelling for dystrophin. A, Normal: dystrophin located at the sarcolemma on all fibres. B, DMD with frame-shift deletion: no dystrophin is present (counterstained with haematoxylin and eosin). C, DMD with frame-shift deletion: single positive fibre ('revertant'). D, BMD with in-frame deletion: dystrophin labelling shows marked variation both between and within fibres. E, Manifesting carrier of DMD: dystrophin labelling shows variation between fibres. Magnification ×250; indirect immunoperoxidase labelling with a monoclonal antibody (Dy8/6C5) which recognizes an epitope at the extreme C-terminus of dystrophin. (Reproduced by kind permission of Dr. Margaret Johnson and the late Dr. Louise Anderson.)

maintained the reading frame (in-frame) were more likely to result in Becker dystrophy.

This so-called *reading frame hypothesis* was first proposed by Monaco with Kunkel and colleagues in 1988[63], and has since been found to hold true in over 90% of cases. Uncommon exceptions of Becker dystrophy with a frame-shift mutation result, for example, from the reinitiation of dystrophin synthesis from an internal start codon further along the gene. Exceptional cases of Duchenne dystrophy with an in-frame deletion seem likely to be due to a defect in protein translation.

Thus, by a combination of dystrophin studies on muscle and DNA studies on peripheral blood leukocytes it was now possible to diagnose accurately a suspected case of Duchenne/Becker dystrophy and to give a good idea of the prognosis in the individual case even before the onset of symptoms. Furthermore, DNA studies on cultured amniotic fluid cells or chorionic villus biopsy material could now provide a precise prenatal diagnosis in an affected fetus.

Some unanswered questions

Although so much has now been learned about the basic molecular and biochemical defects in Duchenne and Becker dystrophies, many questions still remain.

A fundamental question is why, if muscle dystrophin is defective even in the fetus, does weakness not develop until childhood, or much later in the case of Becker dystrophy, and is thereafter progressive? Also, why do certain muscle groups become severely affected early on, such as the quadriceps, whereas others much later, such as the soleus, and yet others never become clinically affected at all, such as the extraocular muscles? Perhaps the delay in onset and the distribution of muscle involvement may be partly related to muscle fibre size. As fibre size increases so the surface-to-volume ratio decreases, and this would lead to greater membrane stress during muscle contraction[64]. Karpati[65] showed that small-calibre muscle fibres are in some way less affected by dystrophin deficiency and more resistant to necrosis.

Although Duchenne muscular dystrophy is clinically well defined, there is nevertheless variation in severity both within and between families. This variability could be a reflection of the *very small amounts* of muscle dystrophin found in some individuals which, it has been suggested, may have functional significance[66]. But why is there such wide variation in clinical features in individuals with in-frame deletions involving the central rod domain of dystrophin? Some have a degree of weakness yet others are symptom-free and may only have a raised serum creatine kinase level. Furthermore, why does pseudohypertrophy occur in Duchenne and Becker dystrophies but is rare in other forms of muscular dystrophy? In addition, there is as yet no clear explanation for certain well documented extramuscular manifestations of Duchenne dystrophy such as macroglossia, thymus hyperplasia, and hyperoestrogenaemia.

Several so-called *isoforms* of dystrophin are produced by the Duchenne (Xp21) locus, each driven by a different promoter, differing somewhat in structure, and having different tissue specificities. Five such isoforms were identified: three full length (brain, muscle, Purkinje) and two shorter (ubiquitous, nervous system)[67,68], and later two further shorter isoforms have been recognized. But there is no simple relationship between these various isoforms and clinical manifestations of the disease.

For example, deletion of the brain promoter does not necessarily result in mental retardation. There is no explanation as to why verbal IQ should be affected significantly more than performance IQ.

Cardiac involvement does not seem to be global but particularly affects the posterolateral wall of the left ventricle. Since dystrophin is presumably absent throughout the myocardium, this is difficult to explain. It may be related to the *longitudinal* distribution of cardiac muscle fibres in this region[69] and therefore to forces directed along this axis. It is even more difficult, however, to explain cardiac involvement in an established case of muscular dystrophy when the individual has no muscle weakness[70].

At this time these and other important questions remained to be answered. It is quite possible that answers to these questions will not only help our understanding of Duchenne dystrophy but also provide clues to the various clinical manifestations and differing severities in other forms of muscular dystrophy as well. The current situation is discussed further in Chapter 13.

References

1. Avery, O. T., MacLeod, C. M., McCarty, M. Studies on the chemical nature of the substance inducing transformation of pneumococcal types. *Journal of Experimental Medicine*, 1944; **79**: 137–58.
2. Watson, J. D., Crick, F. H. C. Molecular structure of nucleic acids—a structure for deoxyribose nucleic acid. *Nature*, 1953; **171**: 737–8.
3. Nirenberg, M. W., Matthaei, J. H. The dependence of cell-free protein synthesis in *E. coli* upon naturally occurring or synthetic polyribonucleotides. *Proceedings of the National Academy of Sciences USA*, 1961; **47**: 1588–602.
4. Agarwal, K. L., Büchi, H., Caruthers, M. H. *et al.* Total synthesis of the gene for an alanine transfer ribonucleic acid from yeast. *Nature*, 1970; **227**: 27–34.
5. Smith, H. O., Wilcox, K. W. A restriction enzyme from *Haemophilus influenzae*. I. Purification and general properties. *Journal of Molecular Biology*, 1970; **51**: 379–91.
6. Kelly, T. J., Smith, H. O. A restriction enzyme from *Haemophilus influenzae*. II. Base sequence of the recognition site. *Journal of Molecular Biology*, 1970; **51**: 393–409.
7. Temin, H. M., Mizutani, S. RNA-dependent DNA polymerase in virions of Rous sarcoma virus. *Nature*, 1970; **226**: 1211–13.
8. Baltimore, D. RNA-dependent DNA polymerase in virions of RNA tumour viruses. *Nature*, 1970; **226**: 1209–11.

9. Cohen, S. N., Chang, A. C. Y., Boyer, H. W., Helling, R. B. Construction of biologically functional bacterial plasmids *in vitro*. *Proceedings of the National Academy of Sciences USA*, 1973; **70**: 3240–4. (For the contribution made by Herbert Boyer, see Aird, R. B. *Foundations of Modern Neurology—A Century of Progress*. New York: Raven Press, 1994: 185–7.)
10. Southern, E. M. Detection of specific sequences among DNA fragments separated by gel electrophoresis. *Journal of Molecular Biology*, 1975; **98**: 503–17.
11. Lawn, R. M., Fritsch, E. F., Parker, R. C., Blake, G., Maniatis, T. The isolation and characterization of δ-linked and β-globin genes from a cloned library of human DNA. *Cell*, 1978; **15**: 1157–74.
12. Jeffreys, A. J., Flavell, R. A. The rabbit β-globin gene contains a large insert in the coding sequence. *Cell*, 1977; **12**: 1097–108.
13. Sanger, F., Nicklen, S., Coulson, A. R. DNA sequencing with chain-terminating inhibitors. *Proceedings of the National Academy of Sciences USA*, 1977; **74**: 5463–7.
14. Maxam, A. M., Gilbert, W. A new method for sequencing DNA. *Proceedings of the National Academy of Sciences USA*, 1977; **74**: 560–4.
15. Botstein, D., White, R. L., Skolnick, M., Davis, R. W. Construction of a genetic linkage map in man using restriction fragment length polymorphisms. *American Journal of Human Genetics*, 1980; **32**: 314–31.
16. Wyman, A. R., White, R. A highly polymorphic locus in human DNA. *Proceedings of the National Academy of Sciences USA*, 1980; **77**: 6754–8.
17. Bell, J., Haldane, J. B. S. The linkage between the genes for colour-blindness and haemophilia in man. *Proceedings of the Royal Society (London) B*, 1937; **123**: 119–50.
18. Philip, U. A note on colour vision and linkage studies. *Annals of Human Genetics*, 1955; **20**: 16–17.
19. Blyth, H., Carter, C. O., Dubowitz, V. *et al*. Duchenne's muscular dystrophy and the Xg blood groups: a search for linkage. *Journal of Medical Genetics*, 1965; **2**: 157–60.
20. Davies, K. E. The application of DNA recombinant technology to the analysis of the human genome and genetic disease. *Human Genetics*, 1981; **58**: 351–7.
21. Davies, K. E., Young, B. D., Elles, R. G., Hill, M. E., Williamson, R. Cloning of a representative genomic library of the human X chromosome after sorting by flow cytometry. *Nature*, 1981; **293**: 374–6.
22. Harper, P. S., Harper, R. M. J., Howell Evans, A. W. Carcinoma of the oesophagus with tylosis. *Quarterly Journal of Medicine*, 1970; **39**: 317–33.
23. Harper, P. S., Dyken, P. R. Early onset dystrophia myotonica: evidence supporting a maternal environmental factor. *Lancet*, 1972; **ii**: 53–5.
24. Harper, P. S., Rivas, M. L., Bias, W. B. *et al*. Genetic linkage confirmed between the locus for myotonic dystrophy and the ABH-secretor and Lutheran blood group loci. *American Journal of Human Genetics*, 1972; **24**: 310–16.
25. Murray, J. M., Davies, K. E., Harper, P. S. *et al*. Linkage relationship of a cloned DNA sequence on the short arm of the X chromosome to Duchenne muscular dystrophy. *Nature*, 1982; **300**: 69–71.
26. Davies, K. E., Pearson, P. L., Harper, P. S. *et al*. Linkage analysis of two cloned DNA sequences flanking the Duchenne muscular dystrophy locus on the short arm of the human X chromosome. *Nucleic Acids Research*, 1983; **11**: 2303–12.

27. Francke, U., Ochs, H. D., de Martinville, B. *et al.* Minor Xp21 chromosome deletion in a male associated with expression of Duchenne muscular dystrophy, chronic granulomatous disease, retinitis pigmentosa and McLeod syndrome. *American Journal of Human Genetics*, 1985; **37**: 250–67.
28. Verellen, C., De Meyer, R., Freund, M. *et al.* Progressive muscular dystrophy of the Duchenne type in a young girl associated with an aberration of chromosome X. In: *Proceedings of the 5th International Congress on Birth Defects.* Amsterdam: Excerpta Medica, 1977: 42 (Abstract).
29. Greenstein, R. M., Reardon, M. P., Chan, T. S. An X/autosome translocation in a girl with Duchenne muscular dystrophy (DMD): evidence for DMD gene localization. *Paediatric Research*, 1977; **11**: 457 (Abstract).
30. Lindenbaum, R. H., Clarke, G., Patel, C., Moncrieff, M., Hughes, J. T. Muscular dystrophy in an X;1 translocation female suggests that Duchenne locus is on X chromosome short arm. *Journal of Medical Genetics*, 1979; **16**: 389–92.
31. Canki, N., Dutrillaux, B., Tivadar, I. Dystrophie musculaire de Duchenne chez une petite fille porteuse d'une translocation t(X;3) (p 21;q 13) *de novo*. *Annales de Génétique*, 1979; **22**: 35–9.
32. Kingston, H. M., Thomas, N. S. T., Pearson, P. L., Sarfarazi, M., Harper, P. S. Genetic linkage between Becker muscular dystrophy and a polymorphic DNA sequence on the short arm of the X chromosome. *Journal of Medical Genetics*, 1983; **20**: 255–8.
33. Kingston, H. M., Sarfarazi, M., Thomas, N. S. T., Harper, P. S. Localisation of the Becker muscular dystrophy gene on the short arm of the X chromosome by linkage to cloned DNA sequences. *Human Genetics*, 1984; **67**: 6–17.
34. Wieacker, P., Davies, K., Pearson, P., Ropers, H-H. Carrier detection in Duchenne muscular dystrophy by use of cloned DNA sequences. *Lancet*, 1983; **i**: 1325–6.
35. Harper, P. S., O'Brien, T., Murray, J. M. *et al.* The use of linked DNA polymorphisms for genotype prediction in families with Duchenne muscular dystrophy. *Journal of Medical Genetics*, 1983; **20**: 252–4.
36. Steele, M. W., Breg, W. R. Chromosome analysis of human amniotic fluid cells. *Lancet*, 1966; **i**: 383–5.
37. Jacobson, C. B., Barter, R. H. Intrauterine diagnosis and management of genetic defects. *American Journal of Obstetrics and Gynecology*, 1967; **99**: 796–805.
38. Nadler, H. L. Antenatal detection of hereditary disorders. *Paediatrics*, 1968; **42**: 912–18.
39. Emery, A. E. H. (ed.) *Antenatal Diagnosis of Genetic Disease.* Edinburgh and London: Churchill Livingstone, 1973.
40. Bakker, E., Goor, N. Wrogemann, K. *et al.* Prenatal diagnosis and carrier detection of Duchenne muscular dystrophy with closely linked RFLPs. *Lancet*, 1985; **i**: 655–8.
41. Kunkel, L. M., Smith, K. D., Boyer, S. H. Human Y-chromosome-specific reiterated DNA. *Science*, 1976; **191**: 1189–90.
42. Kunkel, L. M., Smith, K. D., Boyer, S. H. *et al.* Analysis of human Y-chromosome-specific reiterated DNA in chromosome variants. *Proceedings of the National Academy of Sciences USA*, 1977; **74**: 1245–9.
43. Kunkel, L. M., Monaco, A. P., Middlesworth, W., Ochs, H. D., Latt, S. A. Specific cloning of DNA fragments absent from the DNA of a male patient with an X chromosome deletion. *Proceedings of the National Academy of Sciences USA*, 1985; **82**: 4778–82.

44. Worton, R. G., Duff, C., Sylvester, J. E., Schmickel, R. D., Willard, H. F. Duchenne muscular dystrophy involving translocation of the *dmd* gene next to ribosomal RNA genes. *Science*, 1984; **224**: 1447–9.
45. Ray, P. N., Belfall, B., Duff, C. *et al.* Cloning of the breakpoint of an X:21 translocation associated with Duchenne muscular dystrophy. *Nature*, 1985; **318**: 672–5.
46. Monaco, A. P., Bertelson, C. J., Middlesworth, W. *et al.* Detection of deletions spanning the Duchenne muscular dystrophy locus using a tightly linked DNA segment. *Nature*, 1985; **316**: 842–5.
47. Kunkel, L. M. *et al.* Analysis of deletions in DNA from patients with Becker and Duchenne muscular dystrophy. *Nature*, 1986; **322**: 73–7.
48. Monaco, A. P., Neve, R. L., Colletti-Feener, C. *et al.* Isolation of candidate cDNAs for portions of the Duchenne muscular dystrophy gene. *Nature*, 1986; **323**: 646–50.
49. Burghes, A. H. M., Logan, C., Hu, X. *et al.* A cDNA clone from the Duchenne/Becker muscular dystrophy gene. *Nature*, 1987; **328**: 434–7.
50. Koenig, M., Hoffman, E. P., Bertelson, C. J. *et al.* Complete cloning of the Duchenne muscular dystrophy (DMD) cDNA and preliminary genomic organization of the DMD gene in normal and affected individuals. *Cell*, 1987; **50**: 509–17.
51. Koenig, M., Monaco, A. P., Kunkel, L. M. The complete sequence of dystrophin predicts a rod-shaped cytoskeletal protein. *Cell*, 1988; **53**: 219–28.
52. Hoffman, E. P., Brown, R. H., Kunkel, L. M. Dystrophin: the protein product of the Duchenne muscular dystrophy locus. *Cell*, 1987; **51**: 919–28.
53. Hoffman, E. P., Fischbeck, K. H., Brown, R. H. *et al.* Characterization of dystrophin in muscle-biopsy specimens from patients with Duchenne's or Becker's muscular dystrophy. *New England Journal of Medicine*, 1988; **318**: 1363–8.
54. Sugita, H., Arahata, K., Ishiguro, T. *et al.* Negative immunostaining of Duchenne muscular dystrophy (DMD) and mdx muscle surface membrane with antibody against synthetic peptide fragment predicted from DMD cDNA. *Proceedings of the Japan Academy*, 1988; **64**: 37–9. (See also: Arahata, K. et al. *Nature*, 1988; **333**: 861–3.)
55. Zubrzycka-Gaarn, E. E., Bulman, D. E., Karpati, G. *et al.* The Duchenne muscular dystrophy gene product is localized in sarcolemma of human skeletal muscle. *Nature*, 1988; **333**: 466–9.
56. Bonilla, E., Samitt, C. E., Miranda, A. F. *et al.* Duchenne muscular dystrophy: deficiency of dystrophin at the muscle cell surface. *Cell*, 1988; **54**: 447–52.
57. Campbell, K. P., Kahl, S. D. Association of dystrophin and an integral membrane glycoprotein. *Nature*, 1989; **338**: 259–62.
58. Matsumura, K., Campbell, K. P. Dystrophin–glycoprotein complex: its role in the molecular pathogenesis of muscular dystrophies. *Muscle and Nerve*, 1994; **17**: 2–15.
59. Matsumura, K., Tomé, F. M. S., Collin, H. *et al.* Deficiency of the 50k dystrophin-associated glycoprotein in severe childhood autosomal recessive muscular dystrophy. *Nature*, 1992; **359**: 320–2. (See also: Roberds, S. L. et al. *Cell*, 1994; **78**: 1–20.)
60. Tomé, F. M. S., Evangelista, T., Leclerc, A. *et al.* Congenital muscular dystrophy with merosin deficiency. *Comptes Rendus de l'Académie des Sciences (Paris) (Sciences de la vie)*, 1994; **317**: 351–7. (See also: Sunada, Y. et al. *Journal of Biological Chemistry*, 1994; **269**: 13729–32.)
61. Beggs, A. H., Kunkel, L. M. Improved diagnosis of Duchenne/Becker muscular dystrophy. *Journal of Clinical Investigation*, 1990; **85**: 613–19.

62. Hoffman, E. P. Genotype/phenotype correlations in Duchenne/Becker dystrophy. In: T. Partridge (ed.) *Molecular and Cell Biology of Muscular Dystrophy*. London: Chapman and Hall, 1993: 12–36.
63. Monaco, A. P., Bertelson, C. J., Liechti-Gallati, S., Moser, H., Kunkel, L. M. An explanation for the phenotypic differences between patients bearing partial deletions of the DMD locus. *Genomics*, 1988; **2**: 90–5.
64. Petrof, B. J., Shrager, J. B., Stedman, H. H., Kelly, A. M., Sweeney, H. L. Dystrophin protects the sarcolemma from stresses developed during muscle contraction. *Proceedings of the National Academy of Sciences USA*, 1993; **90**: 3710–14.
65. Karpati, G., Carpenter, S. Small-caliber skeletal muscle fibers do not suffer deleterious consequences of dystrophin gene expression. *American Journal of Medical Genetics*, 1986; **25**: 653–8.
66. Nicholson, L. V. B., Johnson, M. A., Bushby, K. M. D., Gardner-Medwin, D. Functional significance of dystrophin positive fibres in Duchenne muscular dystrophy. *Archives of Disease in Childhood*, 1993; **68**: 632–6.
67. Ahn, A. H., Kunkel, L. M. The structural and functional diversity of dystrophin. *Nature Genetics*, 1993; **3**: 283–91.
68. Schofield, J. N., Blake, D. J., Simmons, C. *et al.* Apo-dystrophin-1 and apo-dystrophin-2, products of the Duchenne muscular dystrophy locus: expression during mouse embryogenesis and in cultured cell lines. *Human Molecular Genetics*, 1994; **3**: 1309–16.
69. Cziner, D. G., Levin, R. I. The cardiomyopathy of Duchenne's muscular dystrophy and the function of dystrophin. *Medical Hypotheses*, 1993; **40**: 169–73.
70. Miyashita, H., Ikeda, U., Shimada, K., Natsume, T., Arahata, K. Becker muscular dystrophy with early manifestations of left heart failure. *Internal Medicine*, 1993; **32**: 408–11. (See also: Siciliano, G. *et al. Neuromuscular Disorders*, 1994; **4**: 381–6.)

Chapter 13

Current trends and the future

From finding a linked DNA marker in Duchenne muscular dystrophy to isolating, cloning, and characterizing the responsible gene and identifying the biochemical defect had taken less than 10 years. This had been a remarkable achievement. The feeling of depression that had previously pervaded studies of the disease, and to which Bud Rowland had referred in 1976, had evaporated. Success in science tends to breed success by attracting more, and possibly better, investigators. This was true in the case of Duchenne muscular dystrophy. But this success would not have been so easily achieved had not the ground been carefully prepared beforehand. Very few advances in medical science are totally original and unique. Most depend to a varying degree on the previous work of others. It is abundantly clear in the recent history of Duchenne dystrophy that scientists have risen to the challenge of molecular diagnosis with spectacular success, and one is reminded of the sentiments expressed by Bertolt Brecht:

> Beauty in nature is a quality which gives the human senses a chance to be skilful.

Clinical and basic research over the past few decades has revealed an ever-evolving panoply of muscle diseases[1]. In this chapter we shall briefly summarize some of the current areas of research and future possibilities with regard to the muscular dystrophies as a group of related conditions.

Genetic and clinical heterogeneity

The identification of the gene for Duchenne dystrophy was soon followed by the clinical and genetic identification of various other forms of muscular dystrophy. These fall into six major groups depending on the distribution of predominant muscle weakness (Figure 13.1). Over 30 different forms are now recognized, and some of the main forms (including congenital muscular dystrophy) and their gene locations and protein products are summarized in Table 13.1.

Pathogenesis

The localization of dystrophin to the sarcolemma clearly placed the basis of Duchenne dystrophy in the muscle membrane. Since then many other

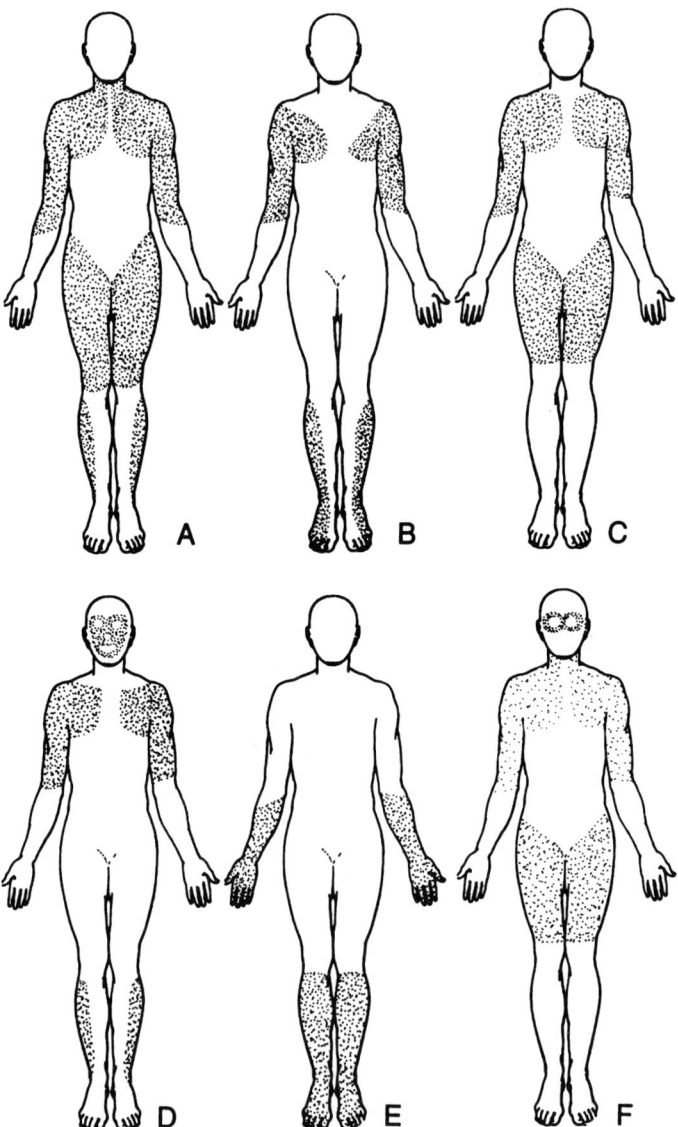

Fig. 13.1 Distribution of predominant muscle weakness in different types of dystrophy. A, Duchenne-type and Becker-type; B, Emery–Dreifuss; C, limb girdle; D, facioscapulohumeral; E, distal; F, oculopharyngeal. Shaded areas are affected. (Reproduced from Emery, A.E.H., (1998), Fortnightly review: The muscular dystrophies, *BMJ*; **317**: 991–995 with permission from BMJ Publishing Group Ltd.)

Table 13.1 Some of the *main* forms of muscular dystrophy, their gene locations, and protein products

Dystrophy	Inheritance	Protein	Gene Location
Duchenne/Becker	X-R	Dystrophin	Xp21
Limb girdle	AD	1A Myotilin	5q31
		1B Lam A/C	1q21
		1C Cav-3	3p25
	AR	2A Calp-3	15q15
		2B Dysferlin	2p13
		2C γ sarcoglycan	13q12
		2D α sarcoglycan	17q21
		2E β sarcoglycan	4q12
		2F δ sarcoglycan	5q33
		2G Telethonin	17q12
		2H TRIM 32	9q33
		2I FKRP	19q13
		2J Titin	2q31
Emery–Dreifuss	AD/AR	Lam A/C	1q21
	X-R (1)	Emerin	Xq28
	X-R (2)	FHL 1	Xq26
Facioscapulohumeral	AD	—	4q35
Distal	AD		
	Laing	Myosin	14q11
	Welander	—	2p13
	Udd	Titin	2q31
	AR		
	Nonaka	Glucosamine epimerase	9p12
	Miyoshi	Dysferlin	2p13
Oculopharyngeal	AD/AR	PABN 1	14q11–13
Congenital*	AR	1A Laminin α 2	6q22
		1B —	1q42
		1C FKRP	19q13
		1D LARGE	22q12
		FCMD Fukutin	9q31

*Other forms of congenital muscular dystrophy also exist (e.g. muscle-eye-brain disease, Walker–Warburg disease). X-R, X-linked recessive; AD, autosomal dominant; AR, autosomal recessive; Lam, Lamin; Cav, caveolin; Calp, calpain; FHL, four and a half LIM; PABN, poly(A)binding protein; FKRP, Fukutin-related protein; FCMD, Fukuyama congenital muscular dystrophy. A computerized and more detailed and comprehensive gene table of monogenic neuromuscular disorders by J-C. Kaplan is accessible at http://www.musclegenetable.org/

proteins, defective in other forms of dystrophy, have also been localized to the muscle membrane (Figure 13.2). However, other proteins have not. For example, those associated with the nucleus (PABN), nuclear membrane (Lam-A, Emerin), or sarcomere (Myotilin, Telethonin, Titin) or a defective enzyme (Calpain-3). In fact, the involvement of various sarcomeric proteins in muscle disease is now well documented[2].

Because of the great variety of protein defects in muscular dystrophy, attempts to provide a satisfactory unifying concept for their pathogenesis have so far failed. Perhaps it might therefore be better not to include all these disorders under the same rubric, but rather consider each group separately under their respective shared defect; for example, dystrophinopathies, laminopathies, and so on. Because of the complex binding relationships between the various sarcolemmal associated proteins[3], this could help explain, in some cases, the efflux of muscle enzymes and the detrimental cascade effects of the influx of calcium ions (see Figure 13.1, page 200, in the first edition of this book). Many other ideas are also being pursued, such as the secondary deficiency of nNOS (neuronal nitric oxide synthase) modulating muscle blood flow, the role of various immune factors and, most recently, the role of certain matrix metalloproteinases (MMPs) [4]. Incidentally, serum levels of MMP-2 may be of value for detecting cardiac involvement in Emery–Dreifuss muscular dystrophy[5].

Clinical variation

Significant clinical variation within groups of affected individuals sharing the same protein defect is becoming clear. In Duchenne dystrophy this has been known for some time. In our own experience of some 150 affected boys followed throughout their lives, the age of onset varied from less than 2 to 9, age at chairbound from 6 to 14, and age at death from 8 to 25 (before assisted respiration was introduced). Admittedly, some of this variation could be due to environmental factors. But it is more difficult to explain the occurrence of at least 12 very different phenotypes associated with LMNA (Lamin A gene) mutations. These include, for example, autosomal dominant Emery–Dreifuss muscular dystrophy and limb girdle muscular dystrophy 1B, as well as autosomal recessive forms of Emery–Dreifuss muscular dystrophy, Charcot–Marie–Tooth neuropathy 2B, mandibuloacral dysplasia, and cases of progeria. Also, a very large family with autosomal dominant Emery–Dreifuss muscular dystrophy has been reported in which some individuals had the complete clinical phenotype, yet in other branches of the same family affected individuals exhibited only the cardiomyopathy[6]. There are many other examples of clinical variation within groups of affected individuals sharing the same protein defect. An important question is how can such variation be explained?

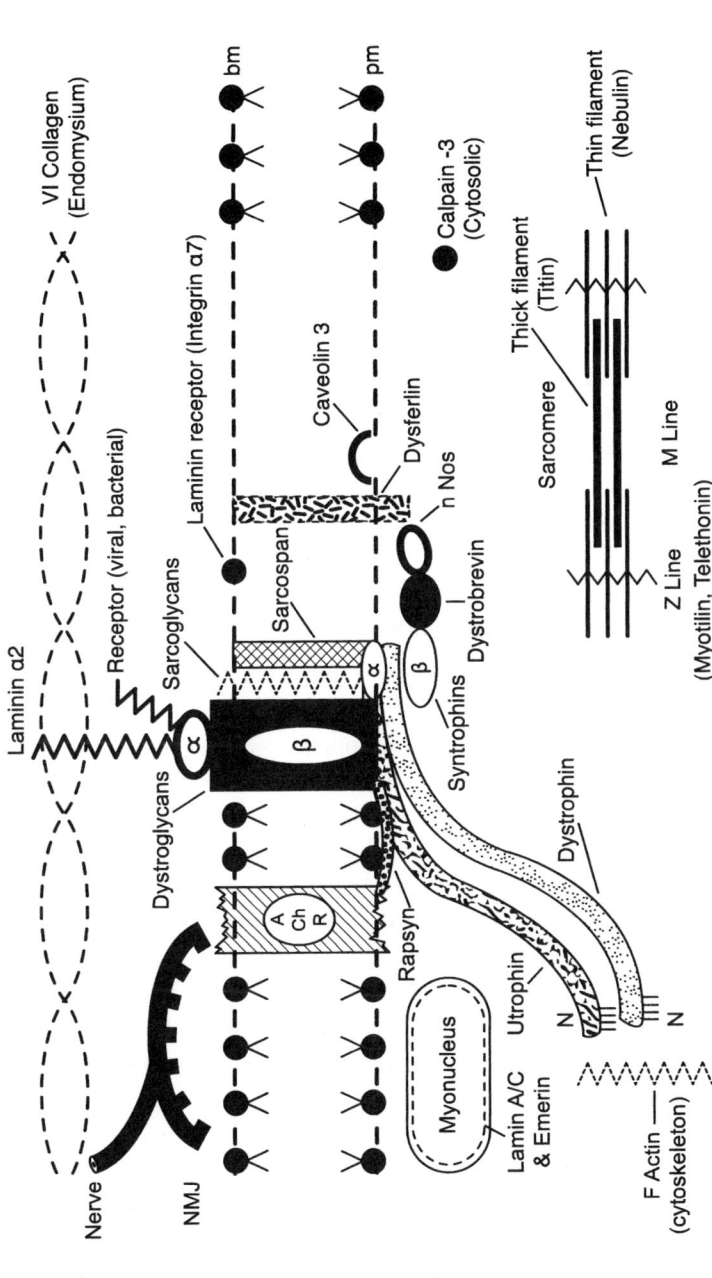

Fig. 13.2 Diagrammatic representation of some of the proteins implicated in different forms of muscular dystrophy. bm, basement membrane; pm, plasma membrane; NMJ, neuromuscular junction; AchR, acetylcholine receptor.

Several approaches to this problem are currently under investigation. These include the possible role of common polymorphisms affecting the phenotype (single nucleotide polymorphisms or SNPs, and copy number variations or CNVs). Certainly there is good evidence now that such polymorphisms can modulate susceptibility to various common multifactorial diseases[7,8]. In fact, a specific copy number variant has now been shown to correlate with severity in unifactorial X-linked mental retardation[9].

Another possible approach to the problem could be the activation of cryptic splicing sites by specific mutations, and the role of heterogeneous nuclear ribonucleoproteins (hnRNPs) which bind single-stranded RNAs. TDP-43 is such an hnRNP involved in specific pre-mRNA splicing and translation, and has now been implicated in several neurodegenerative disorders[10,11]. The possibility that such hnRNPs could be involved in the clinical variability of the muscular dystrophies and related disorders is open to question.

Finally, there could be a possible role for epigenetic factors—heritable changes in gene expression without a change in DNA sequences—which has already been clearly demonstrated in several paediatric syndromes as well as in facioscapulohumeral muscular dystrophy[12].

Infection and muscular dystrophy

The possibility of a link between infection by micro-organisms and the molecular basis of the muscular dystrophies has been summarized[13]. Such a link was first suggested by the work of Badorff and colleagues[14]. They showed that the enteroviral protease 2A of Coxsackievirus B3 specifically cleaves dystrophin in cardiac muscle. This could explain the occasional occurrence of cardiac involvement in healthy people infected with the virus. But from the present point of view could such infections prove particularly serious in those with reduced dystrophin, as in Becker dystrophy? Several other viruses also cleave various muscle cytoskeletal proteins and might therefore account for some of the clinical effects of infections by these particular viruses[15]. There is good evidence of certain muscle proteins being involved in the pathogenesis of particular acquired infections[16]. Perhaps of greatest significance is the involvement of dystroglycans[17].

The α form of dystroglycan (αDG) has a two-fold function: it binds to extracellular proteins such as perlecan, agrin, and the laminins, and most importantly provides a receptor for various pathogenic viral and bacterial micro-organisms[18]. Its binding function depends on effective glycosylation[19]. MMPs cleave the extracellular domain of βDG with the loss of αDG and therefore its binding functions. MMP activity is increased in various infections which thus prevent the invading organism gaining entry into the cell[20] and is therefore an important host defence mechanism. It is now known that MMP activity is significantly increased in the *mdx* mouse, the Japanese dog with muscular dystrophy, and in Duchenne muscular dystrophy[21]. This raises the intriguing question as to whether boys with Duchenne dystrophy are less prone to these sorts of infections than unaffected boys. But there is another matter. The glycosyltransferase LARGE (responsible for congenital muscular dystrophy 1D in homozygotes, heterozygotes being of course normal) is critical for αDG to function as a receptor for several viruses, most significantly for arenaviruses which cause serious Lassa fever in West Africa as well as several related diseases in South America[22]. Furthermore, there is evidence that there has been positive selection pressure in normal heterozygotes for LARGE[23] in West Africa. This could be comparable to the case of resistance of heterozygotes for sickle-cell anaemia to falciparum malaria. Proof of the resistance of heterozygotes for LARGE and Lassa fever could be tested in the field as well as in the laboratory using appropriate animal models[13].

Treatment

Because Duchenne muscular dystrophy is incurable, in the past there was a general lack of interest in the medical management of the condition. But in recent years this has changed[24]. It is now realized that much can be gained from active physiotherapy to delay the development of muscle contractures and deformities. Progressive spinal deformity, which further compromises respiratory impairment, occurs once the individual becomes chairbound. Prolongation of ambulation, by using various orthoses coupled perhaps with surgery, can in some cases be helpful in this regard. In 1982 Eduardo Luque of Mexico introduced a new surgical procedure of spinal fusion which halts the development of scoliosis, and is recommended in some cases. Respiratory care is essential as the disease progresses, and in the later stages some form of assisted ventilation often becomes necessary, a procedure nowadays being considered more frequently and thus prolonging life even into the early 30s. In the more benign forms of muscular dystrophy the importance of maintaining ambulation as long as possible by various orthoses and surgical procedures is particularly important as it often allows the individual to continue with gainful employment and to have many years of productive life. But all these measures, though gaining in importance in the management of dystrophy, are not in any way curative.

Over the past 80 years or so, many drugs have been tried in an attempt to treat the condition (Table 13.2). Unfortunately many of the early trials of drug

Table 13.2 Drugs used in various therapeutic trials in Duchenne muscular dystrophy

Drug	Basis for use	First reported trial
Allopurinol	Increases nucleotide formation believed to be depleted in dystrophic muscle	1976
Amino acids	Deficiency of muscle protein	1953
Aminoglycoside antibiotics	Suppress 'STOP' mutations	2001
Anabolic steroids	Anabolic effect	1955
Aspirin, propranolol, etc.	Counteract proposed defect in biogenic amine metabolism	1977
Azathioprine	Immunosuppression	1993
Calcium blockers	Reduce muscle intracellular calcium	1982
Catecholamines	Counteract proposed defect in muscle sympathetic innervation	1930
Coenzyme Q	Possible benefit in murine dystrophy	1974
Creatine	Deficiency in muscle	2000
Cyclosporine	Immunosuppression	1993
Dantrolene	Inhibit release of calcium from sarcoplasmic reticulum	1983
Digitalis and other cardiac glycosides	Prevent progressive cardiomyopathy	1963
Glucocorticoids	First randomized controlled trials	1989
Glycine	Believed to stimulate muscle creatine synthesis	1932
Growth hormone	Anabolic effect	1973
Growth hormone inhibitor	Growth hormone deficiency ameliorates disease	1984
Ketoacids	Reduce muscle protein degradation	1982
Leucine	Increases protein synthesis	1984
Nucleotides (e.g. Laevadosin)	Replacement of nucleotides believed to be depleted in dystrophic muscle	1960
Oestrogens	Anabolic effect	1972
Oxandrolone	Anabolic effect	1997
Pancreatic extract	Possible benefit in murine dystrophy	1976
Penicillamine	Possible benefit in avian dystrophy	1977
Prednisone	Anabolic and immunosuppressive effect	1974
Protease inhibitors	Possible benefit in murine dystrophy	1984

Table 13.2 *(Cont'd)* Drugs used in various therapeutic trials in Duchenne muscular dystrophy

Drug	Basis for use	First reported trial
Superoxide dismutase	Removal of superoxide radicals associated with membrane damage	1980
Testosterone	Anabolic effect	1955
Thyroxine	Thyroxine depresses serum creatine kinase	1964
Vasodilators	Counteract proposed defect in muscle microcirculation	1963
Vitamins/minerals		
B6	Vitamin B6-deficient rats develop myopathy	1940
E	Vitamin E-deficient animals develop myopathy	1940
Zinc	Membrane 'stabilizer'	1986

treatment were poorly designed with inadequate controls and almost invariably little scientific basis. Currently treatment has centred on the use of corticosteroids, for which there have been many previous trials[25] and a recent extensive Cochrane review[26]. The evidence suggests such treatment can lead to some improvement in muscle strength and prolong walking for a while, though unfortunately often at the expense of side effects.

A novel approach to the problem being explored is the possibility of employing automated drug screening on muscle tissue *in vitro*, thus circumventing all the difficulties and problems associated with clinical trials[27]; however, important limitations to this approach have been voiced[28].

The logic behind all such approaches to treatment is the hope of finding a drug which could interrupt an important pathogenic pathway and thereby be clinically effective.

Meanwhile, various molecular approaches to treatment are being actively pursued[29,30]. There is already a vast literature on the subject. Essentially, these various methods involve:

1. Replacing the mutant gene by a mini-dystrophic gene using some form of viral vector[31,32]
2. The use of a compound such as PTC124 (Ataluren, PTC Therapeutics, New Jersey, USA) to readthrough nonsense (STOP) mutations in the dystrophic gene[33], although at most only around 10% of cases are caused by such mutations
3. Up-regulation of utrophin, a sarcolemmal protein similar to dystrophin with the same binding characteristics, to compensate for the deficiency of dystrophin[34,35]

4. Exon (containing a dystrophin mutation) skipping with antisense oligonucleotides, attached to certain peptides to aid the process (e.g. morpholinos), to restore dystrophin synthesis without the mutated exon(s) [36,37]
5. Stem cell therapy involving injecting stem cells (derived from muscle satellite cells or from other tissues) either from the patient, after appropriately correcting the gene mutation, or from healthy donors but then requiring some form of immunosuppression to prevent rejection[38]. The aim is to encourage normal muscle regeneration.

Each of these different approaches has its advocates as well as critics. For example, in the case of PTC124 and nonsense mutations there could be important limitations to this approach[39]. In all such approaches to treatment the problem exists of devising *systemic* delivery to ensure that all muscles are treated, most importantly the respiratory and cardiac muscles.

So far much of this research has centred on the *mdx* mouse but now clinical trials are beginning, most notably with the use of antisense oligonucleotides to effect exon skipping. The next year or two are going to be critical in assessing the relative values and effectiveness of these various approaches to treatment.

The future

Over recent years clinical studies and genetic research have now made it possible to provide a reliable diagnosis and prognosis for almost all forms of muscular dystrophy. It is also possible to offer prevention through, for example, prenatal diagnosis based on appropriate studies of cultured amniotic fluid cells, obtained by transabdominal amniocentesis, or from chorionic villi obtained by transcervical chorion biopsy. Both are now relatively safe procedures but, of course, if the fetus proves to be affected the mother has to face all the concerns of pregnancy termination.

However, there is now growing optimism that some form of treatment may become available for Duchenne muscular dystrophy in the not-too-distant future. Meanwhile, well planned and coordinated management is essential. This involves physicians, including specialists in cardiology and respiratory medicine with experience in assisted respiration, physiotherapists, and psychologists. Those with specialist training in education and occupational therapy for the physically disabled can also provide important advice and support.

On a wider perspective, there is an important need for clinicians and scientists to collaborate at the national and international level. The European Neuromuscular Centre (ENMC) was set up in 1990, based first in Paris and later in Naarden, The Netherlands. Its clearly defined aims from the outset were to encourage and facilitate internationally recognized clinicians and scientists to collaborate in research into neuromuscular disorders[40]. It was decided that these aims could be best achieved by arranging workshops attended by small groups of internationally recognized experts in a particular field. So far, approaching 200 such workshops have been held. At the conclusion of each a summary of the findings is published online as well as in the journal *Neuromuscular Disorders*. The organization has a readily accessible website: http://www.enmc.org.

TREAT-NMD is an organization funded by the European Union which, through European Centres working with others across the world, aims to harmonize approaches to the treatment and management of neuromuscular disorders, especially muscular dystrophy and spinal muscular atrophy. It too has a readily accessible website: http://www.treat-nmd.eu[24,41]. However, Victor Dubowitz, a renowned authority on the subject, suggests there should now be an open debate (perhaps through his journal *Neuromuscular Disorders*) by those with clinical experience to consider some of the matters raised (or even not mentioned) in TREAT-NMD[42].

Finally, most countries now host charitable organizations providing support for patients and their families. The Muscular Dystrophy Campaign (previously the Muscular Dystrophy Group) in the UK was among the first (http://www.muscular-dystrophy.org), and there are now no less than 45 such organizations throughout the world[43].

There can be little doubt that Edward Meryon would never have imagined that some 150 years after the publication of his brief 11-page article on muscular dystrophy there would be such worldwide interest in the subject. It seems therefore appropriate to conclude with a quotation from William Blake, a close friend of John Linnell who later painted Meryon's portrait:

> What is now proved was once only imagined. (William Blake, *The Marriage of Heaven and Hell, c. 1790*).

References

1. Karpati, G. (ed.) *Structural and Molecular Basis of Skeletal Muscle Diseases.* Basel: ISN Neuropath Press, 2002.
2. Laing, N. G. (ed.) *The Sarcomere and Skeletal Muscle Disease.* New York: Springer Science-Landes Bioscience, 2008.
3. Emery, A. E. H., Muntoni, F. *Duchenne Muscular Dystrophy*, 3rd edn. Oxford: Oxford University Press, 2003: 159–72.
4. Zanotti, S., Gibertini, S., Mora, M. Altered production of extra-cellular matrix components by muscle-derived Duchenne muscular dystrophy fibroblasts before and after TGF-β1 treatment. *Cell & Tissue Research*, 2010; **339**: 397–410.

5. Niebroj-Dobosz, I., Madej-Pilarczyk, A., Marchel, M., et al. Matrix metalloproteinases in serum of Emery–Dreifuss muscular dystrophy patients. *Acta Biochimica Polonica*, 2009; **56**: 717–22.
6. Bonne, G., DiBarletta, M. R., Varnous, S. et al. Mutations in the gene encoding lamin A/C cause autosomal dominant Emery–Dreifuss muscular dystrophy. *Nature Genetics*, 1999; **21**: 285–8.
7. Knight, J. C. Genetics and the general physician: insights, applications and future challenges. *Quarterly Journal of Medicine*, 2009; **102**: 757–72.
8. Conrad, D. F., Pinto, D., Redon, R. et al. Origins and functional impact of copy number variation in the human genome. *Nature*, 2010; **464**: 704–12.
9. Vandewalle, J. Van Esch, H., Govaerts, K. et al. Dosage-dependent severity of the phenotype in patients with mental retardation due to a recurrent copy-number gain at Xq28 mediated by an unusual recombination. *American Journal of Human Genetics*, 2009; **85**: 809–22.
10. Ayala, Y. M., Misteli, T., Baralle, F. E. TDP-43 regulates retinoblastoma protein phosphorylation through the repression of cyclic-dependent kinase 6 expression. *Proceedings of the National Academy of Sciences USA*, 2008; **105**: 3785–9.
11. Buratti, E., Baralle, F. E. The molecular links between TDP-43 dysfunction and neurodegeneration. In: T. Friedmann, J. C. Dunlap, S. F. Goodwin (eds). *Advances in Genetics*, 2009; **66**: 1–34.
12. Rodenhiser, D. M., Mann, M. Epigenetics and human disease: translating basic biology into clinical applications. *Canadian Medical Association Journal*, 2006; **174**: 341–8.
13. Emery, A. E. H. Resistance to infection and the muscular dystrophies: is there a molecular link? *Neuromuscular Disorders*, 2008; **18**: 423–5.
14. Badorff, C., Lee, G., Lamphear, B. J. et al. Enteroviral protease 2A cleaves dystrophin: evidence of cytoskeletal disruption in an acquired cardiomyopathy. *Nature Medicine*, 1999; **5**: 320–6.
15. Lee, G. H., Badorff, C., Knowlton, K. U. Dissociation of sarcoglycans and the dystrophin carboxyl terminus from the sarcolemma in enteroviral cardiomyopathy. *Circulation Research*, 2000; **87**: 485–95.
16. Emery, A. E. H. Muscular dystrophy—an evolving concept. In: A. E. H. Emery (ed.) *The Muscular Dystrophies*. Oxford: Oxford University Press, 2001: 1–9.
17. Emery, A. E. H. Muscular dystrophy into the new millennium. *Neuromuscular Disorders*, 2002; **12**: 343–9.
18. Smelt, S. C., Borrow, P., Kunz, S. et al. Differences in affinity of binding of lymphocytic choriomeningitis virus strains to the cellular receptor α-dystroglycan correlate with viral tropism and disease kinetics. *Journal of Virology*, 2001; **75**: 448–57.
19. Michele, D. E., Campbell, K. P. Dystrophin–glycoprotein complex: post-translational processing and dystroglycan function. *Journal of Biological Chemistry*, 2003; **278**: 15457–60.
20. Lemaitre, V., D'Armiento, J. Matrix metalloproteinases in development and disease. *Birth Defects Research Part C Embryo Today*, 2006; **78**: 1–10.
21. Zanotti, S., Saredi, S., Ruggieri, A. et al. Altered extracellular matrix transcript expression and protein modulation in primary Duchenne muscular dystrophy myotubes. *Matrix Biology*, 2007; **26**: 615–24.

22. Kunz, S., Rojek, J. M., Kanagava, M. et al. Posttranslational modification of α-dystroglycan, the cellular receptor for arenaviruses, by the glycosyltransferase LARGE is critical for virus binding. *Journal of Virology*, 2005; **79**: 14282–6.
23. Sabeti, P. C., Varilly, P., Fry, B. et al. Genome-wide detection and characterization of positive selection in human populations. *Nature*, 2007; **449**: 913–19.
24. Bushby, K., Finkel, R., Birnkrant, D. et al. Diagnosis and management of Duchenne muscular dystrophy, part 1: diagnosis and pharmacological and psychosocial management. *Lancet Neurology*, 2010; **9**: 77–93.
25. Emery, A. E. H., Muntoni, F. *Duchenne Muscular Dystrophy*, 3rd edn. Oxford: Oxford University Press, 2003: 236–7.
26. Manzur, A. Y., Kuntzer, T., Pike, M., Swan, A. V. Glucocorticoid corticosteroids in Duchenne muscular dystrophy (review). *The Cochrane Library*, 2009; Issue 3.
27. Vandenburgh, H., Shansky, J., Benesch-Lee, F. et al. Automated drug screening with contractile muscle tissue energised from dystrophic myoblasts. *FASEB Journal*, 2009; **10**: 3325–34.
28. De Luca, A. Drug screening for muscular dystrophy: from target to function toward patients, is anything lost? *Neuromuscular Disorders*, 2009; **19**: 800.
29. Chamberlain, J. S., Rando, T. A. (eds) *Duchenne Muscular Dystrophy: Advances in Therapeutics*. New York, London: Taylor & Francis, 2006.
30. Bushby, K., Lochmüller, H., Lynn, S. et al. Interventions for muscular dystrophy: molecular medicines entering the clinic. *Lancet*, 2009; **374**: 1849–56.
31. Odom, G. L., Gregorevic, P., Chamberlain, J. S. Viral-mediated gene therapy for muscular dystrophies: successes, limitations and recent advances. *Biochimica et Biophysica Acta*, 2007; **1772**: 243–62.
32. Gregorevic, P., Blankinship, M. J., Allen, J. M. et al. Systemic microdystrophin gene delivery improves skeletal muscle structure and function in old dystrophic *mdx* mice. *Molecular Therapy*, 2008; **16**: 657–64.
33. Welch, E. M., Barton, E. R., Zhuo, J. et al. PTC 124 targets genetic disorders caused by nonsense mutations. *Nature*, 2007; **447**: 87–91.
34. Burton, E. A., Tinsley, J. M., Holzfeind, P. J. et al. A second promoter provides an alternative target for therapeutic up-regulation of utrophin in Duchenne muscular dystrophy. *Proceedings of the National Academy of Sciences USA*, 1999; **96**: 14025–30.
35. Hirst, R. C., McCullagh, K. J., Davies, K. E. Utrophin upregulation in Duchenne muscular dystrophy. *Acta Myologica*, 2005; **24**: 209–16.
36. Wilton, S. D., Fall, A. M., Harding, P. L. et al. Antisense oligonucleotide-induced exon skipping across the human dystrophin gene transcript. *Molecular Therapy*, 2007; **15**: 1288–96.
37. Kinali, M., Arechavala-Gomeza, V., Feng, L. et al. Local restoration of dystrophin expression with the morpholino oligomer AVI-4658 in Duchenne muscular dystrophy: a single-blind, placebo-controlled, dose-escalation, proof-of-concept study. *Lancet Neurology*, 2009; **8**: 918–28.
38. Markert, C. D., Atala, A., Cann, J. K. et al. Mesenchymal stem cells: emerging therapy for Duchenne muscular dystrophy. *Physical Medicine & Rehabilitation*, 2009; **1**: 547–59.
39. Wilton, S. PTC124, nonsense mutations and Duchenne muscular dystrophy. *Neuromuscular Disorders*, 2007; **17**: 719–20.

40. Rüdel, R., Nigro, G., Poortman, Y. Ten years of ENMC—from a patients' initiative to a successful European research institution: the story of the European Neuromuscular Centre. *Neuromuscular Disorders*, 2000; **10**: 75–82.
41. Bushby, K., Lynn, S., Straub, V. Collaborating to bring new therapies to the patient—the TREAT-NMD model. *Acta Myologica*, 2009; **28**: 12–15.
42. Dubowitz, V. Clinical myology at the crossroads. *Neuromuscular Disorders*, 2010; **20**: 95–6.
43. Emery, A. E. H. *Muscular Dystrophy: The Facts*, 3rd edn. Oxford, New York: Oxford University Press, 2008.

Author Index

Page numbers in *italics* represent figures or tables.

Abernethy, John 45
Adams, Joseph 43
Addison, Thomas 29
Alibert, Jean 74
Allbutt, Thomas 29
Althaus, Julius 65–6
Anderson, Louise 23, *199*
Aristotle 41
Askanas, Valerie 167

Babbage, Charles 29
Baily, Catherine (wife of Edward Meryon) 61–2, *67*
Bakker E 6
Baltimore, David 178
Baring, Alexander 60–1
Barker, Thomas 34
Bateson, William 102
Bayes, Thomas 160
Becker, Peter Emil 2, 6, 119, 131–3, *132*
Bell, Charles 6, 13–18, *15*, *16*, 20, 21, 33, 34, 45
Bell, Julia 119
Bernard, Claude 48, 74
Blane, Gilbert 45
Blizard, William 45
Blumenbach, Johann Friedrich 31
Botstein, David 179–80
Boutroy, Barbe (wife of Duchenne) 75
Boveri, Theodor 116
Bowman, William 167–8
Boyer SH (Ned) 189
Bridges, Calvin 116
Bright, Richard 29, 34, 45, 63
Brodie, Benjamin 34, 35, 40, 45
Buchthal, Fritz 147
Budd, William 29
Bynum WF 8

Campbell, Kevin 6, 196–8, *197*
Chadwick, Edwin 45
Charcot Jean-Marie 7, 78
Chung CS 2, 126
Clarke, John 45
Cohen, Stanley 178
Cohnheim Julius F 7, 86–7
Conte, Gaetano 18–19, 34

Cooper, Astley 45
Cruveilhier, Jean 74
Cuthbertson RA 76, 77, 80

Dale, Henry 49
Darwin, Charles 29–30, 41
  and Edward Meryon 32–3
Davies, Kay 3, 6, 7, 180–1, *182*
de Grouchy J 119
de Morgan, Campbell 35
Debré, Robert 154
Dejerine, Joseph Jules 2, 109–13, *112*
Dickens, Charles 29
Dreifuss, Fritz E 6, 133–6, *135*
Dreyfus, Jean-Claude 2, 6, 154–5, *155*
Dubowitz, Victor 6, 139–40, *140*
Duchenne de Boulogne 6, 7
  aetiology and pathology studies 86–8, *87*
  attitude to Meryon's work 82, 88–90
  death 80
  depression 75, 80
  description of muscular dystrophy cases 81–4, *82*, *83*, **84**
  education 73–4
  electrical stimulation studies 76–7, *78*
  German case reviews **84**
  La Salpétrière 77–81, *77*
  life 73–92
  marriages 75, 77
  muscle pathology studies 80, 84–6, *86*
  nervous system examination 86–8, *87*
  opinion of Raphael's *Transfiguration*
  portraits *76*, *79*
  publications 79–80
  recognition in Germany 82
  research 79–81
  return to Paris 76–7
  son 75, 79, 80
  studies in Paris 74
  terminology 81, 84, 89
Dupuytren, Guillaume 74

Ebashi, Setsuro 2, 156, *157*
Emery AEH 6, 133–6
Engel, Andrew G 6, 169–70, *170*
Engel, King 164, 167

AUTHOR INDEX

Engels, Frederick 29
Erb, Wilhelm Heinrich 2, 6, 7, 106–9, *107*
 dystrophia muscularis progressiva 108–9
 electrodiagnosis 108
 juvenile scapulohumeral progressive muscular dystrophy 109

Faraday, Michael 45
Fardeau M 6
Farquhar, W 45
Farr, William 29
Farre, Arthur 36
Fisher RA 126
Fölling, Asbjörn 166
Frampton, Algernon 22
Friedreich, Nikolaus 7, 106
Fuchs, Ernst 145
Fukuyama, Yoko 6, 146–7, *146*

Galton, Francis 41, 44
Garcia, Manuel 29
Garrod, Alfred 45
Garrod, Archibald 165–6
Gateland, Jane (mother of Edward Meryon) 58–9
Gioja L 34
Gowers, William Richard 1, 6, 7, 44, 94–103
 appointment to National Hospital for the Paralysed and Epileptic 94
 clinical heterogeneity 103
 contributions to medicine/neurology 96–7
 death 96
 education 94
 familial cases 102
 heredity studies 102
 honours 95
 illness 96
 inheritance of muscle disease 102
 inventions 97
 marriage 95
 medical studies 94
 medical terms 97
 portrait *95*
 pseudo-hypertrophic muscular paralysis work 97–102
 spinal cord examination 98
 treatment 103
 work with Lockhart Clarke 97–8
Gräfe, Albrecht von 7, 144–5
Graves, Robert 29
Griesinger, Wilhelm 7, 90
Grimm, Tiemo 133, 135
Gull, William Withey 34

Harper, Peter 3, 6, 182–3, *184*
Harris H 166
Helmholtz, Hermann von 29
Herschel, William 45
Hodgkin, Thomas 29, 45

Hodgson, Joseph 35
Hoffman, Eric 6, 7, 194–5, *195*
Holloway, Meryon 60
Holloway, William 58
Holmes, Oliver Wendell 29
Huxley TH 63

Jones, Bence 45
Jones, Wood 31

Kakulas B 6
Kingston, Helen 186–7
Kirke, William Senhouse 47
Klumpke, Augusta Dejerine 110–11
Knapp PC 116
Koch, Robert 29
Kunkel, Louis 3, 6, 7, 188–90, *190*

Laënnec, René 29, 74
Lamy M 119
Landouzy, Louis Théophile Joseph 2, 109–13, *111*
Landseer, Charles 63
Landseer, Edwin 63
Lardé, Honorine (wife of Duchenne de Boulogne) 77
Lewis, Jerry 140, 169, 172
Leyden E von 2, 7, 105–6
Lindenbaum R 6
Lister, Joseph 29
Lister, Joseph Jackson 36
Liston, Robert 45
Little, William J 6, 22–5, *23*, 34
Lockhart Clarke J 97–8
Loewi, Otto 49
Lyon, Mary 153

McKusick, Victor 6–7, 158–61, *158*, 183
Magendie, François 74
Maniatis, Tony 179
Marcet, Alexander 45
Marey, Etienne Jules 29
Marine, David 32
Marx, Karl 29
Maupertuis, Pierre Louis Moreau de 41–2
Mendel, Gregor 41, 115
Meryon, Charles Evelyn 60
Meryon, Charles Lewis 55–7, *56*, 58
Meryon, Charles Pix 60
Meryon, Edward 1, 6, 7, 27–49, 74
 at London University 33, *33*
 birth 58
 and Charles Darwin 32–3
 children 62
 Constitution of Man 30–2
 death 68
 degree 62–3
 education 58, 59–60
 election to fellowship of the Royal Medical and Chirurgical Society 64

engraving by JR Black 68
families described 38–40, *40*
family tree *54*
female carriers 40
first interest in muscle
  disease 33–5, *33*
grave at Brompton Cemetery 68, *69*
heredity studies 38–40, *40*
knowledge of heredity 41–4
librarian of Royal Medical and Chirurgical
  Society of London 45–6
life of 53–69
London Infirmary for Epilepsy and
  Paralysis 65–6
marriage 61–2
membership of Athenaeum 21, 63
microscopic studies 36–8, *37*
muscle disease work 35–41, *37*, *39*, *40*
neglected contribution to muscular
  dystrophy 44–7
obituaries 68
paper to Royal Medical and Chirurgical
  Society (1851) 47–8
paralysis studies 38, *39*
portrait in later years *69*
publications 35, *39*, 48–9
residence *59*, 62, *65*
studies 60–1
study of muscular dystrophy 35–6
The Huguenot 66–7
Meryon, John (father of EM) 57–8
Meryon, Lewis 55
Milhorat, Ade T 6, 116–18, *117*
Möbius P 2, 7, 105–6
Morgan, Thomas Hunt 6, 116
Morton, Newton Ennis 2, 125–8, *127*
Murphy, Edmond A (Tony) 2, 6, 158–61, *158*, *159*
Murray, Joanne 183

Nasse CF 44
Nattrass Frederick John 2, 6, 120–5, *121*
Newsom-Davis, John 8
Nicholson-Anderson L 7
Nigro, Giovanni 19

Oppenheimer G 7
Otto, John C 43–4

Paget, James 35, 45
Parkinson, James 29
Partridge, Richard 20–2, *22*, 34, 63
Pasteur, Louis 29
Pattison GS 61
Pearson, Carl M 167, 168
Pennington R 167
Philip, Ursula 180

Récamier, Joseph 74
Roses, Allen 6, 171–3, *173*
Rowland LP (Bud) 6, 171–2
Ruddle, Frank 191
Rush, Benjamin 44

Schapira, Georges 2, 154–5
Semmelweiss, Ignaz 29
Semmola, Giovanni 19
Shaftesbury, Lord 27–8
Simpson, James Young 29
Smith, Hamilton 178
Smith, Newman 30, 62
Snow, John 29
Sottas, Jules 111
Southern EM 178
Stanhope, Lady Hester 55
Stevenson AC 119
Stromeyer, Louis 22
Sturtevant, Alfred 116
Sugita, Hideo 2, 6, 156, *157*
Sutton, Walter 116
Syme, James 35

Tatum, Thomas 34, 35
Temin, Howard 178
Thompson, Seth 35
Tomé F 6
Trousseau, Armand 74

Verellen, Christine 191–2

Wallace, Alfred Russel 30
Walton, John Nicholas 2, 6, 120–5, *123*
Weismann, August 41
Wells, Spencer 45
Williamson, Robert (Bob) 180
Wolff, Kaspar Friedrich 42–3
Worton, Ron 3, 7, 191–2, *192*

Subject Index

Page numbers in *italics* represent figures or tables.

abiotrophy 97
action potentials 163, 164
adenyl cyclase 171
adhalin 141, 198
aetiology 86–8
agrin 212
albinism 32
aldolase 155, 167
  leaking 160
  serum activity 155
alleles 115
allopurinol 214
ambulation, prolongation of 24, 83, 103, 133, 213
amino acids 214
aminoglycoside antibiotics 214
amniotic fluid cells 188, 200, 216
anabolic steroids 214
ancient Egypt 11, *12*
animal analogues 165
antenatal diagnosis *see* prenatal diagnosis
antisense oligonucleotides 4, 216
arthrogryposis 145
aspirin 214
(Na$^+$ and K$^+$)ATase 171
atrophic, pelvic girdle or pelvifemoral type of Leyden–Möbius 105
autosomal dominant shoulder girdle dystrophy 132
autosomal limb girdle muscular dystrophy 119
autosomal recessive Duchenne-like muscular dystrophy 140
autosomal recessive pelvic girdle dystrophy 132
azathioprine 214

Bar Harbor *dy* mouse strain 165
Barth's syndrome 138
basal lamina 170
Bayesian statistics 2, 5, 9, 158–61
Becker muscular dystrophy 2, 3, 18, 35, 103, 131–3
  allelic with Duchenne dystrophy 148, 185–7
  clinical signs 18
  creatine kinase in 156
  dystrophin 198
  frame-shift mutations 198, *199*
  gene deletions 193
  gene location/product *209*
  landmarks *4*
  locus 136, 185
  point mutations 193
  preclinical *134*
Becker type X-linked muscular dystrophy 119, 131–3
Beggars (Hieronymus Cock) 12–13, *14*
Beni Hasan tomb drawings *12*
biopsy needle/punch 85
biopsy needles 85
Boulogne 73
brachial plexus palsy, partial 90
British Medical Association 29, 122

Ca-ATPase activity 174
calcium blockers 214
calf enlargement 20, 21, 24, 35, *82*, *86*
  female carriers 103
  see also muscle, enlargement
calf pseudohypertrophy 11, 20, 127, 133, 147
  Fukuyama type congenital muscular dystrophy 147–8
  see also muscle, pseudohypertrophy
Calpain-3 defect 210
cardiac failure 20
cardiac involvement 101, 136, 201
cardiomyopathy 136, *139*
  female carriers 142
carrier detection 153–61
  DNA markers 187–8
  Duchenne dystrophy 188
  rate 157
  tests 158
carriers
  dystrophin 142, 198
  female *see* female carriers
  manifesting 40, 103, 142
catecholamines 214
cDNA 178, 193, 194
Charcot-Marie-Tooth neuropathy 2B 210
cholera 28, 29

chromosome
  banding 23, 185, 191
  theory of inheritance 116
  walking 188
clones 178
club foot 11, 22, 23
co-enzyme Q *214*
Cohnheim's areas 87
Communist Manifesto 29–30
conditional probabilities 160
congenital disorders 43
congenital muscular dystrophies 145–8
  gene location/product *209*
  rapidly progressive form 148
congenital myotonic dystrophy 183
Constitution of Man (Meryon) 30–2, 48
contractures 18, 20, 21, 74, 101, 103, 134, 136, *137*, 146
copy number variations 212
creatine *214*
creatine kinase 155
  activity assay 156
  combination with DNA markers 187
  female carriers 156, 158
  serum activity *143*, 147, 156, 157, 160
cyclosporine *214*

dantrolene *214*
Deformities of the Human Frame (Little) 24
degenerative factors 116
Dejerine-Sottas disease 111
deltoid muscles
  changes 20
  fatty degeneration 21
Derbyshire neck 32
diagnosis
  of Morgagni 84
  preclinical 155
  preimplantation 5
  prenatal 5, 187–8
digitalis *214*
discriminant analysis 2, 5, 125, 126
disease delineation 2, 8, 13, 106, 126, 131
distal muscular dystrophy 143
  gene location/product *209*
  types of *143*
distal myopathy 124
DNA 160
  amplification 5
  fragment joining methods 178
  junk 179
  recombinant technology 177–80
  sequencing 179
DNA markers 3
  carrier detection 187–8
DNA-DNA reassociation reactions 190
Doctrine of the Nerves (Spillane) 108
dominance 42

dominant inheritance of muscular dystrophy 118, 119
Drosophila 116
drug therapy *214–15*
DSX7 polymorphism 184, 186, 187
DSX9 polymorphism 183, 186, 187
DSX164 193
Dubowitz score 140
Duchenne gene
  cloning 190
  localization 180–5
Duchenne gene product *see* dystrophin
Duchenne locus, marker error 187
Duchenne muscular dystrophy 2, 3
  clinical signs 20, 24
  gene location/product *209*
  identification of gene defect 5
  landmarks *4*
  manifesting carriers 141–2
  X-linked 127, 139
dystroglycan 212
dystrophia muscularis progressiva 108–9
dystrophin 4, 5, 194–6
  antibodies 7
  cytoskeletal protein 88
  deficiency 88
  deletions affecting central rod domain 195, 198, 200
  discovery 170
  gene product 194–6
  identification 5
  in-frame deletions 200
  isoforms 201
  localization in sarcolemma 196
  manifesting carriers 142, 198
  mutations 198–9
  polyclonal antibodies in identification of 195–6
  quantitation 198
  reverse genetics 4, 174, 177, 195
dystrophin gene 5
  viral delivery 215
dystrophin-associated glycoprotein (DAG) complex 198
dystrophin-associated glycoproteins 196–8
dystrophinopathies 196, 210

echinocyte formation 174
electrical stimulation studies 76, *78*
electromyography (EMG) 123, 137, 147, 158, 163–4
emerin 136, *209*, 210
Emery-Dreifuss muscular dystrophy 133–6
  distinguishing features *134*
  gene location/product *209*
eosinophilic fibres 168
epigenetic factors 212
Epigrams, Epitaphs, Personal Anecdotes (Meryon) 49

epilepsy, musicogenic 97
equinovarus deformity 81
Erb-Goldflam disease 108
Erb's phenomenon 108
erythrocyte membranes 172
  abnormalities in 174
  protein kinase activity 173
Essays on the Anatomy of Expression in Painting (Bell) 15, *16*
Essays on Burns (Duchenne) 75
exons 179, 194
extensor digitorum brevis 164

facial weakness 109, *110*, 113
facioscapulohumeral dystrophies 2
  autosomal dominant 124, 128
  distribution *208*
  dominant 127
  gene location *209*
  inheritance 119
  of Landouzy and Dejerine 109–13
  scapuloperoneal syndrome 136–7
family histories, Meryon's descriptions 38–40, *40*
famine in Ireland 28
female carriers 2
  calf enlargement 103
  cardiomyopathy 142
  creatine kinase 156, 158
fibroblast membrane-associated abnormalities 174
fibroblasts 167
fibrositis 97
Foster Kennedy syndrome 97
frame-shift deletions 23
Franco-Prussian War 80
French Revolution 73, 74
Friedreich's ataxia 106
Fukuyama type congenital muscular dystrophy 147–8

gait 24, 38, 83, 99
gastrocnemius muscle enlargement 21, 24, 83
gemmules 41
gene
  cloning 178
  library construction 179, 180
  locations *209*
  mapping in *Drosophila* 116
  product 5, *209*
  reactivation of genes active in fetal development 167
  specific probes 183–4
  structure 179
gene defects 187
  muscle effects *4*, 171–4
  recombinant DNA technology 177–80

gene deletion 185, 193
  Becker dystrophy 193
  Duchenne dystrophy 190, 193
gene libraries 179
gene therapy 1, *4*, 15
  viral 215
genetic counselling 5, 124, 160
genetic factors 118, 120
genetic heterogeneity 207
genetic linkage 116, 180, 183
genetic markers 124, 180
  linkage studies 180
genotype-phenotype correlation 198–200
germ theory 2, 29, 94
  nosology effects 93
girls, Duchenne muscular dystrophy in 185
glucocorticoids *214*
glutamic oxalacetic transaminase 155
glutamic pyruvic transaminase 155
glycine *214*
glycolysis 155, 172
glycoprotein reduction in muscular dystrophies 198
goitre 32
Gowers' manoeuvre/sign 99, *100*
growth hormone *214*
growth hormone inhibitor *214*

haemophilia 43–4, 102
hereditary diseases 43, 102, 115
heredity 32
  knowledge in Meryon's time 41–4
  Mendel's principles 41, 115
  Meryon's knowledge 41
heredo-familial disease 115–16
heterogeneity 103, 105–13
heterogeneous nuclear ribonucleoproteins 212
historical aspects 1–26
  ancient Egypt 11, *12*
  individual contributions 6–7
  landmarks *4*
  nineteenth-century medical science 7–8
History of Medicine (Meryon) 49
Huguenot, The (Meryon) 49, 66
Huguenots 53–4
Human Biochemical Genetics (Harris) 166
human races 31
Hutchinsonian facies 144
hyaline fibres 168
hyperoestrogenaemia 200

immunosuppression *214*, 216
infection, and muscular dystrophy 212–13
inheritance
  mode of 41
  X-linked *4*, 125, 128, 136–8
inherited disorders 43

SUBJECT INDEX

Institute for Muscle Disease 117
intellectual impairment 81, 84, 164
intracranial abnormalities 25
intramembranous particles 174
introns 179
Ireland, famine in 28
isoforms 201

joint contractures in Fuguyama
    dystrophy 148
joint probability 160
junk DNA 179
juvenile scapulohumeral progressive muscular
    dystrophy 109

Kearns-Sayre syndrome 144
ketoacids *214*
Kinnier Wilson syndrome 97
Klumpke's paralysis 111
knee jerk 97, 108

La Paralysie Atrophique Graisseuse de l'Enfance
    (Duchenne) 79
lactate dehydrogenase 155, 167
Lam-A 210
Lamin A gene 210
laminins 212
laminopathies 210
Lancet 29, 35
LARGE glycosyltransferase 213
Lassa fever 213
l'atrophie musculaire graisseuse progressive de
    l'enfance 109
leucine *214*
limb girdle muscular dystrophy 2, 124, 138–42
    of adulthood 141
    autosomal recessive 141
    of childhood 138–41
    gene location/product *209*
    isolated 127
    recessive 119
limb girdle syndrome of adults 141
linkage studies 116, 180, 183
Little's disease 22
Lives of the Artists (Vasari) 11
lod score method 180
London Infirmary for Epilepsy and
    Paralysis 65
lordosis 11, 24, *82*
lymphocyte membrane-associated
    abnormalities 174
Lyon hypothesis 153

macroglossia 20
mandibuloacral dysplasia 210
manifesting carriers 40, 103, 142
Manual of Diseases of the Nervous System
    (Gowers) 97

mast cells, increased function 88
matrix metalloproteinases 210
Mbo 1 restriction enzyme 190–1
mdx mouse/human/dog 4, 165, 213, 216
Méchanisme de la Physionomie Humaine
    (Duchenne) 79
Medical Act 1858 28
medical science, developments in 1–4
membrane glycoproteins 198
Mendelian inheritance 5, 33, 41, 44, 115
    acceptance of principles 115, 116
Merchant Taylor's School 55, 59, 60
merosin 198
Meryon's disease 2
messenger RNA 178
metabolic block 166
microscopy 36, *37*–8
mini-dystrophic gene 215
mitochondrial disorders 144
motor nerve supply abnormality 164
motor units 163, 164
muscle
    biochemistry 165–7
    biopsy 85
    contractures 18, 20, 21, 74, 101, 103, 134,
        136, *137*, 146
    cytoskeleton 38
    de-differentiation 167
    Duchenne's pathology studies 80, 84–6, *86*
    electrical stimulation 76, *78*
    enlargement 21, 24, 83
    enzyme activity 160
    fibrous connective tissue hyperplasia 85–6
    function 164
    glycolysis 155, 172
    granular degeneration 35–41
    hypertrophy 21, 24
    hypotonia from birth 145, *146*, 147
    microscopical study 36, *37*–8
    pathology 84–6
    pseudohypertrophy 99, 105, 113, 124, 134,
        139, 141, 200
    see also calf enlargement; calf
        pseudohypertrophy
muscle disease
    inheritance 44
    Meryon's interest in 33–5
muscle fibres 85, 87, 170
    contraction 76
    degeneration 115
    hypercontracted 169
    necrosis 165
muscle membrane 210
    defects 160, 171
    leaky 171
muscle wasting 18, 21, 99, 115, 136, 164
    associated diseases 108
    Meryon's descriptions 35, 39

SUBJECT INDEX

muscle weakness 20, 23
    associated diseases 108
    from birth 145
muscle-eye-brain disease 145, *209*
muscular dystrophy
    Bell's observations 18
    classification 2, 120–5
    clinical heterogeneity 103, 105–13
    clinical variability 119, 212
    discriminant analysis 2, 5, 125, 126
    Duchenne's cases 81–4, *82–4*
    dystrophin-associated glycoprotein reduction 196–8
    early clinical description 18–19, 21–2, 24
    facial weakness 109, *110*, 113
    genetic classification 128, *138*
    genetic differences 118–20
    genetic factors 118, 120
    history 4
    membrane defects 160, 171
    Meryon's contributions 35–6, 44–7
    neurogenic basis 163–4
    onset 200, 210
    pathogenesis 163–74, 207–10
    progression 5, 20, 101, 103, 118, 124
    serum enzyme levels 154–6
    sex-linked recessive inheritance 118, 132
    transmission 5
    see also specific types
Muscular Dystrophy Association of America 117, 171
Muscular Dystrophy Group of Great Britain 121, 122
musicogenic epilepsy 97
mutation rate 124, 128, 194
myasthenia gravis 97
myoblast transfer 4
myopathy
    with autophagy 138
    congenital 120, 144
    distal 124
    ocular 124
    Xp21 196
Myotilin 210

NADP-linked dehydrogenases 167
nasal smile 97
nerve root lesion localization 108
nervous system, examination 90
Nervous System of the Human Body (Bell) 17, 18
neurogenic basis of dystrophy 163–4
neurogenic hypothesis 171
neurological development scoring system 140
neuronal nitric oxide synthase 210
nosology 93, 115–28
nucleotides *214*

ocular muscular dystrophy 144, *144*, 148
ocular myopathy 124
oculopharyngeal dystrophy 2
    gene location/product *209*
oestrogens *214*
olivopontocerebellar atrophy 111
On the Functions of the Sympathetic System of Nerves (Meryon) 48
one gene-one enzyme concept 165
ophthalmoplegia 144
    progressive external 144
ovarian agenesis 125
oxandrolone *214*

pancreatic extract *214*
pangenesis hypothesis 41, 42
paralysie hypertrophique de l'enfance 81–4
    clinical features 81, *82*
    German cases 82, *84*
    intellectual ability 84
paralysie musculaire pseudo-hypertrophique 84
pathogenesis
    Duchenne muscular dystrophy 163–74, 207–10
    Duchenne's views on 86–8
Peacock School (Rye) 57
penicillamine *214*
perlecan 212
PERT 87 probes 191, 193
PERT probes 191
phenol-enhanced reassociation technique (PERT) 190
phenotype
    Becker dystrophy 198
    Duchenne dystrophy 160, 198
phenylketonuria 166
photomicrography 36–7
Physical and Intellectual Constitution of Man Considered 62
plasma membrane defects in muscle fibres 160, 171
plasmalemma 170
plasmid vectors 178, 191
point mutations 177
    Becker dystrophy 193
    Duchenne dystrophy 193
poliomyelitis 11, 88, 108, 147
    acute anterior 88
polymerase chain reaction (PCR) 5
population in Victorian times 27–8
Practical and Pathological Researches on the Various Forms of Paralysis (Meryon) 38, *39*, 44, 60
preclinical diagnosis 155
prednisone *214*
preimplantation diagnosis 5
prenatal diagnosis 5, 187–8
prevention 216

prior probabilities 160
probability 160
progeria 210
progressive bulbar palsy 90
progressive external ophthalmoplegia 144
progressive muscular atrophy 88, 89, 90, 101
propranolol *214*
protease inhibitors *214*
proteases 167
proteins *209*, 210, *211*
proximal muscular dystrophy 143
pseudo-hypertrophic muscular paralysis 98–102, *100*
 cases reviewed 98–9
 clinical heterogeneity 103
 contractures 101
 gait 99
 Gowers' lectures 98–9
 Gowers' manoeuvre/sign 99, *100*
 heart effects 101
 lordosis 99
 mental handicap 101
 survival 101
 treatment 103
Pseudo-hypertrophic Muscular Paralysis (Gowers) 18
PTC124 215
Public Health Act 1848 28
publications *3*
puerperal fever 29, 75
Punt, Queen of 11, *12*

quadriceps myopathy 133

reading frame 198–9
recombinant DNA technology 177–80
Registration Act 1836 28
research funding/teams 6
respiratory care 213
respiratory infection 101
restriction enzymes 178
restriction fragment length polymorphism (RFLP) 3, *4*, *5*, 179–80, 182, *183*, 184, 185, 188, 193
 Duchenne gene location 188
reverse genetics 4, 174, 177, 195
reverse transcriptase 178
ribosomal RNA 193
RNA
 messenger 178
 ribosomal 193
Royal Medical and Chirurgical Society 44–7, *46*
 Meryon's election to *64*
Rue de l'Ecole de Médecine (etching by Charles Meryon) *75*
Rye 53, 54, 55, 57, 58–9
 Mermaid Street *59*

Sanders School 55, 57
sarcolemma 38, 170, 196, *199*
 breakdown 90, 160–1
 defects 86, 169, 170
 Meryon's observations 168–9
scapuloperoneal syndrome 136–7
 clinical features *139*
 distinguishing features *138*
scoliosis 24
seated position, rising from 97
segregation analysis 42, 125–8
Sequential Tests for the Detection of Linkage (Morton) 126
serum enzyme levels 154–6
severe childhood muscular dystrophy, autosomal recessive 38, 103, 140
severity variation 113, 200
sex-linked characters 116
sex-linked recessive inheritance 118, 132
sex-linked recessive pelvic girdle dystrophy 132
shoulder girdle weakness 24
Sick Boy, The (Karl Schmidt-Rottluff) 13
sick motor neurone 164
single nucleotide polymorphisms 212
slum dwellings 27, *28*
smallpox 28
soleus muscle enlargement 21, 24
somatic cell hybrids 191
Southern blot 178, 181, 184
spastic spinal paralysis, chronic 108
spectrin band II phosphorylation disorder 172, 173
spinal cord
 Duchenne's study 86–7
 Gower's examination 101
 Meryon's study 36, 38, 87
spinal deformity, progressive 213
spinal fusion surgery 213
spinal muscular atrophy 88, 141, 155, 181, 196, 217
stem cell therapy 216
sternomastoid muscles
 changes 24
 fatty degeneration 21
sticky ends 190, 191
superoxide dismutase *215*
surgery, development 29
sympathetic nervous system 48, 49
System of Dissections (Charles Bell) 14–15

Telethonin 210
tendon knee reflex 108
tenotomy, subcutaneous 22, 23
testosterone *215*
thalamic syndrome 111
Thomsen's disease 106, 132
thymus hyperplasia 200
thyroxine *215*
Titin 210

Transactions of the Royal Medical and Chirurgical Society of London 45, 46–7
transcription 178
Transfiguration (Raphael) 11, *13*
translation 178
transmission of inherited traits 42
transport 27
treatment 103, 213–16, *214–15*
trick movements 24
tuberculosis 28
Turner's syndrome 5, 125, 185
typhoid 28

Ullrich disease 146
utrophin, up-regulation 215

vascular hypothesis 164–5
vasodilators *215*
venereal disease 28
Victorian times 27–30
viral vector 215
vitamin B_6 *215*
vitamin E *215*

Walker-Warburg syndrome 146
Windmill Street School of Anatomy 15, 20, 21

X chromosome 125, 153
  gene map 181, *183*
  library construction 179
X-linkage 44, 102
X-linked Duchenne muscular dystrophy 127, 139
X-linked inheritance *4*, 125, 128, 136–8
X-linked mouse mutant (*mdx*) 165
X-linked muscular dystrophies *139*
X-linked traits 180, 189
X/autosome translocation 185
  with Duchennne dystrophy 191
Xg blood group 124, 135, 136, 180
XJ probe 193
XO, Turner's syndrome 5
Xp21 myopathies 196
Xq28 locus 136, *209*

zinc *215*